Geriatric Dentistry

GATEWAY TO LONGEVITY
AND LIFE-LONG HEALTH

Geriatric Dentistry
GATEWAY TO LONGEVITY AND LIFE-LONG HEALTH

Eric Zane Shapira, DDS, MAGD, MA, MHA
Dental Practitioner; Author; Educator;
Professor of Geriatric Dentistry, Medicine and Nursing

edra
PUBLISHING

This edition first published 2024

ISBN: 978-1-957260-51-8
eISBN: 978-1-957260-71-6

Editor: **Paola Sammaritano, Edra S.p.a.**

edra
PUBLISHING

Edra Publishing US LLC
3309 Northlake Boulevard,
Suite 203, Palm Beach Gardens,
FL, 33403
EIN: 844113980

info@edrapublishing.com
www.edrapublishing.com

Printed by "Printer Trento" S.r.l. (Trento), September 2023

Dedication

The author would like to dedicate this book to the following people with my gratitude and thanks for: your inspiration; information; diligence; assistance with my education; teaching me about life and humanity and for allowing me to learn how to integrate my family values with my scientific studies; allowing me to treat people as Human Beings with not only clinical concerns, but emotional feelings as well; and in turn, respecting and encouraging humanity in working with people, ultimately caring about and for them.

Thank you to:

My parents: Irving and Betty Shapira foremost for being my first teachers.

My instructors... all of them for giving me the goals of learning knowledge that no one can take from me.

Temple University Kornberg School of Dentistry, for the opportunity to achieve a Doctorate in Dental Surgery and allowing me to be in such a great profession.

My patients, who taught me humility: how to care for them and others, and for helping me learn about the limits of my own abilities in order to show empathy and care. To those who have become my friends throughout life (you know who you are); who have encouraged me to succeed in the face of adversity by keeping my "nose to the grindstone", learning all that I could absorb and understand.

My students, who have taught me in turn about how to learn better and how to ask questions and answer them honestly and forthrightly; about truth and desire and the knowledge that I am not alone in this world and that I am not alone in my aspirations.

My wife, Susan, who has encouraged me, nurtured me, and supported me in all that I do for myself, for us and for others. We learn together how to be better Humans and partners for each other as we age like so many others.

My granddaughter, Emily Erickson, RDAEF, who has continued to carry "the torch" in Dentistry.

My son, Zane, and twin daughters, Desi and Sabrina, both RDAs, for your support and understanding and love.

Debbie Wong for her assistance with transcribing my slides and illustrations.

Professor Bernd Stadlinger, Clinic of Cranio-Maxillofacial Surgery, Red Cross Hospital, Kassel, Germany, whom I met at an American Dental Association/FDI World Dental Congress in 2019 in San Francisco. He has inspired me to write this book by showing me a book that he wrote.

I am grateful to all of you for your support, knowledge and inspiration. May we all age with grace, be teachers and communicators to our patient's and empathic practitioners as well, who ultimately assist patients in making valid decisions for themselves with respect to their geriatric dental journeys.

Geriatric Dentistry: Gateway to Longevity and Life-Long Health is just the beginning of an unknown journey. Life is full of change. We must be able to cope with it, embrace it, try to understand it, and sculpt it into a beautiful entity that older people will find beneficial in some way. Geriatric dental care will stand as a beacon of light, preserving the knowledge that we gain over time in order to help us, help them, preserve their dentitions; restoring them to optimum health and, in turn, prolonging life itself, giving our older patients hope for continued happiness.

Eric Zane Shapira

Prolog

*"Age is state of mind. Being old is thinking old.
Being older implies chronological age but thinking older is mental.
Older persons, who are infirm in some way, think they are really
old-Geriatric! It is when the mind thinks that the body cannot do what
it used to do, that one is old. Do-Be, Do-Be, Do-Be Do... Be Young at Heart."*

Geriatric Dentistry has not been recognized as an official dental specialty by the American Dental Association, yet. In my personal experience with other dentists, it seems that most dental practitioners have had the mindset that "people are people" and what applies to one person is good enough for the next. However, this is a misnomer when it comes to both Geriatric and "special needs" patients. In my thinking, Geriatric Dentistry is a subspecialty of Geriatric Medicine, which is a recognized specialty by the American Medical Association.

Geriatrics usually refers to medical care for older adults, an age group which is not easy to define precisely. "Older" is preferred over "elderly", but both are equally imprecise; 65 is the age often used, but most people do not need geriatrics expertise in their care until age 70, 75 or even 80 years of age.[1]

In my book, *A New Wrinkle: What I Learned from Older People Who Never Acted Their Age*,[2] I have enumerated a "New Aging Paradigm" which I have included in this book for reference purposes in defining the Aging Process.

Geriatric patients are a special breed of person, with a whole gamut of issues to cope with as their minds and bodies are subjected to the aging process. These issues include a diminished ability to fight disease; cope with stress and fend off loneliness and subsequent depression, to name a few. All these entities have specific effects on each of our bodies and personas over time, by accelerating the aging process itself on specific individuals. These issues are usually not inherently visible in the younger population for the most part.

Aging, over time, has its way of changing one's oral health conditions: systemic diseases; physical traumas; emotional stressors; depression; memory loss and cognitive decline; acute disease situations, such as habits developed over time or lack thereof, such as brushing and flossing on a regular basis or visiting a dental office for routine care. These issues can and do diminish the oral health of any individual, especially an older, more compromised person. These things can exacerbate and accelerate aging and possibly hasten one's demise.

The aging process is one in which there is a mixture of metabolism, as well as catabolism. Some scientists, as well as this Author, have advocated that aging is a *disease process* that begins with the building blocks that make us viable humans, and then the subsequent destruction of metabolic processes that begin to cause our decay over some period of time occurs, ultimately causing a major change in our overall health, ending in death as we know it.

At the turn of the 20th century, the average age at death was 45 years[3] compared to that statistic today, which is almost two-fold that age in our American society as it is in the more well-developed countries of our World. The variables that confound this figure are many and dependent upon one's manner of living, genetics, general health and the ability to survive and cope in a world fraught with disease, hunger, poverty, stressors and more.

Chronic disease is the major cause of death in our population more so than acute disease (not taking into consideration a pandemic of acute disease such as today's COVID-19).[4]

An older person who presents at a dental office with a toothache is much more than a "walk-in tooth" with a "hole" in it. I can remember many years ago when my dental assistant came to tell me that there was a "broken denture in the reception room, and what did I want to do about it?" I told her: "Please make the denture comfortable and bring in the person they came with for me to speak to about her situation". We are missing the point here when we reduce people, especially older people, to just teeth or dentures in this case; not remembering that "attached to every tooth is a person!" We are treating *people*. Although the Constitution of the United States says in basic terms "that we are all created equal"..., we are not equal with respect to the changes that happen to us along life's path and our individual set of experiences that we imbibe as well that make us what we are in total. These identifiers, accompanied by a complex set of genetics, predisposing us to a myriad of things that can cause our Beings to fail, as well as what physically befalls us as we move along life's path define our Beings.

Older people have much more to be aware of than younger people do when considering any kind of dental or major medical treatment. When considering any kind of dental treatment, we need to take into consideration all of each person's respective histories and dental knowledge. There is more than one history we should be looking at, not just their previous dental history. I have dedicated a chapter in this book to this topic alone because it is so germane to the issue of treating our older patients.

In today's world, I know that we are supposed to "inform, before we perform", regarding any intended dental procedure. But, in both hindsight and future sight, we, dental practitioners, as well as all dental professionals, need to "*know, before we go*". Communication is the "key" here and I have dedicated a chapter in this book to this important topic as well.

The joys of treating our older population are many. I have met extremely interesting, enjoyable, educated and encouraging people, from one end of the spectrum: some of which have become my personal friends. In turn, I have treated those people who were angry, sad, distraught, hopeless and down-right mean spirited at the other end of the spectrum. I have learned from all of them that the Human *species* is most complex. Treating our *species*, for lack of a better word to categorize it, is most educational indeed. I have taught my students that good judgment comes from experience and experience comes from "bad judgment". This is how we learn. Therefore, there are no mistakes in life, as far as I am concerned, only experience. We learn by doing. So, in order to be a more versatile, educated and proficient dental practitioner, it behooves us all to study the many facets of dentistry, not just the treatment modalities themselves, but the patients for whom our treatment is designed. Learning how to communicate is the first hurdle. Asking appropriate questions is another hurdle. Putting all the information you receive together and making sense of it is another hurdle. Making a treatment plan from the assimilated information is a big goal. Presenting the information is a major function of being an astute and concerned practitioner. Presenting both a recommended treatment plan and several alternate treatment recommendations is a necessary step in the process. Communicating to get positive feedback is *a priori* in getting to "Yes".

This takes not just communicating through verbalization, but active listening as well, something most dentists do not learn in dental school. This will be covered in one of the chapters of this book as well as "Case Studies" involving different treatment modalities for different patients and instances.

Considering all the factors involved in treating an older patient, the financial considerations may make or break treating the patient. It is important to assist your patients' needs with this issue, in order to give them the treatment that they not only need, but desire. The most difficult entity we have to cope with as practitioners is getting our patients to want what we think they need. And we do this from start to finish with: an appropriate examination, a clear plan, alternate treatment plans, active communication (listening and speaking in an empathic manner) and taking an interest in the patient, so that they know we "care" about them. "No one cares how much you know, until they know how much you care!" Geriatric Dentistry is not just about repairing aging teeth, but re-instilling a sense of pride, good health and a continued good quality of life for those who might not have been aware that their "hopeless" teeth and aging sense of self were not hopeless after all. Allowing an older, more compromised patient to understand the ramifications of their actions, their unknown destructive habits, how their medical conditions affect their mouths and vice versa, will allow the patient to understand how both oral and systemic disease processes will affect their overall health and longevity. It will also give them the needed information to make an adequate and acceptable treatment acceptance in the end. *Carpe Diem*... Seize the day!

References

1. *Oxford English Dictionary*, 3rd Edition, 2020.
2. Shapira, Eric Z. *A New Wrinkle: What I Learned from Older People Who Never Acted Their Age*, 2009; 2nd Edition, 2011. iUniverse Publishers, Bloomington, Indiana, USA.
3. NCHS, National Vital Statistics System, Historical Data, 1900-1998 (see https://www.cdc.gov/nchs/nvss/mortality_historical_data.html).
4. Agus, David B, MD. *The End of Illness*, 2011. Free Press Publishing, a division of Simon & Schuster.

Table of Contents

Chapter 4

Geriatric Periodontal Disease or Why Aren't Your Teeth in a Jar?

Chapter 5

Considerations in Treating the Older Compromised Patient: *«Who Am I and What Am I Doing Here?»*

Chapter 6

Just in Case You Want to Talk "Turkey..." Truth and Consequences

Chapter 7

Communication: Can you Hear me? Are you listening? Can you Understand What it is I am Saying? "Please take your fingers out of your ears!"

Chapter 8

Sex and Oral Disease in the Compromised Older Patient: May be a "Touchy" Subject!?

Chapter 9

Habits and Other Factors that Lead to Oral Disease in the Older Population

Chapter 10

Case Construction and Presentation: It Is Not All That You Say... It Is How You Say It. It Is Not What You Bring, It is How You Show It...

Epilog

Appendix

Chapter 1

Will We Live Longer than Our Teeth?

DEFINITION: ***Statistics*** *is the practice or science of collecting and analyzing numerical data in large quantities, especially for the purpose of inferring proportions in a whole from those in a representative sample. Statistics is the science that deals with large amounts of data and methodologies that reviews and analyzes and draws conclusions from this data for the purpose of stimulating useful data and theories based on mathematical probability, which imposes order and gives some representation of information of our human interest.*

> ***"Statistics are to baseball what a flaky crust is to Mom's apple pie. An hour sitting with a pretty girl on a park bench passes like a minute, but a minute sitting on a hot stove seems like an hour."***
>
> *Unknown author, 2017*

1.1 The Importance of Statistics in Geriatric Dentistry

Statistics is a crucial and important process behind how we make discoveries in science, make decisions based on data, and make predictions, such as "Will we live longer than our teeth?". It is a major beacon that assists us in lighting up a SWOTT analyses, based upon statistics, when dealing with "strengths, weaknesses, opportunities, threats and trends", in any discipline such as the practice of Dentistry.

Without this modality, we would not be able to adequately equate the processes by which we function within our profession: by reading and measuring from exacting radiographs, three-dimensional tomograms, CAT scans, medical tests of all kinds; mixing techniques, utilizing dental materials and just about anything else we do in clinical dentistry today, to name a few.

Geriatric Dentistry utilizes statistics when it comes to predicting outcomes of treatment. Based on mathematical numbers we can predict the success or failure of a procedure coupled with other statistics about aging, death and dying, general health, dental history, habits, desire, attitude and a set of choices one must make about our care based on these entities. Essentially, it gives us information that is useful in treating our patients.

Therefore, in order to understand what we face in the future with respect to accomplishing dental treatment on our patients, we need to know statistical data that will enlighten us about our older generation. Knowing what our strengths are, our weaknesses and such, we can look for opportunities in providing dental care to those in need, especially the older patient. Threats that pose a danger to practitioners are the lack of information and knowledge about what this cohort of patient brings to us. So, we need to educate ourselves in every facet of the aging process, medically and dentally, as well as socially and economically. We can look at the trends and figure out how the increasing numbers of patients over the age of 65 years will be an important asset to our practices. But "we" must be prepared, as dental practitioners, to face these patients with an armamentarium filled with not only appropriate and good treatment, but

Table 1.1 Population >65 years – World Health Organization (WHO)

1998	2025
• **390 million** people >65 years	• **780 million** people >65 years
	• **300% increase** in >65 population in developing countries

U.S. Department of Health and Human Services, 2018.[1]

hope, desire, understanding and communication about preserving the dentition and ultimately one's longevity at the same time. Hopefully, we will live a longer, healthier life with a full complement of teeth to get us there!

A statistical fact is that over 10,000 "boomer babies" a day turn 65 years of age. By 2030, all boomers born in the years 1946-1964, will have turned 65 years of age.[2] The 2020 statistics from the U.S. Census will be used to determine how Federal Government monies will be spent initially to provide public services for our elderly into the next decade. By utilizing Census statistics and geographic information in the system that are a direct result of the information collected, communities can plan and refine a picture of where older Americans live and how close they are to services they need, such as healthcare facilities, senior citizens centers, markets, adult day health centers, hospitals and other necessary services germane to their ultimate survival. One can also look at statistics to determine how many older people are living alone, who are more than 10 miles away from any healthcare facilities and access to care. We need to learn how to provide access to care for such a burgeoning population of people.

The number of people aged 65 and over in the United States, similarly as in other wealthy nations, has grown rapidly over most of the 20th century from 3.1 million in 1900 to 35 million in 2000. In 2018, there were 52 million people aged 65 years or older. Their share of the population grew as well, from 12.4% in 2000 to 16% in 2018. Life expectancy at age 65 went from 11.9 years (1900-1902) to 19.1 years in 2010, according to *An Aging World*, a Census Bureau report.[3] Persons aged 85-100 years of age are in the fastest growing cohort of people in the world (Table 1.1 and Figs. 1.1 to 1.4).

All in all, older adults are projected to outnumber children under the age of 18 for the first time in U.S. history by 2034, according to the U.S. Census Bureau statistical projections. This is due in part from a declining birth rate amongst younger individuals. Therefore, we can extrapolate from this statistical data that a given conclusion will be an increase in older patients frequenting our practices for treatment and extended care in the future, more so than younger patients. We need to be prepared to treat everyone, but especially, the older segment of our society, who carry with them a great deal more information, with respect to their social, economic, medical and dental histories. These histories are the important pieces to everyone's "Human Puzzle". These "puzzle pieces" are the key to the sum total of what the patient brings with them to our practices, which in turn, allows us, with the assistance of an appropriate examination and discussion, to figure out our individual treatment plans for each patient. This act of knowing our patient can help us "know, before we go".

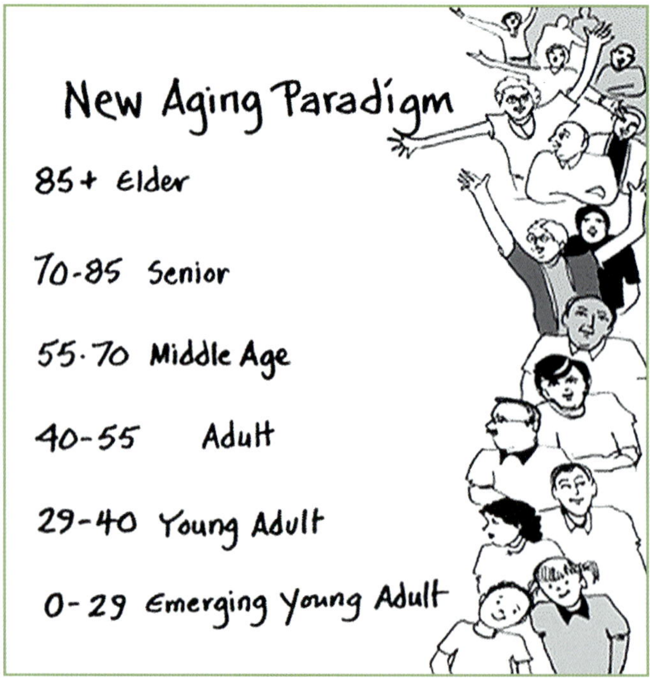

Fig. 1.1 New Aging Paradigm. *(Shapira, Eric Z. A New Wrinkle: What I Learned From Older People Who Never Acted Their Age. iUniverse Publishers, 2009; 2011 ©.[4])*

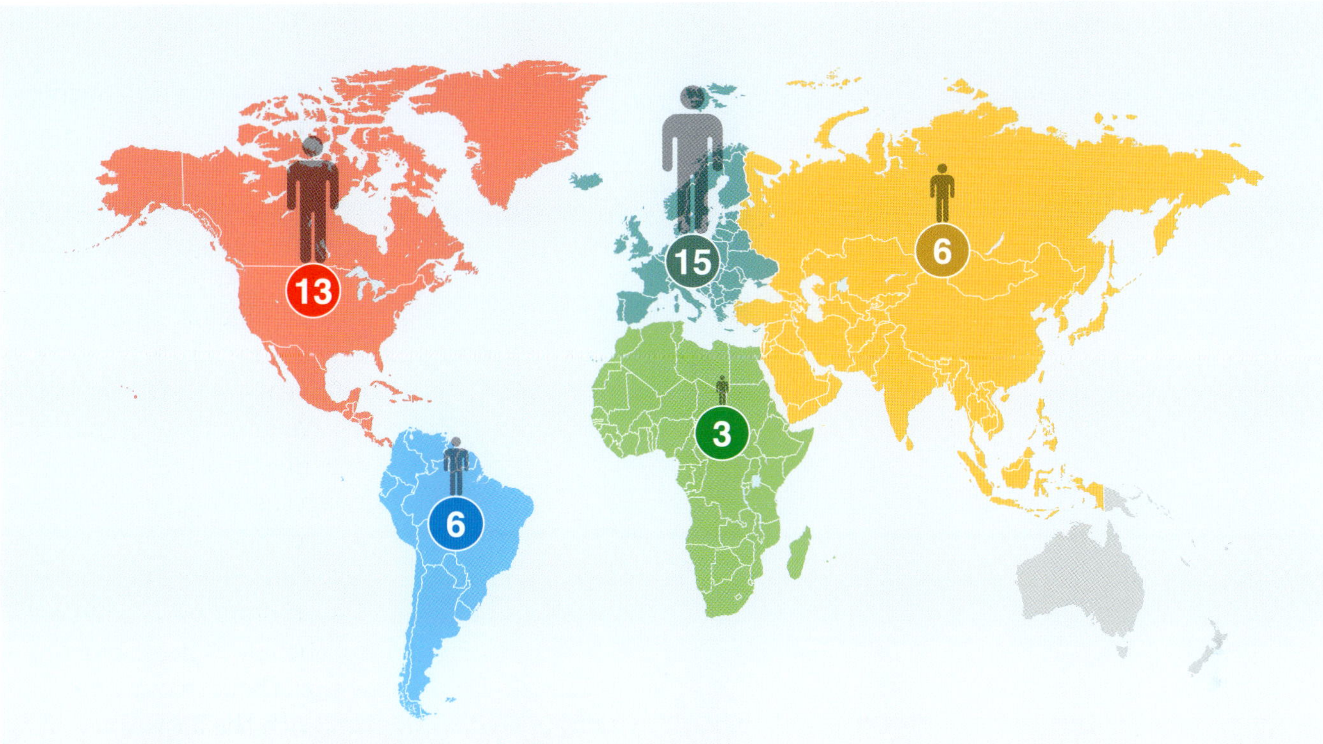

Fig. 1.2 Percentage of the senior population by continent and date (2000).[5]

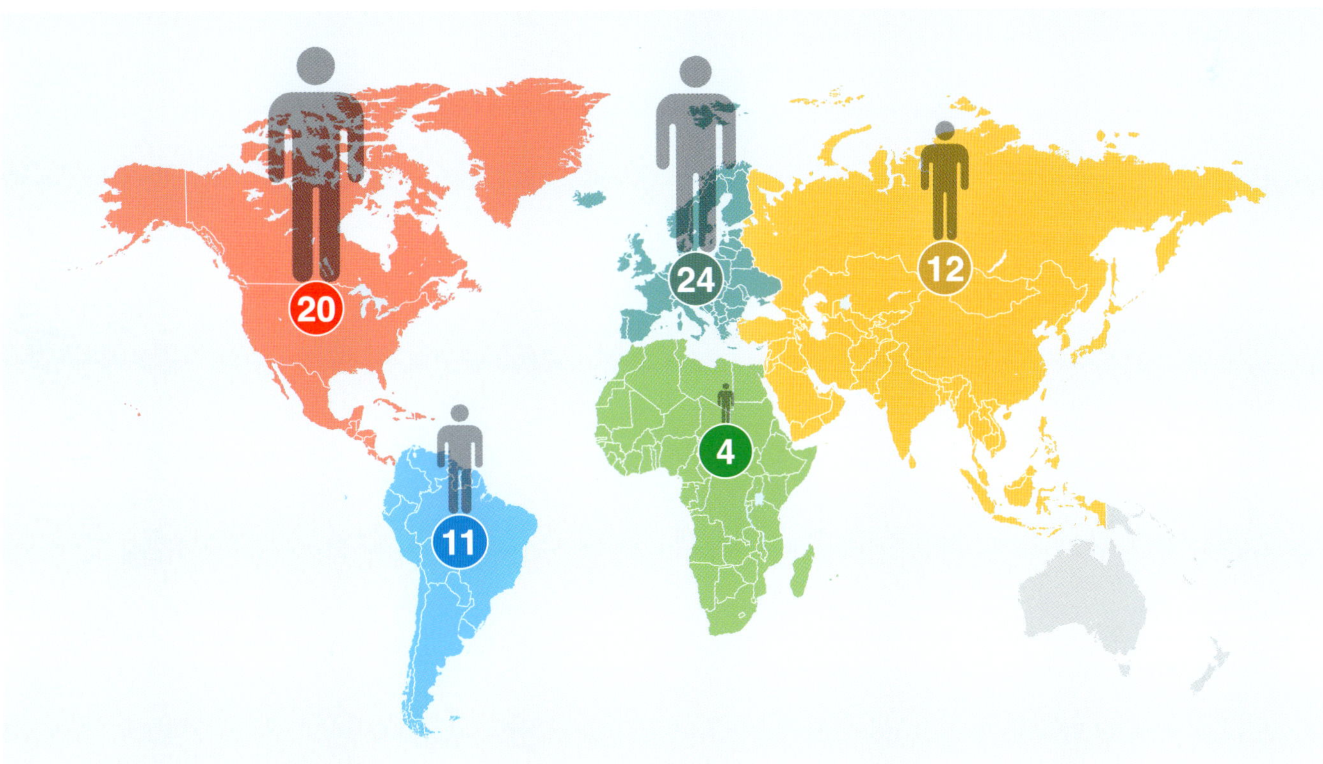

Fig. 1.3 Percentage of the senior population by continent and date (2030).[5]

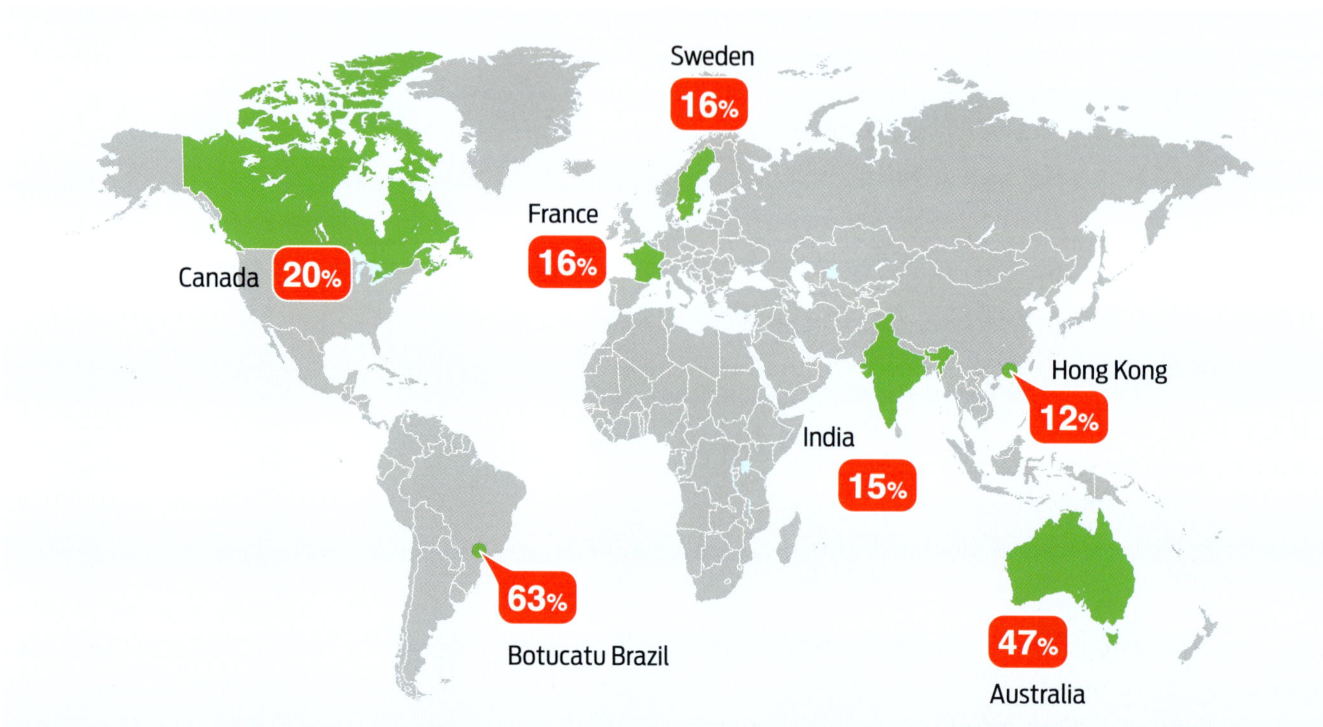

Fig. 1.4 Percentage of edentulous people worldwide.[5]

1.2 What is Geriatric Dentistry

Geriatric Dentistry is an amalgamation of all disciplines in the field of Dentistry, as well as Clinical Dentistry, as we know it. It also includes the knowledge of Medicine, with respect to diagnosis, disease processes, treatment, prevention and physiological manifestations of disease in the Human body and embodies people over 65 years of age, for the most part. There are younger persons who harbor "Geriatric Dentitions", and by this, I mean, have dentitions that are aged looking or in an advanced state of disrepair, something a dentist might find in an older individual.

> **DEFINITION:** ***Geriatrics*** *is the branch of Medicine concerned with the diagnosis, treatment and prevention of disease in older people and the problems specific to aging.*

> **DEFINITION:** ***Dentistry*** *is the evaluation, diagnosis, prevention and/or treatment (non-surgical, surgical or related procedures) of diseases, disorders and/or conditions of the oral cavity, maxillofacial area and/or the adjacent and associated structures and their impact on the human body; provided by a dentist, within the scope of his/her education training and experience, in accordance with the ethics of the profession and applicable laws.*

"Attached to every tooth is a person". So, we know that we are not just treating teeth, we are treating a specific person who has teeth or needs teeth to function. Never lose sight of this fact because it can save you from despair in the future. Just because you may have a person in your dental chair, who may look homeless and aged, does not mean he/she should be treated any the less than a younger, more kempt individual. Sometimes, looks are deceiving... and passing judgment can come back to bite you where it hurts.

"We know that oral disease can lead to systemic disease and that systemic disease can lead to oral disease". All disease processes can be either chronic or acute in nature. Until the onset of COVID-19, an acute disease process, more people have been dying from chronic diseases since 2010.[6]

Chronic illness, as we know it, is long-term in the scheme of things. It can be confounded by an acute disease, such as COVID-19, and change the status to an acute exacerbation of a chronic disease; whereby, the end of life may be eminently in the forefront of these specific individuals' eyes. In January 2021, according to the CDC (Centers for Disease Control in the U.S.), 10% of the senior population, 65 years or older, have died from complications of COVID-19; an example of people who had one or more chronic disease issues and contracted this virus on top of it.

With respect to Geriatric Dentistry one might look at the accompanying New Aging Paradigm (Fig. 1.1) to see the shift in age categories that can further define the word "Geriatric" for us. In many instances, local governments have helped define age group dissemination with financial benefits, social security benefits, and discounts for seniors at age 50 years and not on the merit of the age of the person. So there is a broad spectrum connoting "Geriatrics" today. The most likely definition parallels the onset of social security benefits at 65 years. However, in the next chapter, a discussion on a broader theme about "Geriatric Dentition" will ensue.

1.3 The Immune System and Oral Health

The immune system is the guardian of our bodies. With precision, timing, energy, direction and a sense of neurologic urgency to both time and place, our immune systems keep us in check. Socrates once stated, "The eyes are the windows to the Soul". This author advocates that "**The mouth is the pathway and the key to Healthy Aging**".

It's not just what we put in our mouths with respect to the types of foods we eat and the kind of diet we maintain for ourselves, but how we take care of our mouths that protect us and bolster our immune systems. Enzymes found in the salivary glands break down our food into nutrients, which in turn are ultimately converted into energy for our cells and organs to function in a normal, healthy manner.

Saliva plays a huge part in this process due to its ability to provide enzymes and other proteins that help fight bacteria and virus and the possibility of subsequent infection from occurring. We will discuss more about these issues in Chapter 3.

More pertinent in this discussion about immunity for our bodies, especially the geriatric population, is a marker that can tell us about the presence of inflammation in our bodies, including the mouth. This is C-reactive protein (CRP) and/or high-sensitivity C-reactive protein (hs-CRP). CRP is an extremely sensitive and nonspecific acute-phase marker for inflammation that is produced by the liver in response to many forms of injury and disease in one's body. CRP contributes to host defense and is part of the innate immune response. Plasma levels of CRP can rise to more than 1000-fold within hours after acute inflammatory response and infectious disease processes. It has a short half-life and makes for a good marker for follow-up of patients with infectious disease and the like who may be under antibiotic therapy for their infection.[7]

A simple blood test can determine the efficacy of C-reactive protein, or high-sensitivity C-reactive protein, as a marker for periodontal disease and oral disease, as well as systemic disease. Clinical correlation should be made with the results of the specific blood test for this marker.

C-reactive protein is regulated by cytokines like interleukin-6 (IL-6), interleukin-1β (IL-1β) and tumour necrosis factor-α (TNF-α). These are major building blocks of one's immune system. C-reactive protein is currently considered a key biomarker of systemic inflammation.[8] However, there are no signs or symptoms that are specific for an elevated C-reactive protein level, because it is not a "specific test". The symptomology, if present, would depend upon any underlying inflammatory conditions, like periodontal disease or oral and systemic infection that would be the cause of an elevated level of C-reactive protein. Consequently, this would be diagnosed by a simple blood test for CRP.

Many older individuals may be "stuck" in their ways and not take stock in a professional opinion from a dental practitioner, if nothing "hurt" them or bothered them in the face of an oral or head and neck infection. This test, if the patient would consider it, would help the believability of the issue at hand and, subsequently, give the dental practitioner more credibility as both a good diagnostician and caring and knowledgeable dentist. This simple test could be the difference in saving an older persons' teeth and eradicating their oral disease, as well as possibly saving their life.

Being a good geriatric dental practitioner means wearing many hats. For instance, it is always a good idea to understand the dietary habits of our patients and make recommendations about "eating healthy". It is also incumbent upon us to ask more meaningful questions about an older individuals habits in order to ascertain those that might be deleterious to their over-all health. When I ask a patient if they smoke at all, I usually ask "What do you smoke? How long have you had this habit? How many times a day do you smoke? And what do you enjoy about it?" This gives me an idea of whether I think I can help correct this habit in my patient or not. But it sometimes takes a lot of persistance with a well-seasoned habit in an older individual. Habits die hard. If we can help a patient with their negative habits, then we have achieved something worthwhile.

Statistically speaking, habits are learned responses to negative stimuli. Sending a patient to a counselor who can better deal with the patient and their habit is sometimes a good bet. Getting the patient convinced they should go is another story altogether, as many of you reading this book already know. I remember a patient that I was questioning about a specific action that they took regarding their dental care, or lack thereof, and I was pushing hard to get into the patients mindset to find out why they did not like to floss the one or two teeth they had. The patient became extremely angry and told me to my face that they did not need a "shrink", but they wanted a dentist to make them some teeth! I found this a bit startling at first until I understood what I did and who I was dealing with. Some people are incorrigible and inflexable. Therefore, we have to know our limits. I advocate that "We cannot undo what the patient will not let us do". I learned a valuable lesson, way back when, and it has "stuck" with me for the rest of my career. We can only try. As practitioners, we know that we cannot assist everyone. We need to "know before we go", who it is, exactly, that we are working with. It is okay to say "No, I don't think I can be of service to you", if your values do not coincide with the issues the older, more "set-in-their-ways" patient brings to you. Another valuable lesson in life.

Table 1.2 Chronic illness

• Nearly 1 in 2 Americans (160 million).
• By 2025, about 160 million will be affected.
• Projected to increase by 1-2% yearly and by 2030 an estimated chronically ill population of more than 180 million, more than ½ of our society.
• 60% are between 18-64 years.
• 90% of seniors have at least one chronic illness and 77% have two or more chronic illnesses.

U.S. Department of Health and Human Services, 2018.[1]

Because the world's population is living longer and subsequently there are more people in the world as we know it, there will be more chronic and acute diseases affecting people to a larger degree in the future (Table 1.2). This includes tooth issues and the maintenance of one's teeth and oral structures. In a report given in the year 2000 by the U.S. Surgeon General to the National Institutes of Health, he stated that at that time "chronic oral diseases, such as periodontal disease coupled with dental caries, were two of the top pandemic disease entities encountered worldwide".[9] These diseases are both endemic to all countries and all inhabitants of the world and as chronic diseases they remain a major cause of tooth loss in all Humans.

It behooves us, as practitioners, to be aware of these issues and to emphasize prevention in our practices, not just treatment. Without the proper education of our patients about dental disease, it will never be eradicated. I dare my patient's to "put me out of business", by learning all there is to learn about themselves physically, orally and medically, using this information as a platform to change their actions. Essentially, I would like them to be proactive in caring for themselves, not reactive when they have a disease. I am the teacher, and they are my students...

So, one of the main issues in working with older individuals as our patients would be to instruct them and encourage them to practice good oral hygiene and to show them how to maintain a healthier oral cavity, not just "fixing something" that does not work right in their eyes. Many older patients I have encountered over the years have told me that they were "too old to learn". Not true. We need to go behind their words to see what created this attitude they brought into the office with them. Denture wearers especially will need to be educated about not wearing their dentures 24/7. I inform them that it is "like sleeping with their shoes on". The oral tissues need to rest. Force causes change and subsequent bone loss, making the dentures eventually ill-fitting. Consider the numbers of edentulous people in the world and look at how they could have kept their teeth, if someone had taken the time to educate and really care for them instead of just taking out their teeth to solve an immediate unmet need.

1.4 The Immune System

> **DEFINITION:** ***Immunity*** *is defined as the ability of an organism to resist a particular infection or toxin by the action of specific antibodies or sensitized white blood cells. Essentially the immune system is a complex network of cells, tissues, organs and the substances they make that helps the body fight infections and other diseases. The immune system includes white blood cells and organs and tissues of the lymph system, such as thymus, spleen, tonsil, lymph nodes, lymph vessels and bone marrow.*[10]

The human organism, *Homo sapiens*, begins life with a somewhat genetically weak immune system and evolves into a more resistant organism initially through its mother's milk and subsequent diet, exposure to air and the particulate surrounding it from all sides. It is this so-called immunity, or resistance to disease, that protects it from the harm of unknown bacteria, virus, and unknown harmful protein molecules that can pierce its vail. However, there is only so much our bodies can do against these intruders without the aid of drugs, medicines and vaccines that have come to the fore over the ages.

The average age at death in the U.S. at the turn of the 1900's was 47 years.[11] In 2020, the life expectancy for males was 77 years and for females it was 81 years, almost double the number over 100 years ago.[12] The explanation lies in many facets of our living environment and in genetics, when one thinks of the "survival of the fittest" law.

Today, people are living longer not only because of their protective longevity genes, but because of better healthcare, better technology, improved diets and healthier foods on the menus, as well as modern research efforts to improve all facets of the general living conditions of most people, especially those in wealthier nations. Access to care is much better than 100 years ago, as is the care itself. However, there is an endpoint to all these things when our "internal clocks" tell us that it is the end of the day for us, forever.

Considering patient health factors as we age involves many different modalities in order to make sure all the bases are covered. And these are only a small part of why people may or may not live longer in the scheme of things called *LIFE*.

1.5 Geriatric Patient Health Factors[13]

- **Age**: as one ages, their ability to fight infection diminishes. This is termed *immune senescence*.
- **Genetics**: this plays an important part in both the long-term health benefits of the patient and lifelong deleterious effects it may cause.
- **Diet**: poor nutrition affects the overall health of an individual. Drinking water and hydrating oneself is also a priori, due to the inactivity and diminishment of pituitary hormones and enzymes that stimulate the desire to drink as one ages.
- **Exercise**: is important to maintain strength and stamina. Walking is the best exercise averaging 10,000 steps daily and for at least 30 minutes, five times a week with constant cardiac output.

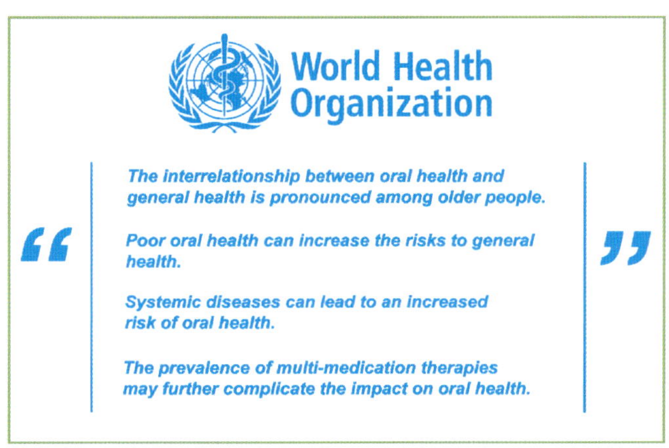
World Health Organization
The interrelationship between oral health and general health is pronounced among older people.
Poor oral health can increase the risks to general health.
Systemic diseases can lead to an increased risk of oral health.
The prevalence of multi-medication therapies may further complicate the impact on oral health.

Fig. 1.5 U.S. Department of Health and Human Services, 2018.[1]

- **Attitude**: a good attitude is half the battle in overall personal health, especially mental health. We cannot change our past or how people will treat us. Life can hand us things we do not expect, which we may not be able to cope with. If that is 10% of what happens to us, then the other 90% is how we react to it in a positive manner... our attitude.
- **Knowledge**: is a necessity in order to survive the journey and to maintain proper care of oneself-*self-efficacy*.
- **Persistance**: being forward directed allows older individuals to increase their coping skills, in order to challenge life and stay in the mainstream.
- **Time**: affects one's ability to seek out care, work and carry out dreams, as well as procure one's needs.
- **Money**: without this modality, care of any kind may be limited or non-existent.
- **Medically or mentally challenged**: can affect a person's ability to get care or seek out care on their own, as well as understand the why's of what they need health-wise.
- **Healthcare providers**: necessary for ongoing care, which includes access to geriatric care and the prevalence of facilities and providers for medical and dental services in general.
- **Products**: necessary to assist in both providing care, ADLs (Activities of Daily Living), and maintaining oneself.
- **Understanding**: being able to interpret information, process it and discuss it through adequate, open and honest communication. Without understanding there may be continued poor health or no care of any kind forthcoming.

Our immunity depends upon so many factors to keep us viable organisms. One may find that these confounding issues previously mentioned create a great deal of difficulty for the older individual; especially, if that person is infirm, alone, has cognitive decline of one form or another and many other physical and mental factors which can cause one's demise.

We know that oral disease can cause systemic disease issues and vice versa (**Fig. 1.5**). We know that the body is an integrated network that works in sync with all its parts. However, when something is broken in the system that promotes health and there is a decline in physical as well as mental resistance, the body will fail to keep its good health status. The many patient health factors listed here are dependent not only upon the older person's ability to manifest them or put them in place, but also their physical and mental ability to make them work for themselves. It is also incumbent upon us to be able to resist the negative effects of all these factors.

Our circadian rhythm is one thing that keeps us going, but it is the actual ability of the older individual, that is, their energy, their drive, their willingness to move forward, their resistance and coping skills and more, which gets them to their end-goal: good oral and physical health.

1.5.1 Systemic and Oral Disease with Respect to the Aging Process

When the body reacts to a disease process in one's youth or in old age, there is a chain reaction that happens. The physiologic chemicals inside of us, such as epinephrine, cortisol, cytokines, endorphins, as well as lymphocytes, monocytes, eosinophils, various tissue factors, such as interleukins and high-sensitivity C-reactive protein, to name a few, move at full force. Our organ systems also kick-in to produce these entities to help bolster our immune systems and help quell whatever it is that is creating the immune response over time. In older and more medically challenged individuals this reaction process is much slower, if it exits at all. Physiologic breakdown can be a chronic disease that happens over a long period of time, or it can be swift if that chronic disease process is exacerbated by an acute disease process. Chronic periodontal disease, for example, is a long-term disease. It can happen in one's youth and continue until the gingival tissue and bone loss are so diseased that teeth just fall out on their own. "Supervised neglect" has a way of aiding this process. More about this process will be discussed in Chapter 2. I mention it here because I want the reader to start thinking about all the entities that go into making our systems healthy and, likewise, unhealthy as we age. If one gets a good practitioner or many practitioners when they are young who are instructive and motivating, then they may not have to suffer the chronic infections in their mouths and subsequent loss of teeth or eventual systemic related disease.

Again, *"Attached to Every Tooth is a Person"*, and when a tooth is lost, so is a vital part of that person's identity, make-up and function, which may or may not be able to be regained in good order. It will all depend upon the *Patient Health Factors*, the age of the person who is affected by these issues and their individual coping skills, education and desire to replace what is missing or repair what is damaged. Adequate finances will be a major factor as well.

In Figure 1.6 you can see one that is filled with inflammation and disease. The patient is an older individual, in their 70's, who has both chronic and acute disease processes going on. Periodontal disease symptomology is quite evident clinically, but it is the chronic disease, other than periodontal disease, that is not. Clinical patients who present with these types of findings should be encouraged to seek out medical diagnosis of their clinical findings and beyond. A simple C-reactive protein test might elucidate a subclinical inflammatory situation. This would then lend itself to further investigation into what is the exact cause through other tests and examinations. This patient has a blood dyscrasia, such as lymphoma or leukemia and, as such, it changes the entire spectrum of treatment both orally and systemically. If one were to biopsy a piece of gingival tissue from this patient, they might find leukemic infiltrates within the tissue, confirming a systemic disease diagnosis.

The aging process can bring on *immune senescence*: simply a decline in one's ability to fight infection, which, in turn, places an older person's overall health in a state of major compromise. Having a low dental IQ would also be a cause that is termed "supervised neglect", and a patient who might not have the ability or know-how to see a dentist on a regular basis, as well as not know how to take care of their dentition. The resultant periodontal disease and bone loss could be a direct result of these factors. The onset of an underlying systemic disease only exacerbates the obvious issues that one can see.

I have coined a new type of periodontal disease under the heading of *"Geriatric" periodontal disease*. This periodontal disease classification is associated with a systemic disease as well as an oral disease. This type of inflammatory situation puts the immune system into overdrive; however, with the body being so overwhelmed with both oral and systemic

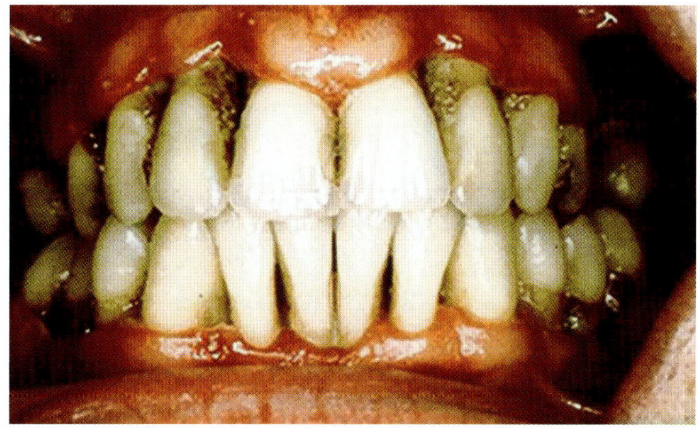

Fig. 1.6 Chronically ill middle-aged adult with periodontal disease.

inflammation it can only handle so much before there is a massive breakdown of multiple systems, as evidenced in Figure 1.6. This makes it difficult in the long run to treat this patient effectively or at all. The underlying disease needs to be arrested before the oral disease can be repaired; the extent of which is unknown due to multiple factors: seriousness of the systemic disease and ability to see it in remission; time of treatment; degree of the oral disease and the body's ability to maintain the dentition in the face of mobility and oral infection; the overall effectiveness of the patient's immune system and the patient's ability to survive in total throughout treatment, if any.

Immunity basically implies wellness for the most part. **Wellness** constitutes the following:

- Physical
- Emotional
- Intellectual
- Social
- Spiritual
- Environmental
- Occupational

One must exhibit at least the first five components to be considered well. *Wellness is the act of practicing healthy habits on a regular basis in order to not just survive, but to thrive.* Without the ability of one's *immune system* to participate in the physical aspects of this process, total wellness may not be achievable. Therefore, it is so important for dental practitioners to encourage their patients total body health. We need to consider counselling our patients in: proper nutrition; assisting them to understand the importance of proper dental homecare;

emphasize self-efficacy in all directions; show that we care about them, not only as their practitioner, but as their friend; help improve their dental IQ by giving them the health information they might need to help themselves in the long-run; refer the patient to ancillary healthcare practitioners as needed; and, provide them with excellent dental care overall.

"**No one cares how much you know, until they know how much you care**". When assisting our older patients, it is so especially important to take the time to spend with them before, during and after treatment, because of the invisible bonds that this will create for us ultimately, resulting in the patients' better adherence to personal care; increased patient referrals and increased care options accomplished over an extended time and a happier and healthier patient overall.

As scientists in Dentistry, it might be somewhat difficult for us to relate the immune system, with all its physiological properties, to a healthy thought process. The brain controls our ability to think, and our thoughts are extremely powerful in heightening the ability of the immune system to be effective against "foreign invaders" to our bodies, without even a conscious thought at all. The enemies that attack our bodies can and do create inflammation, infection and disease; perhaps, which will ultimately cause our demise. As Humans, we can help our immune systems by practicing good oral health, maintaining a good diet and practicing *Wellness* in all respects with our patients and ourselves.

1.6 Comparing the Past with Present-Day Dentistry

We have the luxury of looking back some 5000 years into history to see that all types of ethnic groups, in all parts of the world, had some version of Dentistry that they practiced. Each successive generation passed on their ideas and their improvements in treating dental "pain" and disease.

This practice of the past has led to today's practitioners and a profession that is more productive, less painful and one in which patient's come willingly for treatment; not simply frightened or anxious about having treatment done that creates more pain, angst and fear in the long run.

One hundred years ago, there were much fewer "older" people living in our society, as there are today. Dentists like "Painless Parker", in the early 1900's in New York, saw people who were middle-aged for extractions along with some younger patients who, for one reason or another, needed a tooth repaired or taken out. He had a travelling "side-show", with his office in a wagon, pulled by a horse from city to city. People, who were considered *Geriatric* patients, were pretty much in their forties and fifties, because people did not live much longer than that in those days. We have come full circle since then and have made great strides in improving dental care in all respects.

> *"The circle is a reminder that each moment is not just the present but is inclusive of our gratitude to the past and our responsibility to the future."*
>
> *Kazuaki Tanahashi*

The circle of life, starting with the past, is a steppingstone to the future from which we learn. If it were not for the *pioneers* in Dentistry, we would still be "stuck" just taking out teeth, rather than saving them, as well as eliminating disease. Comparing the past to the present and beyond, one must look at the following entities that have changed over the last 200 years:

- The kinds of equipment that we had available to use for our profession: no X-rays then and three-dimensional films now.
- The sterility, or lack thereof, compared to today's stringent standards.
- The simple materials dentists used or had available to restore teeth and mouths: wooden dentures and wired-up teeth versus today's implant retained overdentures made of lifelike acrylic or porcelain.
- The technology of the past that was primitive, compared to today's space-age equipment, such as robotics in Dentistry.
- The techniques of yester-year that were primitive and somewhat barbaric compared to the luxuries of today's relatively comfortable treatment: alcohol or cocaine used as a pain killer versus medications,

local anesthetic and general anesthesia and sedation of today.

- Knowledge of science and dental treatment and care was minimal, at the least, in the past and always the basis for new and improved discoveries, such as lasers in Dentistry.
- The perception of pain in the past regarding dental treatment versus the comfort and prevention of pain in today's society.
- Specialties of Dentistry did not exist in the beginning as they do today. At least seven specialties in Dentistry are recognized by the American Dental Association: the exception being Geriatrics.

These are the objective and sometimes subjective markers of our successes and failures of treating our patients and promoting our profession.

President John F. Kennedy once stated: "Change is the law of life. Those who look only to the **past** or the **present** are certain to miss the **future**". There is certainly room to grow, with respect to our knowledge base of dental science. Things are always in flux and there are always new advances that come about as a result of something that is needed and most definitely in response to change itself.

Today's treatment of our older generation of adults is much different than in the past; even as far back as 20 years ago. The advances in Medicine, as well as Dentistry, have given dental practitioners a new lease on treating those persons of an older ilk who are medically or mentally compromised. Through the constant curiosity, inventiveness and change in knowledge itself, "we" as the practitioners of today are in one of the most sought-after and respected professions in our culture. Dentistry has been ranked second as one of the most trusted professions in the United States.[14] It would be nice if we could replicate that attitude and desire in the older population of today, thereby stimulating patients for and toward our practices.

Trust is a major factor in going to see a dentist. Trust must be earned and does not come easily to an anxious or "set-in-their-ways" older individual. I think because of the primitive nature of Dentistry, going back to the 19th and early 20th centuries, patients generally had no trust for a dentist because usually the pain they received from previous treatment was worse, or perceived worse, than what they brought with them to a dental office in the first place.

Case Study 1

Supervised Neglect in a 70-Year-Old Patient

In **Figure 1.7** of an older individual, from a Sicilian ethnic background, brings with him a set of values that must be determined before any treatment is discussed. How did this person get to this point in his life? What are his habits and why did he let his mouth get to this state of disrepair? These are good questions to ask yourself when you see this type of oral condition. Did he have discomfort or pain? Yes, but mostly psychological pain for the most part. Unfortunately, he had years of conditioning about ***not*** going to a dentist for oral care, because his parents and grandparents, each from the "old country", had a different set of values that did not put much faith in going to a dentist for prevention. This gentleman's daughter, a patient of mine, brought him to my practice because she ***trusted*** me. Her father, who spoke broken English, was a hard-working man who usually did not go to a dentist, although there is some evidence that he did go to see a dentist at some point in his life, but not often enough to salvage his remaining teeth. He sought a second

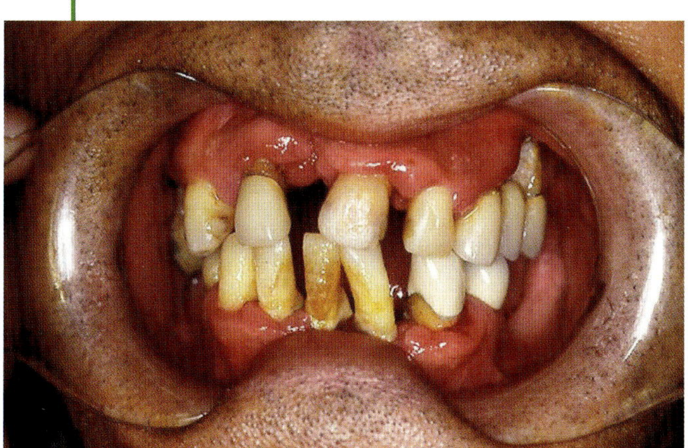

Fig. 1.7 Deceased 70-year-old man.

opinion from me regarding getting dental implants in his mouth, many years ago. He had seen an oral surgeon on his own, not knowing who to see, and was told he could have 9-12 implants placed immediately, after his full mouth extractions! I was in shock and took a moment to reflect on what this man was telling me. I suggested that he let me take a thorough history and do an examination on him, including whatever X-rays and models I needed to ascertain the depth of his issues, because the oral surgeon he visited did nothing but talk to him after looking in his mouth. This told me a lot about the oral surgeon he had seen and the lack of information that was ascertained before making a treatment plan for this patient. I also think because the patient was older, had poor English skills and had no insurance (he only paid his bills in cash), the surgeon was eager to give the patient what this patient had wanted: teeth he could "eat" with. All this, without doing a full work-up and giving this man alternative treatment plans to go along with the diagnosis of chronic periodontal disease, poor homecare, generalized mobility and sub-acute pain associated with gingival and bone inflammation. Unfortunately, this kind of thing is seen all too often with older people that frequent dental offices looking for assistance but knowing not how they got to that point or how to care for themselves.

The result showed that this genuinely nice person was depressed about his condition, his inability to eat, due to his loose teeth and pain, his lack of a smile and not being able to socialize and the lack of dental knowledge he had. I informed this gentleman that he could have implants, but it was risky doing immediate implants due to his infection and generalized bone loss. I told him he was not a candidate for implants at this juncture in time and that if he opted for a more judicious, less costly and simpler treatment plan first, that he could subsequently have implants in the future if he still wanted them once he was in good health and re-evaluated.

We discussed needed extractions and bone grafting. We discussed extensive periodontal therapy and regular recall. We discussed keeping the teeth we could salvage and using them as anchors to hold a set of overdentures (**Figs. 1.8, 1.9**). In the end, I told him that once his progress continued into a healthy mouth and he still wanted implants after a

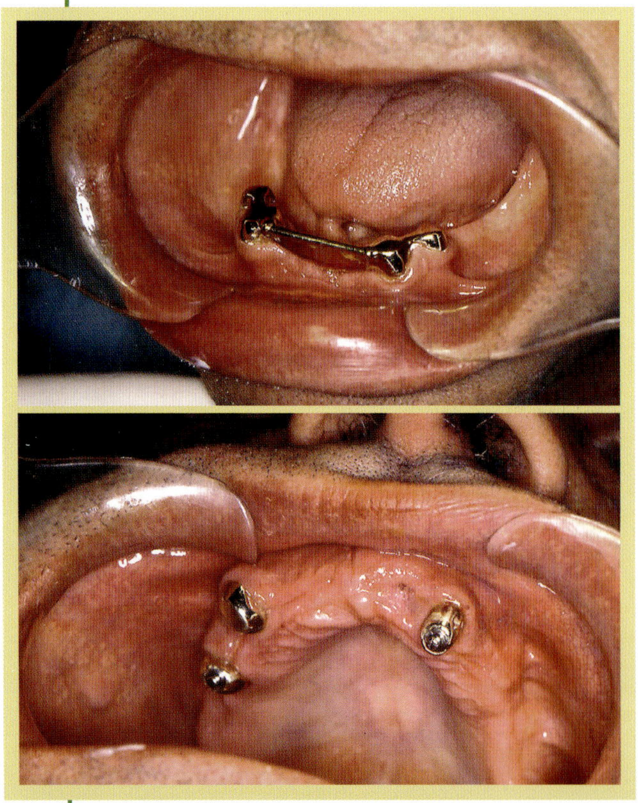

Fig. 1.8 Post-treatment overdentures.

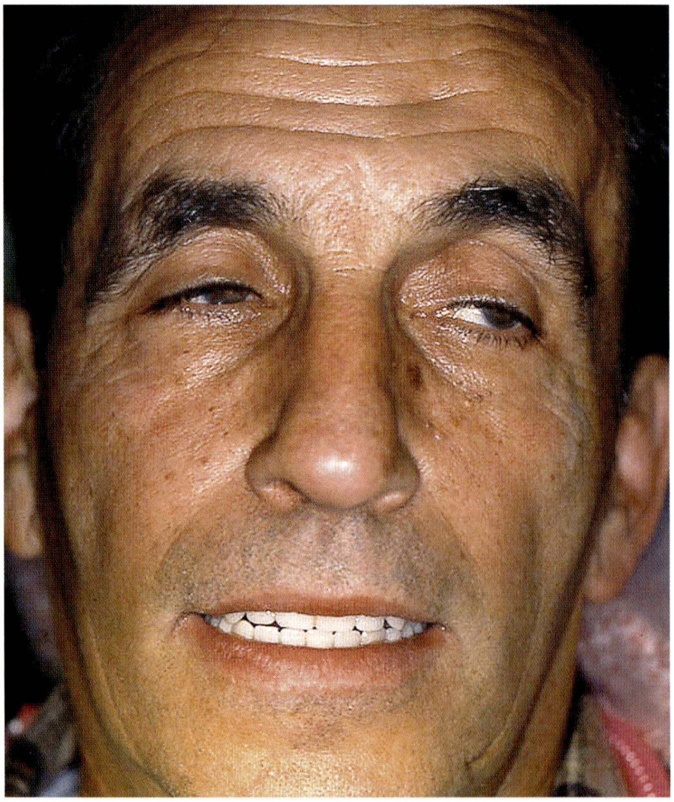

Fig. 1.9 Overdentures.

year, we would oblige him. I wanted to make sure he was compliant in every respect. Subsequently, we made his visits educational and fun. We made him responsible for his own oral health, but we were the guardians of his care. He liked that fact. His entire life changed after this treatment for the better!

A year later, he made an appointment to come in to discuss what I had told him when we first started his treatment; however, I did not know that he had had an accident: a fall from a third story ladder while doing work on one of his buildings, in which he fractured many bones and lost the upper left cuspid from his maxillary overdenture, but not the upper or lower overdentures themselves! He was so impressed with the work I had done and the comfort and stability of his overdentures that he opted out of having any implants whatsoever.

The modalities in Box 1.1 have shaped Dentistry into what it is today. It is a profession that is in a state of constant flux. New materials, for different situations of repair, are germane to the myriad of dental issues that patients bring with them to the dental office. Geriatric patients require more patience, communication, explanation and visual reinforcement of what the dentist intends to perform on them and with them. Showing someone the evolution of materials and explaining in simple terms how something works in one's mouth is creating a bond between the patient and the practitioner consisting of trust and understanding. Silver diamine used today to arrest dental caries in older patients is a boon to eliminating dental caries. The only issue here is that silver diamine turns the teeth black, a possible esthetic issue for some people. Dental fluoride is necessary for older patients to use to protect the enamel and dentin, as is synthetic saliva substitutes for xerostomia, all evolving through trial and error to use with our older and some younger patients as well.

We should not underestimate the presence of dental inventions in **history** when it comes to these explanations. They were and still are the gateway to the present and the future care of our patients-at-large.

BOX 1.1

200 Years of Dental Related Modalities

- A toothbrush was a piece of wood with animal bristles on it or just a piece of wood to scrape the teeth.
- Toothpaste was made from salt and sodium bicarbonate, if available; otherwise, it was a medium of soap and/or herbs and salt.
- Disinfectants consisted of alcohol (various types, some of which were very poisonous to Humans, such as Methanol-wood alcohol).
- Dental chairs varied from wooden stools to wooden chairs (Fig. 1.10). Evolving into metal chairs with truly little room to move; eventually made with arms to hold onto during surgery (Fig. 1.11). Modern chairs are contoured, soft, comfortable and fully adjustable.
- Topical anesthetics were used, such as cocaine and then a mixture of cocaine and grain alcohol. In the early 1800's, Ether was founded and used by William Morton, MD in 1845 for general surgery and in 1846, Dentist, Horace Wells, used a gas he discovered: Nitrous Oxide, for light sedation of his patients having tooth extractions. The first dental extraction using this "new" gas was given to himself. Wells reported "feeling nothing at all". It was considered an "Amnalgesic" type of drug. One that basically numbs the brain and one's ability to feel pain, let alone remember it.
- Gowns were not worn usually to treat patients, only street clothes and no gloves. Later, gowns made from sheets of linen were used. Who knows how often they were washed?
- Hand-washing and sterile technique had not been known yet to dentists.

(continued)

(continued)

- Dental Hand pieces or "Drills" were of the wheel and treadle type and had to be pumped by foot until electricity changed all that later in the late 19th and early 20th centuries.
- Hand pieces run by air turbine came into the fore in the latter part of the 1900's.
- Restorative techniques have evolved through the entire two centuries discussed here with the use of amalgams, cast metals, and eventually porcelain to replace teeth in part or in total. Today we see bonded restoration's taking the place of cemented restorations.
- Lasers for treating both hard and soft tissues evolved in Dentistry over the past 50-75 years and are now a normal part of the dentist's daily armamentarium.
- Dental implants have been improvised for many years and evolved into a viable entity for replacing missing teeth in the 1950's, with the advent of the blade implant and then modified to various forms of cylindrical implants, most of which now osseointegrate with surrounding bone. Techniques have evolved using CBCT (Cone Beam Computerized Tomography)-3-Dimensional CAT scans and "Guided surgeries", utilizing acrylic appliances for exact placement of the implant referencing three axis points: horizonal, vertical and oblique.

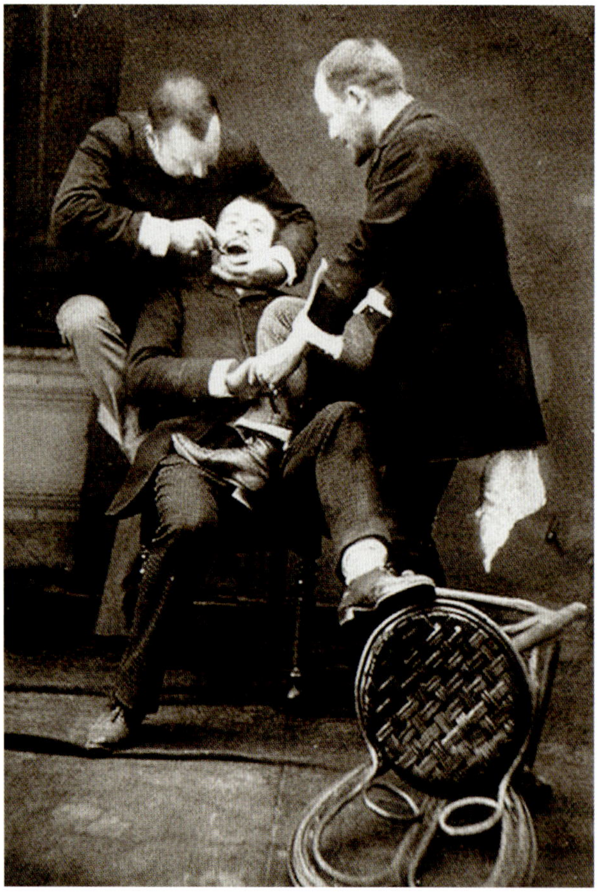

Fig. 1.10 Historical dental photo circa late 19th century. *(Pinterest.com.)*

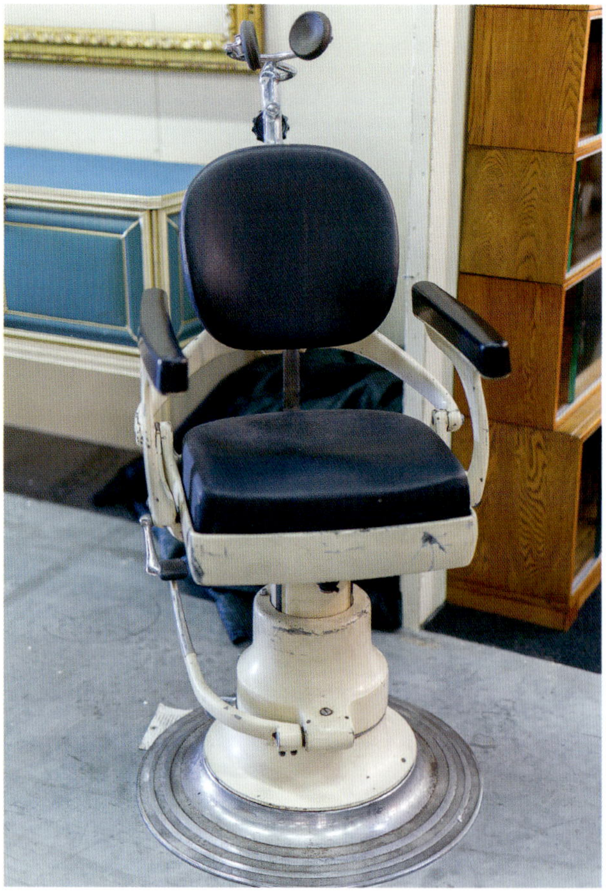

Fig. 1.11 Typical dental chair of the mid-1930's-1960's. *(Temple University Dental School Dental Museum, Philadelphia, PA.)*

References

1. U.S. Department of Health and Human Services, 2018.
2. Citation on statistics: *New Oxford American Dictionary*, Oxford University Press, Inc. 3rd Edition, 2016.
3. U.S. Census Bureau, 2020.
4. Shapira, Eric Z. *A New Wrinkle: What I Learned from Older People Who Never Acted Their Age.* iUniverse Publishers, Bloomington, Indiana, USA, 2011.
5. Petersen PE, Kandelman D, Arpin S, Ogawa H. *Global oral health of older people--call for public health action.* Community Dent Health. 2010 Dec;27(4 Suppl 2):257-67.
6. Agus, David, MD. *The End of Illness.* Free Press Publishing. A division of Simon & Schuster, 2011.
7. Chang HY, Kim AR, Pi SH, You HK. *A Study on the Correlation between C-Reactive Protein Concentration and Teeth with a ≥5 mm Periodontal Pocket in Chronic Periodontitis Patients.* Int J Dent. 2020 Dec 23;2020:8832186.
8. Bansal T, Pandey A, Deepa D, Asthana AK. *C-Reactive Protein (CRP) and its Association with Periodontal Disease: A Brief Review.* J Clin Diagn Res. 2014 Jul;8(7):ZE21-4.
9. U.S. Surgeon General Reports. Department of Health and Human Services, 2000.
10. National Cancer Institute, National Institutes of Health, 2021, www.Cancer.gov.
11. Senior Living.Org, July 25, 2019. Jeff Hoyt, Editor-in-Chief.
12. www.Statista.com, January, 2021.
13. Shapira, Eric Z, *Geriatric Dentistry Clinical Lectures*, 2021.
14. www.ADA.org; *ADA News*, 2020-archive, Jan 14, 2020. ADA.org/en/publications/ada-news/2020-archive/January/dentists-rank-2-in-news-and-world-report-best-jobs-report.

Chapter 2

Don't Step on the Cracks, or Bite Their Backs, Time will tell if One's Teeth will last a Lifetime?

"Attached to every tooth is a person.
People do not last a lifetime,
but hopefully our teeth will...!"

2.1 Introduction

Technical differences in our teeth, over the years, are a result of various factors that influence their make-up and include a variety of causes, such as forceful abuse, neglect, supervised neglect, diminished immunity, accidents, lack of funds, and a low dental IQ, to name a few.

> **DEFINITION:** ***Anthropometrics**, the measurement of the human individual; with respect to the dentition in this case, can be valuable in maintaining a complete dentition of at least 28 adult teeth throughout a person's time on Earth (sans four wisdom teeth). One must study cause and effect when considering longevity of teeth.*

I get the feeling, after practicing for almost 50 years, that most people take their teeth for granted, as well as their overall health for the most part. The teeth will last for a lifetime, says the brain! If something should happen to a tooth, like a fracture and the need for an extraction or endodontic procedure is eminent, many people become resigned to the fact that this now "injured" tooth is going to be lost anyway, so why not just settle for the extraction without thinking of the ramifications of their decision: "cause and effect". What do we do about the change in my mouth, as I now have a big hole there, says the psyche? Money becomes a factor here, especially without dental insurance of some sort, as endodontic procedures on teeth are usually the first step in salvaging a fractured tooth; unless it is so irreparably damaged that it really does have to be extracted. Either way, it can be costly.

Secondly, after having a root canal procedure, the possibility of placing a post and core into the tooth root and remaining crown structure for support and then covering it with a crown, made of some sort of material that will be strong, making for a cohesive restorative procedure that is both supportive and functional, is the treatment of choice most of the time. These steps all cost money. If a person is not insured, or of the mindset that "I'm going to lose my teeth anyway in the future; then, why not just take the tooth out now and be done with it is the prevalent choice, then so be it!" (The thinking here is that the tooth is not worth saving for the monetary price I must pay). But are they done with it? Most recently an older neighbor of mine stated that she was going to have her back molars taken out as they were periodontally involved. She alluded to the fact that she had spent thousands of dollars in the past on periodontal treatment, which did not seem to work for her. Her upper molar teeth had become severely loosened over time and the bone around them had subsequently disappeared. Unbeknownst to me that she was going to speak about her teeth to me, I brought her and her husband a book on Avocados, which they grow, and placed several new, in the wrapper, hand toothbrushes on the package. When I gave her the gifts, she replied, "Why are you giving me these brushes we don't brush our teeth!" Again, "for every action there is an opposite and equal reaction: "cause and effect". This is Newton's First Law of Physics. Need I say more?

This person did not want to be educated, talked into anything or even consider what was going to happen without her molars, such as a bite shift to her anterior teeth, stress and subsequent issues with her temporomandibular joints, increased wear, inability to chew properly with the possibility of some future digestive system issues, as well as a significant change in diet. There was no way I could reason with her or begin to educate her as her mind was made up. "We cannot undo what our patient's (or friends and neighbors) won't let us do". She told me her age, yet she looks close to 80, rather than the 57 years that she says she is. She has youth on her side but looks and acts old. One can be young and sport a "geriatric dentition".

The older one gets, the more this type of scenario takes place. It is the rare patient that understands what we, as dentists, are trying to do to assist them with their issues at hand.

"**Inform before you Perform**" is of ultimate importance for all patients, especially our older geriatric patients. Understanding only comes from effective communication in these cases. One caveat being that the mind can only absorb what it wants to hear. Old habits die hard, and many patients leave our offices because we do not give them enough good choices to do what we think needs to be done to solve an issue at hand, or something in the list of issues I previously discussed: lack of money, dental insurance, disinterest, fear and anxiety, and a myriad of other reasons the patient can come up with to not agree to treatment that benefits them.

2.2 Anatomy of a Tooth

A tooth germinates from a "Bud" within the confines of the jawbone. The "Bud", or "tooth bud", is genetically destined to be a specific type of tooth depending upon its location in the mouth and the probability that its ability to erupt a normal tooth is exacting. The tooth bud develops in the 8th week of intrauterine life. At this point, the tooth bud grows around the ectomesenchymal aggregation, taking on the appearance of a cap, and becomes the **enamel** (or **dental**) **organ** covering the **dental papilla**. A condensation of ectomesenchymal cells called the **dental sac** or **follicle** surrounds the enamel organ and limits the dental papilla (Fig. 2.1).

Enamel is the hardest substance in the human body. It is harder than bone, but it is not impervious to wear from various sources, including abrasion against other teeth. Enamel becomes fused rods running perpendicularly within the bud as they grow into a tooth form. Dentin, a softer underlayment, contains tubules as well, but they run horizontally outward from the

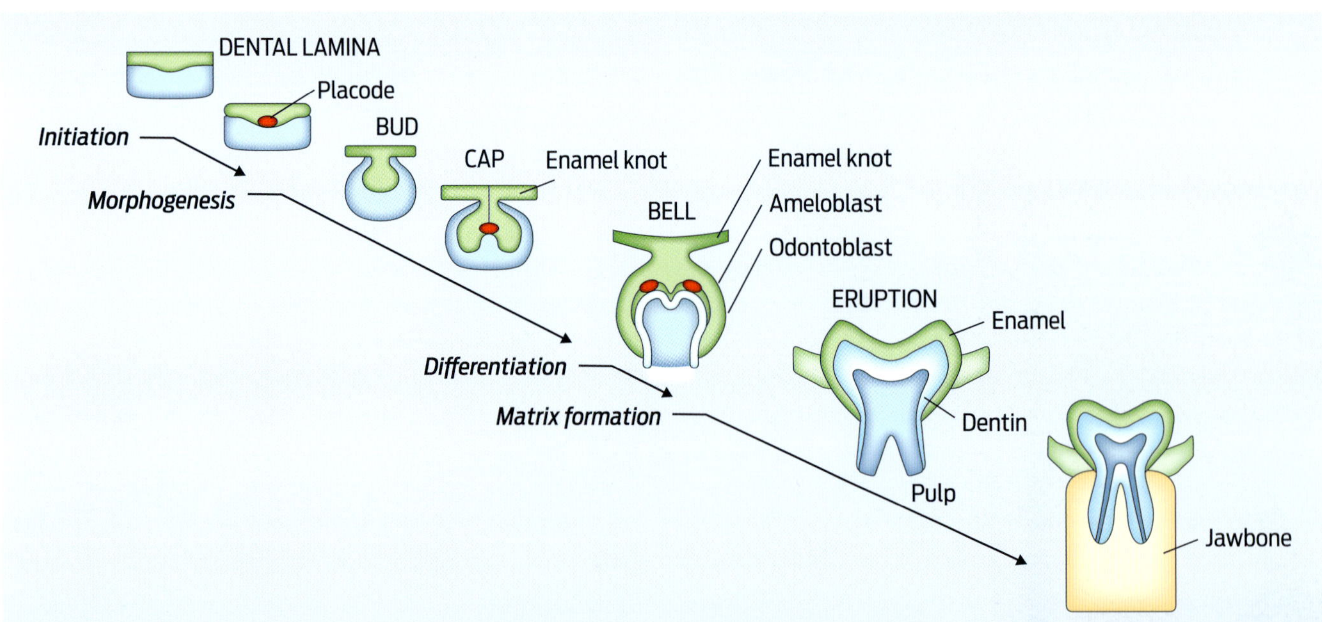

Fig. 2.1 The evolution of a tooth.

pulp of the tooth carrying the blood vessels, nerves and lymphatics inside the tooth to the periphery meeting the enamel shield. Once the enamel has been breached through cracks, chips, decay, wear and other abnormalities, the tooth can break down further causing sensitivity to hot or cold or overt discomfort. The roots of teeth are made of dentin and covered with a protective soft shield called cementum. Cementum can be easily worn away if exposed, leaving a sensitive root surface with exposed dentinal tubules.

Case Study 1

A 104-year-old patient of mine presented with pain in the upper left maxilla, where he had a fractured tooth down to the root (Fig. 2.2). He had existing implants with crowns and was no stranger to dentistry. His X-ray showed a calcified root on his first upper bicuspid. There was inflammation around the gingiva of his fractured tooth, telling me that this gentleman did not possibly perform the appropriate homecare, but he also had inflammation and swelling from the fractured root situation itself with tissue ingress. The patient had an involved medical history, including previous heart issues and blood thinners that he took. Treatment in this case would be minimal and I made a concerted effort to get him out of pain before doing anything long-term. Of course, he did not want to spend a lot of money on "fixing" anything, nor did he want me to do anything really involved in the first place, other than telling me what he thought he did not need. He continuously complained that his teeth were not holding up and was angry and frustrated, as this was not the first time this had happened to him. At his tender age of 104 years, he was hampered by arthritis, which affected his ability to floss and brush.

I ended up removing some inflamed gum tissue around the neck of the root with a Diode laser. There was no bleeding from this action. The laser also seals the blood vessels and nerve endings in the area, which promotes healing and allows for no post-treatment discomfort. The root was solid and somewhat "ankylosed" to the adjacent bone. I removed minor decay and elevated the root to the level of the alveolar ridge using a dental handpiece, thus, allowing him to keep his remaining bone and promoting growth of the gingiva on top of the bone, which would eventually heal over the retained root. This was a very conservative procedure called a "Root Burial" and it is basically painless with little to no post-treatment discomfort or problems.

I felt it would be more traumatic to remove the root and cause the patient both destruction of the existing bone and prolonged physical trauma getting the root out. If I had taken the tooth out without first checking with his medical doctor to take him off blood thinners completely, he might have bled profusely. Ultimately, he would have had more extensive problems than what he presented with in the first place. The patient was most thankful and happy for the care he had, paid his bill and stood for a photo with me, even though he is not smiling (Fig. 2.3).

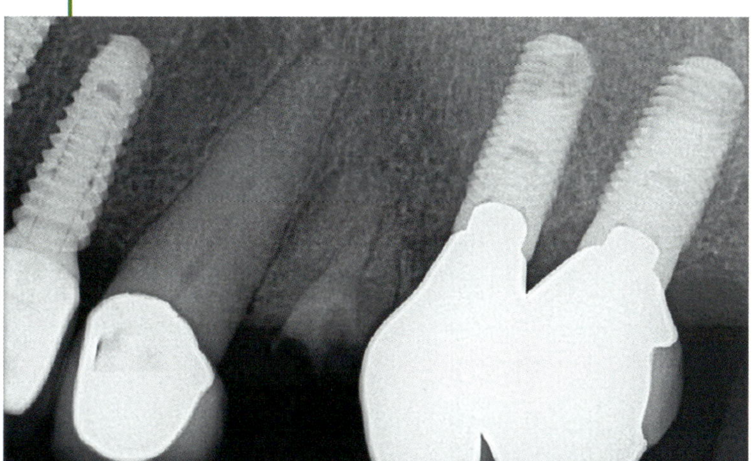

Fig. 2.2 Fractured retained root.

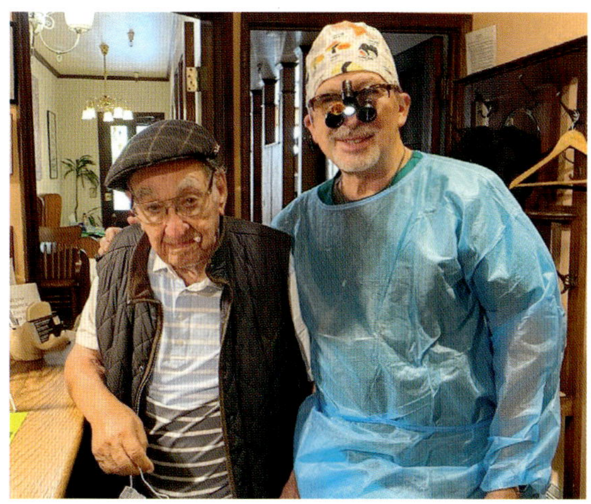

Fig. 2.3 104-year-old patient post-treatment with this Author.

Situations like this one require a lot of listening, thought and communication. It requires teaching the patient about himself and his apparent habits and showing pictures and explaining what I found through the radiographs he allowed me to take. His hearing was not very good, and I found myself almost "yelling" at him during my discussion of treatment and the treatment itself, trying to explain what he brought into the office with him and what I recommended he do about it. He kept checking with his caregiver, who had accompanied him to the office, and who was standing alongside of him during treatment. I had previously explained to the caregiver what my intentions were and what I wanted to do for this patient, and he understood and agreed. Once the patient got the nod of the caregiver, whom he trusted, he went ahead with the intended treatment.

All in all, after a lot of discussion he was very amenable to having me do what I did to make things better for him. However, he never stopped mumbling about how his teeth were failing him at this age. So, in the long-run, people's expectations need to be communicated and either validated or elucidated as being unrealistic. If this had happened to this patient, he would probably have left with a smile on his face instead of the look of pensiveness or unsureness about things. On the other hand, I had to evaluate my behavior in periodically raising my voice to discuss my treatment recommendations with him and assuage my own guilt about wanting to be civil, yet possibly not appearing to be.

The first "rule of thumb" with respect to Geriatric Dentistry is: **To Do No Harm.** In essence, I think that being cognizant of the patients' well-being, their histories (both medical and dental), the crux of the issue(s) they bring with them, the social factors they discuss, their attitude in general about dentistry for sure and their willingness to listen to reason in the face of an adversity and, possibly, a traumatic event in their mouth, this all-encompassing information which is their "puzzle", they bring with them to our offices, will allow us the ability to treat them with the utmost of respect and care and, essentially, doing them no harm. This holds true for all our patients as well.

Geriatric Dentistry, one will find, is fraught with many situations which require much thought and purpose on the side of the practitioner. There is always the unexpected and then the more unexpected we might encounter in terms of what it is we are called upon to "fix". Being conservative in care, being cognizant of a patient's mental disposition, being fair to all concerned parties, being respectful no matter the patients position in life and always being communicative with an open mind and heart will help us as practitioners to "do no harm".

We, as practitioners, will need to be logical, inventive, prepared for anything and everything and sometimes we may have to involve a guardian, a translator, an interpreter, and an overly concerned relative who may hamper our best intentions, or refer the patient to someone else. Therefore, it is important to always *listen* more than we *speak*. This is what my grandfather always said of why we have two ears and one mouth, so we can listen more than we speak!

> *"Wisdom is the reward you get for a lifetime of listening when you would have rather talked."*
>
> *Mark Twain*

2.3 Geriatric Dentition

For the most part, I define a Geriatric Dentition as follows:

> **DEFINITION:** ***Geriatric Dentition*** *is the complement of remaining teeth in the mouth of an older person that remain in a person's mouth; which have been subjected to a decline or deformity in shape, form, function and usage and suffering from caries; periodontal disease; attrition; abrasion; fracture; loss of a tooth or teeth; internal pulp infection; mobility and the inability to function in a "normal" manner.*

This modality can be seen with age and the subsequent use of ones' teeth leading to wear through years of using teeth as "tools", a vehicle to eat with, which results in many physiologic and physical changes, such as the collapse of the bite and masticatory system, as well as temporomandibular joint issues and chronic pain. Subsequently, one sees these intraoral changes, in and among themselves, eventually leading to the subtle structural collapse of the jaws and face, with the onset of an appearance of an aged person in both older and younger individuals.

This phenomenon is also found in people of any age who may have abused their mouths along life's path, or had the occasion to use illicit drugs, alcohol in excess or exhibited lack of oral care and self-efficacy. Many young patients of all ages I have seen over the many years of my practice have exhibited a "Geriatric Dentition"; and yet, they are not of that ilk physiologically or chronologically. I have also seen many older people in their 80's, 90's and 100's who have a full complement of teeth in good health, who have taken the best of care of themselves throughout their lifetimes and who do not carry the label of a "geriatric dentition".

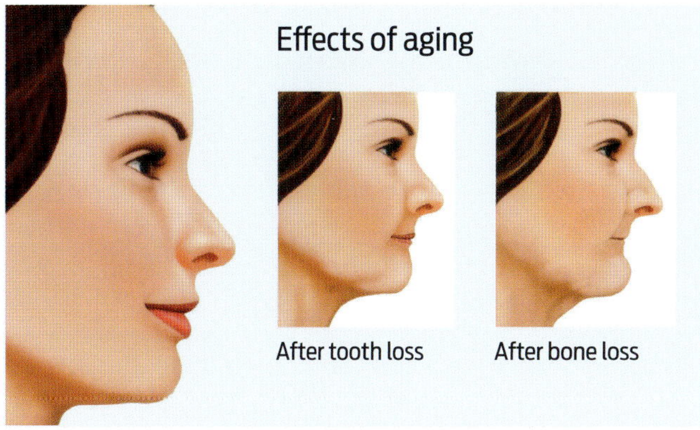

Fig. 2.4 Facial profile changes. *(Pinterest.com.)*

The scenario in Figure 2.4 shows the progressive aging of a young patient's face with the subsequent loss of teeth over time. By not replacing the majority her total complement of teeth, this person would be creating a loss of bone structure and a subsequent collapse of her vertical dimension. This in turn would cause her appearance to be the result of accelerated aging of her facial features and anatomy, being characterized as her having a "geriatric dentition". This same phenomenon can be seen in older people as well over time, whereby the loss of teeth over the years, the collapse of the bone and jaw profile, as well as collapsed bite from wear or worn dentures, create the look of an aged or aging person.

Restoring this kind of mouth takes much forethought, planning, willingness on the patient's part to undergo a lot of treatment over an extended period, stamina and a commitment of both the patient and the dentist, as well as the financial ability to afford this care to bring back a dentition that is esthetic and functional. The result being that of a more youthful and healthy-looking person. Essentially full mouth rehabilitation can and does change a person's life forever.

Figures 2.5 and 2.6 show supervised neglect, a collapsed bite, caries, periodontal disease, and lack of vertical dimension. I was the 7th dentist to see this patient that no one else wanted to care for when he broached their offices. He was not on drugs but did have a multitude of issues to cope with at the time.

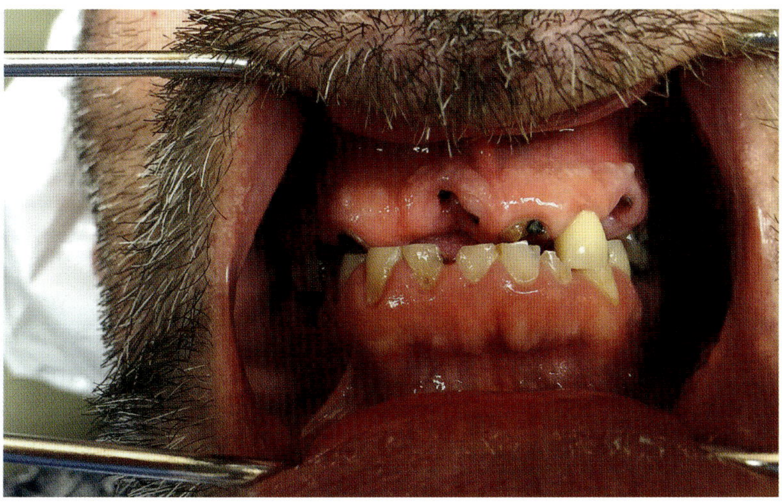

Fig. 2.5 A 55-year-old man in centric occlusion with a "Geriatric Dentition".

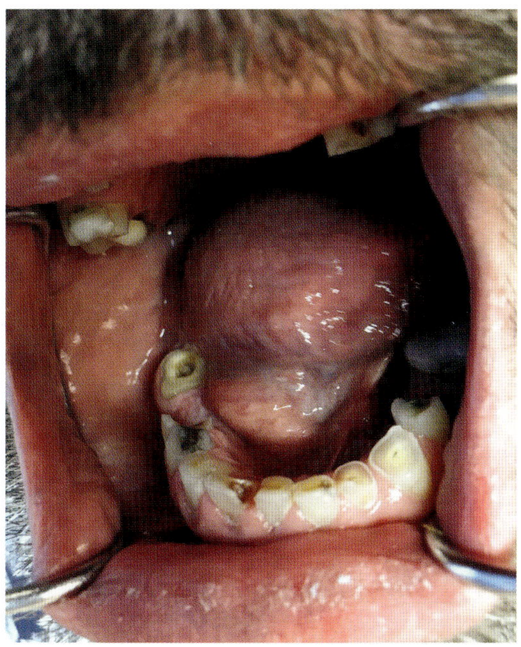

Fig. 2.6 A "Geriatric Dentition" in a 55-year-old man.

2.4 The Importance of Saving Teeth in the Medically/Dentally/Mentally Compromised Patient

2.4.1 Dealing with Loss, Grief and Anxiety

As one ages, it is a given that "loss" is evident in one's life. Loss in older individuals creates much *grief*, which in turn can lead to depression and the possibility of suicidal tendencies. Grief is intense suffering, sorrow or mourning, usually due to loss of some sort.[1] *Mourning* is the array of psychological processes that are set in motion by bereavement in order to moderate and integrate grief by coming to terms with the loss and reorienting to a world without our loved one in it or to the loss of something that was owned, or included as part of our make-up or being.[2] Many people may experience anxiety as a result of grief. Our reaction depends upon different factors including the specific loss itself; our age at the time of the loss; our closeness to the person who we are or may be grieving over and our dependence on the person. If anxiety is self-imposed, we may find ourselves in a state of sadness. Unresolved sadness then can lead to depression over time, as does extended grieving, through a circle of feelings connected with anger, guilt and loss of self-esteem. These, in among themselves, will also add to the grief one may feel and potentiate the anxiety involved. It is a vicious circle and needs to be broken in a timely manner using counseling and a lot of *tender loving care* (TLC). Grief and subsequent mourning can be found in most people undergoing the loss of teeth as well. It is quite common and sometimes overlooked by the dental practitioner, who should be able to recognize these symptoms during the process of discussing the intended treatment.

The risk factors for suicidal behavior can be found in older people who have become widows or widowers, having mental disorders, chronic physical illnesses and inability to cope with bereavement and loss in general.[3] Various clusters of suicide factors included patients aged 80 and older who died by suicide; the first cluster included married or widowed patients, the second was composed of individuals who were living alone or socially isolated, and the third one included people suffering from dementia or depression.[4]

Single men who live alone are most prone to suicide more so than single women who live alone in later life it seems. Being single and alone can lead to an older individual's lack of social activities and a great deal of alone time in general. Older, single women tend to be more social than men and therefore, can cope better, in general, with loss. All these entities coupled together, affect the brain and change the neural chemistry in the brain, in turn, causing a change in attitude, demeanor, and ability to function in a normal manner on many fronts, as well as with associated depression of one sort or another. One such symptom I have found in my older patients who live alone, 65 and above who may also be suffering from some sort of cognitive decline, is the lack of dental homecare with little self-efficacy, as well as not going to a dentist on a regular basis. Low dental IQ may account for this denial and the lack of importance in doing so, stunted by inherent dementias of all kinds. Too much introspection or lack of communication coupled with the lack of socialization, company, work, play, unreached goals, fun and continuous loss, to name a few, can lead to one's demise.

People with dementia of one sort or another, people with prolonged symptoms of grief and mourning and who may obsess about being a "victim" are exposing themselves to something called a *Complicated Grieving Process* (CG). This has been recognized as a condition that occurs in about 7% of bereaved people. People with this condition are caught up in constant fixation about circumstances of their loss, about consequences of death or excessive avoidance of the reminders of loss itself in any shape or form.[2] Those persons with specific personality disorders, which are akin to a disease process, such as obsessive-compulsive disorder or OCD as it is referred to, tend to be hypersensitive to conditions such as complicated grief as well as grief itself. Obsessing over anything, such as oral issues, can be deleterious to one's well-being; however, the potentiation of the grieving process by being obsessive can lead to a depression or a state of *dysthymia*, normally called "the Blues". This condition can go on and off over a lengthy period with the patient, or anyone else, not realizing that it is a condition that is an offshoot of sadness. Sadness can then create depression and is potentiated by OCD and the initial loss experienced.

In clinical settings, up to 75% of individuals with Dysthymic Disorder will develop a Major Depressive Disorder within 5 years.[5] Suffering and sadness that bereaved people often have can confuse clinicians of all kinds. On the one hand, it can seem inane not to treat their concerns; however, on the other hand, if we regard grief as a normal human response to loss, then this suggests it may not be the right thing to focus on for clinical treatment.[6] If one attempts treatment, then how do we determine the who, what, where and how of treatment, if this condition is supposed to be normal in the first place? The use of good communication again as a tool is first and foremost on the top of the list of mechanisms to use when confronted with a grieving person, no matter what the cause of their grief. Once the practitioner has elucidated that the patient has a depression issue, it should be brought out in the open, if it has not already occurred, and discussed. It is best to forego dental treatment until the patient can be rational around his or her intended dental treatment knowing that they will be better suited for it in the end. Moving forward without addressing these types of issues only places the patient in jeopardy, the practitioner at risk and moving backward with intended care; ultimately exacerbating the patients' symptoms and angst. An example follows.

Case Study 2

A patient presented to my practice for treatment about 20 minutes late one day. She was a married, middle-aged person, highly educated and overly involved with anything and everything in the community, to the point of being obsessive with her life. I believe she had a difficult time coping with loss and things that were not "perfect" in her day and her life as she knew it. This placed a great deal of subliminal pressure on her to achieve her goings on and goals daily. She sat in the dental chair and apologized for her lateness, knowing that I was on a schedule. I asked her if she knew what was planned for her morning with her dental visit. She responded, "Yes, a filling". I said, "That's right and it is the last molar on the bottom right section of your jaw. It is alright that you were late; rest assured we still have plenty of time to do the job and do it well". I told her that I was going to give her some anesthetic and was handed the topical to place first and then I was given the syringe to get her totally anesthetized. As I wheeled around toward the front of her face, her hands, feet and arms started shaking. She grabbed her arms and held them tightly crossed over her chest and opened her mouth, as if to invite me in with my anesthetic. I stopped moving toward her and asked if she was alright. She started to cry and apologized profusely for "wasting my time!" I handed her a tissue and told her that it was okay to cry and if she felt like talking about it, I was there to listen to her. I did not address her negative comment about wasting my time.

The rest of the appointment time was taken up with her talking about her guilt: she woke up late; she had to see her husband off to work and he had left without her making his breakfast; she had to see her kids off to school and make their lunches, but missed them as well; and then she said she got dressed, forgot her make-up and rushed to her car to come to her appointment, but forgot to open the garage door. She got out and opened it, jumped back into her car and put it in reverse and "stepped on it!" She heard a thump and stopped. Got out of her vehicle to see what the noise was all about and then realized that she had let the cat out into the garage the night before, which was sleeping under her car in the garage, and she ran it over unintentionally, causing its immediate demise.

This woman was grieving filled with remorse and mental anguish, as well as self-flatulating her ego for killing her beloved cat, not to mention letting her family down with her morning routine. There was no way that my treatment on this woman would have been successful in any way, shape or form had I attempted to force her to have the needed treatment, which I would never do under these circumstances. Her obsessive-compulsive disorder, which I had not studied until now, was in overdrive. Her grief compounded this disorder, and she was now going into a depression over her day, which was just getting started. I listened for over the next 30 minutes, not saying anything except an occasional "I hear your concerns" or "I sense your pain". I wanted her to know that I heard what she was saying and that my listening to her emotions, and not so much the story, would put her at ease. She finally calmed down enough to thank me for my understanding and left, but not before making another appointment. I asked her to forgive herself and to try not being so hard on herself. She smiled...

With patients who are handicapped in some way, but do not realize it, it is necessary to listen intently to all their senses with all our senses. I did touch her hand as I listened to her story and concerns. Touch is our most intimate form of communication, and I am sure that she knew I was present for her, thus reassuring her in the end that she would be alright. If I had acted any differently, I doubt she would have made another appointment to see me. Over the years, she referred me hundreds of patients, for which I attribute to how I treated her that day in my office.

Other factors to consider in treating the compromised patient that feed into the grieving process coupled with depression and obsessions of one form or another are: heredity; habits; abuse; disease in general; immune deficiency; finances; wants and desires; attitude; cognitive decline; dementias and Alzheimer's disease and post-traumatic stress disorders.

Case Study 3

An interesting situation happened to me in my office with a Medical Doctor who was a patient of mine, being of Filipino extraction. She presented for an anterior restoration one day. I had treated her for years, having made her a partial denture on her lower arch and some crowns and restorations on the upper arch. She had poor homecare habits and did not come into the office to have her teeth cleaned on a regular basis. When broached about her habits, she always had the same excuses that it was hard to find the time to come in due to her busy schedule and both her commitments in the community and at home had kept her away. So here she was, sitting in my chair, quiet and reserved. I sat down next to her and asked her if there were any changes to her health in any way and she said "No". She and I had been friends for many years, and she was also my primary care physician at the time. She was a very quiet and reserved woman, demure one might say. She had a sweet smile and was soft spoken and an almost subdued personality. She asked what I was going to do, and I explained it to her. She agreed to treatment. I placed a Q-Tip with topical anesthetic under her lip and I was going to do a small composite resin on her upper lateral incisor. I told her that the anterior injections could be sensitive, but I would try to make her not feel it. As I lifted the syringe and placed it ever so gently into the mucosa, she opened her eyes, which suddenly were the size of silver dollars, grabbed my right wrist and thrashed my hand down into the side of the chair, while screaming "bloody murder", "don't kill me, don't kill me!". As one can imagine, I was horrified and scared and did my best to calm her down.

At that point, I reached behind me for an ampule of Ammonia that I kept taped to my dental unit behind me and single handedly broke it and waved it in front of her nose causing her to stop ranting. My brain went into "high gear" thinking of all the possible things this might be. Anxiety was on the top of my list, but she had never had this type of reaction before when I treated her. There was nothing in her history about any anxiety disorders or anything that she had previously told me about her that would have indicated this type of dental phobia. I was at a loss. I told her I would like to give her some oxygen mixed with a small amount of nitrous oxide just to relax her, and she agreed. After about 20 minutes, I asked her if she wanted to talk about what happened. She said "Yes". I asked what she thought prompted her to act out like she did. She wasn't sure, but then she started to tell me a story about when she was a little girl: "I grew up in Manilla, in the Philippines. When I was around seven years old, my mother told me that the Japanese had invaded our Island and that we needed to be prepared for their arrival. I had no idea about who they were, why they were coming to our home or what they wanted from us. But just before they came to our village, my mother told me that I had to be brave and strong, that I had to listen to her every word and obey her. I was frightened and scared and felt alone. My mother placed me inside an empty rice bag and while I stood very still next to a lot of other rice bags, she filled it with rice that had been harvested from the fields around our house. She then tied the bag and told me that I should stay as close to the bottom of the bag as I could and to not make a sound, no matter what happened; no matter what I heard outside the bag. The Japanese soldiers came. There was a lot of commotion, talking and noise and then screaming. Suddenly, out of nowhere the bag I was in was being shaken and then a long knife blade, a Bayonet, was thrust in front of my face at the level of my eyes! I was not sure what it was, but I did not move and did not utter a sound. The blade went in and out a few times and then the soldier who placed it there left. Tears rolled down my cheeks in silence and I found myself trembling; yet, not trying to move. It seemed like an eternity before my mother opened the bag and let me out. I never heard her words. I stood there with her holding me for a long time". My patient, obviously at this juncture, was suffering from Post-Traumatic Stress Disorder (PTSD).

I asked my patient if she had these attacks before and she said, "not really". However, I do not think she ever acknowledged what she had and sublimated it. As a physician, it is sometimes difficult to "heal thyself". I listened to her story intently and then asked her to describe what she was feeling when she saw my syringe and needle, which she had seen before in my office and was the catalyst for her terrifying memory. My patient has used syringes and given many injections to her patients in her own office on many occasions; yet this never seemed to conjure up a reaction like she had in my dental chair. She said she was frightened of feeling pain while having her tooth filled and when she saw the needle, she had a flashback to being in that rice bag and lost it, going into a different state of mind, transporting herself back to her childhood frightening event in her village: another time and place, when that Japanese bayonet went by her eyes. I told her that it was in her best interest to seek out some psychological counseling specific for this issue, as it would continue, as well as escalate if she did not. She never made another dental appointment with me, and she never socialized with me again either. I only hoped that my words registered with her in a good way and that she sought out some help for her issues. She eventually retired and no one has seen or heard from her since.

Denial is a difficult thing to understand. It may be a combination of guilt coupled with fear that creates a taciturn individual. My patient was in her mid to late-sixties when this happened in my office. I believe that she suffered from PTSD her entire adult life, which transformed itself into dementia as she aged; thus, giving her eventual freedom from this terrible memory and life-long experience, even though she kept this malady hidden from herself and others, like myself, until this "flashback" occurred in my office.

PTSD is a mental health condition that is triggered by a terrifying event, either experiencing it or witnessing it. Symptoms may include flashbacks, nightmares and severe anxiety, as well as uncontrollable thoughts about the event. PTSD symptoms may start within one month of a traumatic event, but sometimes may not appear until years after the event. These symptoms cause significant problems in social or work-related situations and in relationships. They can also interfere with one's ability to go about their normal daily tasks.[7] Like having dental treatment.

It is interesting to note that such *intrusive memories* can cause such unwanted, recurrent and distressing thoughts which can alter how you respond in what I might label "a normal everyday non-threatening dental visit". As practitioners, we must follow the Boy Scouts of America's motto: *Be Prepared.* And that means being able to handle any adverse surprises that come our way during treatment. I had no idea that this would happen to me with this physician. My thoughts were keeping her from harming herself and disarming her by staying calm and collected and assuring her that she would be alright.

2.4.2 Dementias and Memory Loss

Another example of dealing with a medically or mentally compromised patient, who may surprise us at or during treatment, is in treating dementia patients. One never knows how they will respond, or if they will allow the practitioner to treat them dentally in a somewhat "normal" manner or at all. It is always a surprise. Three systemic or genetic spawned diseases where I have found dementia components in the scope of treating patients are with Parkinson's disease, Multiple Sclerosis and Down's syndrome patients. During the aging process, the brain is encumbered by multiple modifications from the age of 60 years, which causes it to shrink in size.

Essentially, dementia is a significant sign of *progressive neurodegeneration*. In turn, this causes the death of brain cells as well as tissue loss. Those most frequently affected are the memory center, the cerebral or thinking areas, the behavioral areas and the area that gives us the ability to do certain tasks. Dementias are insidious and tend to have a slow progression over time. Mild Cognitive Impairment (MCI) is a precursor to most dementias. It has a slow onset, and one may be aware that they cannot remember simple things, like finding their toothbrush or car keys. They do have enough memory to know that they are forgetting things more and more and this in itself may cause frustration, leading to anger, guilt and sadness (Fig. 2.7). This dysfunction can evolve into any of the dementias, but there is a good bet that it may be associated with vascular dementia; whereby, the blood flow to the brain is lessened and memory is affected leading to bad decision making and executive thinking skills becoming diminished.

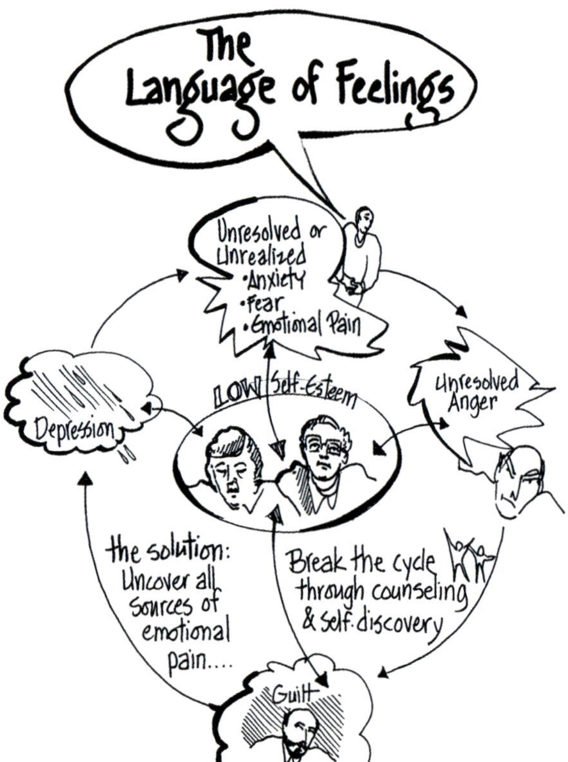

Fig. 2.7 The Language of Feelings. (Shapira, Eric Z. *A New Wrinkle: What I Learned from Older People Who Never Acted Their Age*. iUniverse Publishers, 2009, 2011©.)

Alzheimer's disease is probably the best known of the dementias. I think that people probably "lump" a lot of the other dementia categories into this one, due to the lack of being able to discern the differences or knowing that there are other kinds to choose from. Alzheimer's disease shows an abnormal shrinkage of the brain and the invasion of *Tau protein* particles, which form a fibrous network over the cerebral tissue. It is thought, from what I have learned in the past, that this protein causes an interruption of the neural pathways, thus affecting memory, behavior, action and function. This disease wreaks havoc with interpersonal relationships. Its first signs include difficulty remembering things. It is a progressive disease and eventually leads to the death of the person who has it. Most all Down's syndrome patients get Alzheimer's disease between the ages of 30 and 40 leading to the cause of their death as well. This disease has been thought of akin to how a virus attacks our systems and changes the RNA and DNA, as it mixes with our own; therefore, literally changes who we are genetically. This disease has a genetic component and if one of your parents has or had it, you have a 50% chance of getting it. If both of your parents have suffered with it, then there is a good chance that you will get it sometime in your lifetime. There is a genetic test that can be performed to determine if you have the marker on the gene for it: Gene 19. All you need is a blood sample to find out. Many people I have assisted both dentally and in geriatric work I have done with them have refused this test out of fear.

A second dementia is called **Lewy Body Dementia**. It is like Alzheimer's disease, but also features Parkinsonian like tremors and stiffness. It comes with sleeping disorders and visual hallucinations. In late-stage Parkinson's disease, one may see tremors and stiffness and well as memory loss and a stare. In many of my patients like this, looking at their eyes with this stare is both haunting, daunting and difficult to read, with respect to how the patient is feeling. Many of these patients have a heightened sensitivity to pain, when one might think it should be just the opposite.

Vascular dementia can come from a stroke, TIA or Transient Ischemic Attack and atherosclerosis of the vessels. The symptoms elicited by this dementia are much the same as Alzheimer's disease. Memory disorders, bad decision making and difficulty planning things (diminished Executive Functioning Skills). There is also a "slowing down" in physical activity as well as difficulty in breathing and anemia, should there be internal bleeding as in Heyde's syndrome connected to gastrointestinal bleeding associated with angiodysplasia in the presence of aortic stenosis (hardening of the arteries).

Frontotemporal Lobe Dementia is another dementia affected by neurodegeneration. This dementia causes changes in behavior, language difficulties, difficulty moving and memory loss. The first symptoms appear in the early 60's.

Mixed Dementia is where someone is affected by two types of dementia. The most common combination is Alzheimer's disease and vascular dementia. This dementia has many symptoms that mimic either one or the other of these dementias both physiologically and in appearance.

Lastly, a new form of dementia considered a rare disease, but like Alzheimer's disease, is VT or **Vacuolar Tauopathy Dementia**. Recent research in September of 2020 at the University of Pennsylvania School of Medicine found that the VCP gene in the brain, Valosin-containing protein, causes a buildup of Tau protein. It is considered a neurodegenerative disease characterized by an accumulation of neuronal vacuoles and Tau protein aggregates. Its symptoms are like Alzheimer's disease in all respects causing acute memory loss.

All patients with some form of cognitive impairment tend to exhibit their symptoms most all the time and that means when visiting a dental office. Being aware of the dementia patients' symptoms is an advantage for the practitioner so that he or she can prepare to cope with the expected or unexpected behavior that may be present during their dental visit. It behooves the practitioner to have emergency oxygen and a medical kit nearby. It also helps to practice emergency drills in the office so that when confronted with a situation of any kind, especially an irate dementia patient, you are prepared to handle that emergency with care and expertise.

Figure 2.8 shows "supervised neglect", gross caries and chronic geriatric periodontal disease. The patient's son wanted all her teeth restored and not extracted. He would not listen to reason about her oral condition. His mother had an advanced stage of Alzheimer's disease and did not talk. She could not function and was very combative, making it impossible to treat her without general anesthesia, which the son did not want her to have. No treatment was rendered. Trying to clean her teeth or even take the accompanying photo was difficult as she had her jaws locked down ever so tightly and liked to bite. It was a very precarious situation that was a no-win for both of us.

The pursed lips and the solid, blank stare as well as rigid body structure were outward signs of this patient's dementia (Fig. 2.9). She did not speak, nor did she look directly at me. Her distressed look tells a story that we, as practitioners, need to learn to read in order to understand who we are working with and what we have in store for us if we are challenged by this opportunity.

I label this type of a patient "The Silent Sufferer". There is no way to elicit from her what she is feeling emotionally, the amount of discomfort, if any, she is feeling and what she would like us to do for her. We are at the whim of her son, who has placed his own judgment onto his mother' wishes for the kind of treatment he thinks she should have. He would not listen to reason about her condition, nor the treatment recommendations made on her behalf by me, the practitioner. And so, she will continue as is, until this oral disease process affects her systemic system exacerbating her pre-existing physical

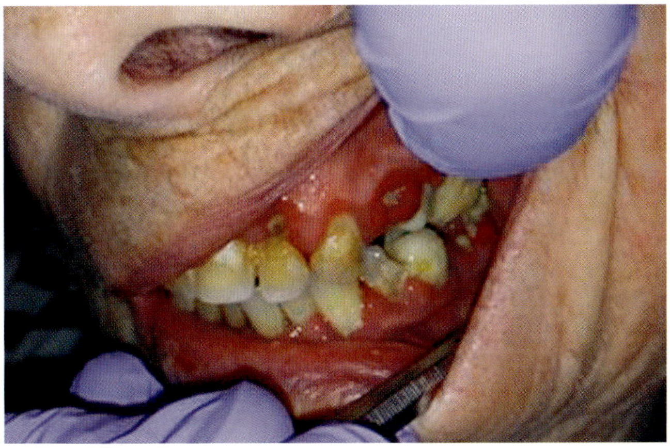

Fig. 2.8 Deceased dementia patient.

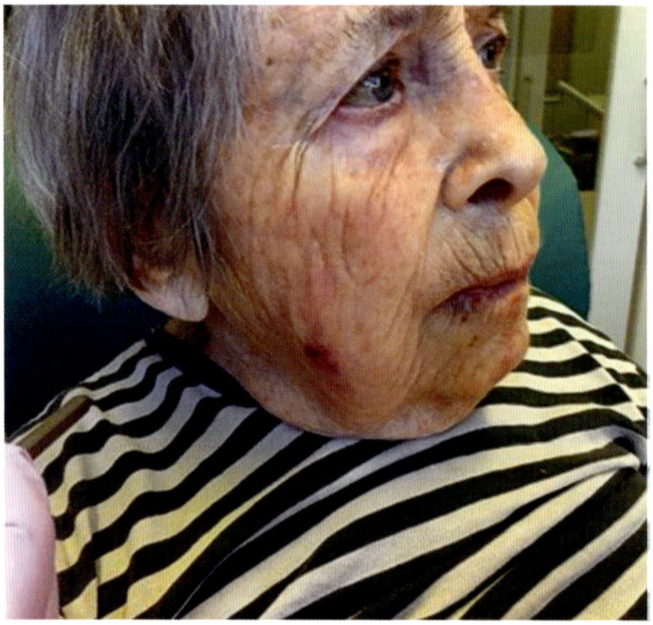

Fig. 2.9 Deceased dementia patient.

issues, she has brought with her in both combined acute/chronic infections, heart disease and more, placing her at risk for a life-death scenario.

Parkinson's Disease is a neurodegenerative disease and effects one's ability to function fully due to subsequent muscle weakness and muscle loss, as well as other physical and mental changes. Most all these afflicted and inflicted patients end up with dementia and face eminent death a short time afterward. They tend to have a specific stare or gaze, have difficulty walking and their hands shake as well as the thumb and forefinger show a "pill rolling effect", which does identify this disease, in part. Most of these patients end up not having the ability to do dental hygiene, which in turn causes issues with gross caries, tooth loss and periodontal disease. These then cause subsequent issues of not eating properly and general loss of overall good health.

Case Study 4

Several Case Studies with Parkinson's Disease Patients

This 70+ year-old male (Fig. 2.10) with advanced Parkinson's disease also had a dementia. He has the typical stare of a dementia patient, yet he can talk and function to some extent with gross tremors. He allowed some simple restorative treatment and cleanings using local anesthetic as he was hypersensitive to pain. He had gross periodontal disease due to lack of care on his part and his wife's part as well. She would not clean his teeth, nor would she floss him, as he would bite her periodically. So, she did not try to assist him with his homecare. It was a constant battle to keep his mouth clean and to help him with his rampant caries. Situations like this are most difficult to handle, making communication with this patient especially important, as well as working quickly intraorally.

I had him come back every two months for cleanings to try and maintain his oral cavity in relatively good health. It took a lot of discussion with this patient's wife. She had taken me out of the operatory on the first visit with her husband and informed me that her doctor had told her **"Not to do any involved dental treatment on your husband because he was going to die soon, and I am trying to save you money"**. At the onset, the patient had an infected lower anterior incisor with a periapical abscess. The radiograph showed caries into the pulp and an extensive radiolucency at the apex. I discussed that fact that this kind of infection can be a nidus for bone destruction, tooth loss, difficulty in eating and a systemic infection as well, which could cause an early demise should it go unchecked. His wife allowed me to do an endodontic treatment on this lower anterior tooth and the lesion eventually resolved. The tooth tightened up and was functional. The patient had no residual pain from the tooth or the procedure.

Figure 2.11 shows the completed endodontic treatment on the lower anterior tooth with a large radiolucency. In treating this patient, I thought it important enough to keep the remaining teeth of this person. There was no way to justify what the medical doctor told the wife and no way to determine exactly "when" this patient would die. My goal was to get him healthy orally and make him functional in the time he had left. I imparted this upon the wife of this patient, and she understood my rationale and thinking, eventually coming around to paying for the treatment he did have. It was difficult for her, to say the least. As the patient started to fail physically and mentally, his wife

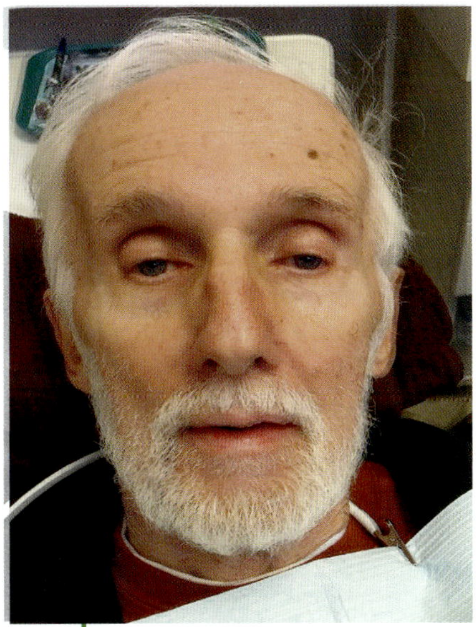

Fig. 2.10 Deceased 70+ year-old dementia/Parkinson's patient.

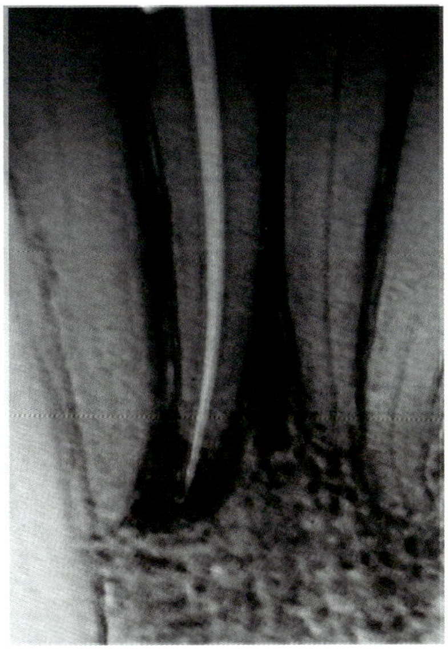

Fig. 2.11 Completed endodontic treatment on the lower anterior tooth with the large radiolucency created by infection from caries.

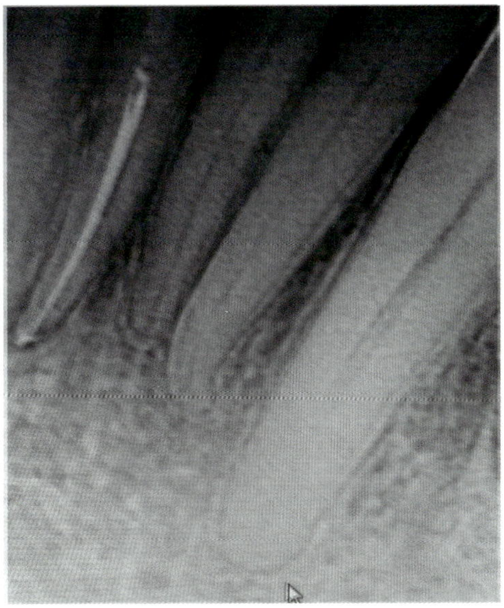

Fig. 2.12 Post-endodontic treatment with healed peri-apical abscess and complete bone fill at the apex of the tooth.

was at her wits-end. She had no help in her home and no respite. I recognized the strain she was under and her desire to stop all dental treatment. I suggested she place him in an assisted living/memory care facility, which she eventually did.

Figure 2.12 was taken several months post-endodontic treatment, showing the periapical lesion and infection are almost totally gone, as well as the bone fill in the lesion being filled in. Keeping the patient safe from future disease was the goal due to his compromised immune system. Risking the periapical infection to continue without proper treatment would have been a mistake, costing the loss of bone, destruction of the buccal or lingual plates of bone and the eventual traumatic loss of the tooth, as well as pain and suffering. This, in turn, would have altered the patient's ability to eat, bite into his food, and function properly. In the end, this may have caused the loss of his self-esteem. We have no way of knowing these facts about his self-esteem, but we can surmise.

Figure 2.13 shows the results of rampant, chronic Geriatric Periodontal disease in this medically and mentally compromised patient. The patient had an acute exacerbation of a chronic disease enhanced by the decline of his immune system and his systemic disease of Parkinson's disease, as well as his mental decline and indifference to doing his own homecare daily, mostly because of his dementia.

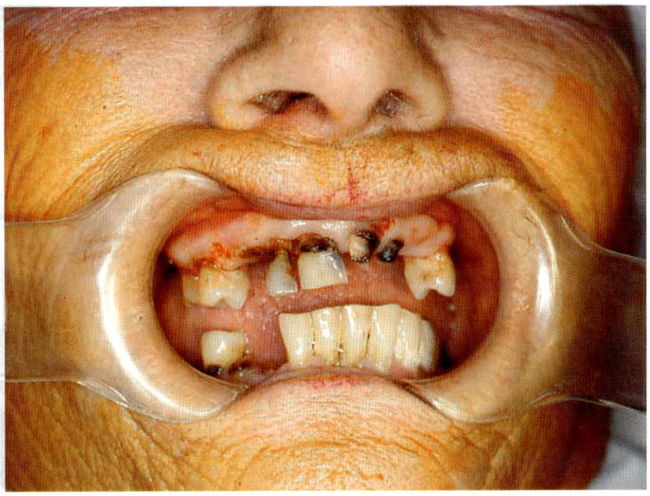

Fig. 2.13 It shows the results of rampant, chronic Geriatric Periodontal disease in this medically and dentally compromised patient. The combination of Parkinson's disease, a lowered immune system and dental neglect due to dementia has created a difficult dental situation. I made a commitment to the patient, his wife and family to try and keep the patient pain-free, functional, and as healthy as I could under the circumstances.

BOX 2.1 **Some Rules of the Road with Patients Who Need Special Assistance**

- ✘ Do not reason.
- ✘ Do not argue.
- ✘ Do not confront.
- ✘ Do not remind them they forget.
- ✘ Do not question recent memory.
- ✘ Do not take it personally.

- ✔ Do give short, one sentence explanations.
- ✔ Do allow plenty of time for comprehension and then "triple" it.
- ✔ Do repeat instructions or sentences, exactly the same way.
- ✔ Do eliminate "but" from your vocabulary; substituting 'nevertheless.'
- ✔ Do avoid insistence. Try again later.
- ✔ Do agree with them or distract them to a different subject or activity.
- ✔ Do accept the blame when something is wrong (even if it is a fantasy).
- ✔ Do leave the room, if necessary, to avoid confrontation, but do not leave them alone.
- ✔ Do respond to their feelings, rather than their words they speak (EBW-Emotions Before Words©. 2021 Dr. Eric Z. Shapira).
- ✔ Do be patient and cheerful and reassuring. Do go with the flow.
- ✔ Do practice 100% forgiveness. Memory loss progresses daily.
- ✔ Do increase and apply your generosity and graciousness, especially with compliments, whether needed, warranted or thought about.

These small tips will save you hours, days, months and years of grief. Dementia patients thoughts and perceptions are their "reality". You cannot change them, but you can acknowledge and validate them. I will discuss these issues in the remaining chapters, especially in Chapter 7.

2.5 The Evaluation Process Leading to Successful Treatment

What is successful treatment when working with a geriatric or younger patient? This all depends on your definition of the word "successful", and yours and your patient's perception of what successful means to each of you.

Being successful means the achievement of desired visions and planned goals. Furthermore, the word *success* can be a certain social status that describes a prosperous person that could have gained fame from a favorable outcome. The dictionary defines or describes *success* as the following: "attaining wealth, prosperity and/or fame".[8] I do not feel *success* can be defined in one sentence. It is comprised of many different facets, and it depends upon what one bases it on, with respect to the expectations each party may bring with them to the table.

Firstly, one must have a set of goals around the patient once the history is taken and the patient states what they want from being in the dental office. If the patient is old and infirm and cannot speak well, then a family member or caregiver must be the one to speak of goals from the point of view of the patient. This is difficult because we do not know in what capacity this person has played in the life of the patient and how well they know the wants and desires of the patient; again, look out for a different perception from someone like this.

Secondly, the illumination of Who, What, Where and the Why of the patients wants and desires of treatment should be considered fully, taking into account the patient's realistic ability to have the treatment they seek. We must look at the patient's overall physical, emotional and psychological ability to follow-through with projected treatment at the time of examination and planning. The most difficult aspect of proceeding with treatment is **to get our patients to want what we think they need**. To accomplish this, we need to take into consideration the facts of the examination results, the medical, social and dental histories, as well as our abilities to meet the expectations of the patient and our own physical dexterity in performing the treatment with an all-encompassing eye.

Once we finish getting all the relative clinical data we think we need, such as radiographs, study models, complete measurements of periodontal pockets and recession, occlusal measurements including protrusive, overjet, overbite and opening, we then need to sit with the patient and his/her caregiver or relative in a private setting to discuss the treatment findings and projected plan in depth. If you want to be effective, in earnest, with your treatment plan and findings, it is important to cover all your bases and make sure that the patient is involved and understands every nuance of what you are saying and proposing.

It is important to know that much of the time, when dealing with older, possibly memory impaired, hearing impaired or vision impaired patients, they may not remember what you discussed with them or what they agreed upon, either because they did not hear you correctly, see the material being presented or understand it at all. Therefore, it is imperative to discuss this information with them more than once in a repetitive fashion and then have them sign the treatment plan showing that it was discussed, understood and agreed upon in advance. This does not mean that it should not be discussed again; it should be discussed all through whatever treatment is elected. If the treatment plan recommendations are amended, then the patient needs to sign or re-sign a consent form for the amended treatment plan, as well as a consent form for each procedure to be done at the time of treatment. This also does not mean that they will not argue with you about their treatment or attempt to bring a legal action against you should something go wrong during treatment. Dementia or cognitively impaired patients are immersed in their perception of their world. Their perceptions are their reality, and we cannot change that perception without first trying to educate them; even then, this may not be enough. That is when one must involve a family member or a relative who is responsible for the patients' welfare. Again, these persons have their own set of values and perceptions that may not align with yours or the people they represent, making things complicated.

2.5.1 An Outcome Assessment

Form follows function. I think that it is important to put together an outcome assessment at the beginning of the evaluation process. Use this as your goal and make steps to check off as you move down the lists of things you need to adequately propose in a treatment plan that fits each individual older patient. No two patients are alike. Each treatment regime is unique unto itself and may even involve referring this patient to someone else who is better equipped to handle them.

An outcome assessment involves the following: a **clinical outcome assessment** (COA) *is a measure that describes or reflects how a patient feels, functions, or survives.* Types of COAs include Patient-reported **outcome** (PRO) **measures**, Observer-reported **outcome** (ObsRO) **measures** and Clinician-reported **outcome** (ClinRO) **measures**.[9] At the onset of treatment, it would be best to look ahead utilizing a timeline and determine the length of the projected treatment, the type of result expected and an educated guess as to whether the treatment will be successful based on experience and facts, as well as the possibility of failure as a percent of chance. These things can be used as a marker of your care of the patient. Trying to predict, at each step of the way how the patient will fare and whether the patient reports as well how he/she is doing, will enhance your overall treatment and give you a base from which to determine the overall success of your treatment with this patient. Having a patient-reported outcome at each step will give you much needed information as to how you, as a practitioner, are doing with your direct treatment on this patient. This can be factored into the overall outcome assessment to determine the increase or decrease in treatment goals. It is a new way to think; however, it is a good bet when working with compromised, elderly patients where one does not know how they will respond to treatment or whether they will make it to the end of their projected treatment based on their continued health and commitment to dental care, we may need to "fill-in the blanks".

Case Study 5

I did an outcome assessment on the patient aged 55+ years shown previously (see pre-treatment photos in Figs. 2.5, 2.6). His mouth was basically destroyed, and I knew from the get-go that it was not just a dental issue. There were medical issues involved as well and through my detection and referral for what I thought he had, he was treated medically before I saw him dentally, except for a complete dental examination and work-up for future care. After doing a consultation with him that lasted several hours, he made a commitment to rehabilitate his mouth. I told him at the onset that I would commit to assisting him with this major rehabilitation if he made a commitment to show up, pay his bills and improve his homecare, which he did. He was very anxious and had a low self-esteem. This was something that he had to get over for a successful outcome of his dental treatment.

He was divorced and continued to be very depressed after this experience for many years after the unhappy and stressful event. He had a bad opinion about himself as well. Counseling helped him, as well as my slow and definitive treatment plan enabling him to come to grips with the metamorphosis he was about to make. I did numerous outcome assessments with him to determine if my treatment was beneficial to him, if there were changes in his attitude and personality and if he was improving with his mastication after opening his bite up, as well as him gaining a better handle on his general opinion of himself. Once his vertical dimension was established through trial and error and several tomograms to determine the position of his condyles, I was able to embark on the restoration plan for the maxillary arch, which took at least one year. His parents helped him financially with the restoration of his mouth and we managed to finish the upper arch in good form; however, his father became seriously ill, and his mother said that they could no longer afford to help him with his dental care. This threw a "monkey wrench" into the gears of completing his dental rehabilitation, so I thought. But the patient was so excited at the change in his appearance, his improved health and self-esteem, he told me that he would find the money to pay for the restoration of his lower arch, which he did over time. However, it extended treatment another year.

The patient was in regular recall and would come back every three to four months for his dental cleaning and check-ups for the next year and then out of nowhere, without a warning or sign, he disappeared. This was a sad day for me because I had put so much of myself into working with him on getting to wellness. I know that I helped him immensely, yet it is difficult to undo what your patients will not let you do. So always expect the unexpected in your treatment plans and subsequent dental treatment and plan for contingencies. Your periodic assessments should give you some hint of these fall backs and you can make changes to care accordingly. At least I finished the full mouth rehabilitation and assisted him in changing his life (Fig. 2.14).

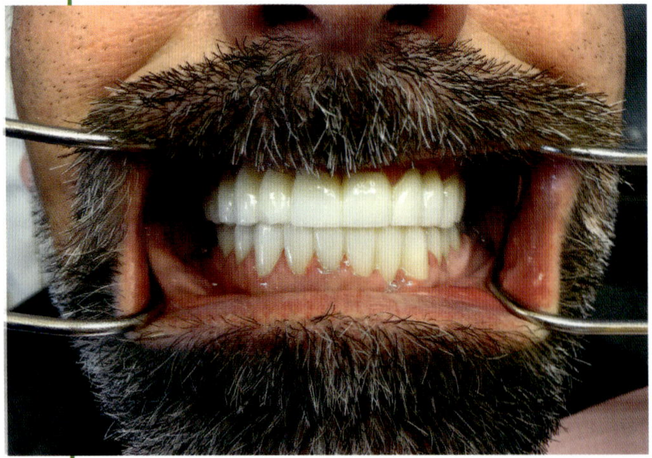

Fig. 2.14 The 55-year-old-Oral Rehab patient completed treatment after 2 years (at 57 years).

This life-changing treatment changed this patient's entire outlook, disposition, personality, function, lifestyle and future. He could not believe that after two years of treatment and both our commitments to improve his well-being and health, that he was given back what he had lost… himself.

> I am not sure what his actual expectations were during treatment as they changed so often. He was a quiet and reserved individual and did not say much, as far as words were concerned; but his eyes told the whole story most of the time. He could not look at me in my eyes nor could he look at himself in the mirror after the completion of his treatment. It was only sometime later after his metamorphosis, when he came into the office to tell me that he was dating again, had gone on a strict diet and stopped smoking, that he looked at me; eyes welling-up with tears and in a soft tone of voice saying, "thank you for changing my life".
>
> *Expect the unexpected*, believe in the *unbelievable*, and achieve the *unachievable*...

"Organization is not about perfection, it is about efficiency, reducing stress and clutter, saving time and money as well as improving one's overall quality of life; for ourselves and ultimately for our patients."

Dr. Eric Zane Shapira

"If you don't know where you are going, any road will take your there..."

Yogi Berra

2.5.2 Function Follows Form(s)

The evaluation process that takes place after all your examinations, histories, radiographs, second opinions, study models and the like, is probably the most important step that you can take with all your patients, especially, your aging, geriatric patients. The second most important step is to have a treatment conference to explain what you have found in an orderly fashion and then to discuss your treatment recommendations based upon several plans.

Putting all the myriad of information and facts together is a chore, but I know that when I see things come together for both the information that I organize, as well as the treatment plans that I wish to present, it is all worth it. I know that these things will do the following:

- **a.** Save me time, effort and money in the long run.
- **b.** Allow me to present the information of my findings in an organized fashion. Thanks to my examination forms, models and diagrams.
- **c.** Allow the patient to understand what they brought in with them for me to see and learn what oral issues they have and what they can do to rectify these issues that may be deleterious to their overall health.
- **d.** Give me a chance to educate my patients about dentistry in general, optimum health, as well as disease processes that they may have going on in their mouths.
- **e.** Allow me the opportunity to show the patient my examination forms, which contain the findings of my examination. As we are in a "visually oriented society" people like to see things straight-up in front of them.
- **f.** Allow me to present multiple treatment plans, recommending one that may fit the patients' budget and/or blending treatment plans that will cover all the bases as a compromise to any one treatment plan which may be readily affordable.
- **g.** Allow me to have the appropriate documents as a legal record of the examination process, includes all the forms; intentions for treatment; the patient's acknowledgement about the proposed treatment and subsequent future treatments, and the patient history for your present and future review.

As a practitioner, **you can never document enough**. Unfortunately, we live in a litigious society. The more documentation one has, the more protected you are legally, and the more information the patient will have in order to understand his/her dental needs.

It is also important to have a staff person sit in with you and the patient during your consultation with the patient, taking notes about your discussion. The more information you have to back up what is discussed, the better the outcome. You can bet there will be misconceptions and denial at times about what was discussed and the written backup from a coworker, such as a treatment coordinator, who will ultimately be working with the patient throughout treatment, is a good support system and ally.

For example, many years ago I had a middle-aged professional woman come into my practice for a cleaning and exam. She had received some of the first composite bonding produced in the United States by a well-known New York, self-proclaimed, "Cosmetic" dentist. The dentist did not leave any embrasure space when he built-up the facial surfaces of teeth numbers 7-10. This created a gross, chronic gingivitis around the front teeth. These four upper front teeth were also out of proportion to the upper canine teeth, which went unrestored previously.

After her examination, she was informed about the periodontal condition caused by the restorations that she previously had done; at which time, she started yelling at the top of her voice at me about how this dentist was the best in the country etc., etc., etc. And "how dare you malign his work!" I sat quietly listening to her through all this noise. I then stated that I heard her anger and frustration and asked if I could show her some photos and measurements of her periodontal pockets. She could see the difference between her oral condition and the healthy gingiva in the photos I presented. I recommended that she consider redoing the composites, which were some 25 years old, and including the canines either with new composites or porcelain veneers to even out her smile. She refused. She continued to come into the office irregularly to get her teeth cleaned, thinking that this would solve her periodontal condition, but it did not.

About 5 years later, she came into the office stating that she was going to be on the program, "60 Minutes", to discuss her new creation and she wanted to get her upper front teeth redone with porcelain veneers. We had a consultation about the treatment, at which my treatment coordinator took notes, and we scheduled her. I had a lot of trepidation about treating her due to my first introduction to her "mean streak" and anger. But I did not listen to my inner voice telling me to "refer". After preparing her teeth for veneers, cuspid to cuspid and luting on processed custom temporaries, she left with a nice smile with cleansable embrasure spaces. I had a substitute staff person that day and dental assistant that day as they both got conveniently ill. My assistant did not give her the consent form I found out after-the-fact, and I asked my patient to sign it, which she promptly refused. She called me two days later on a Friday from somewhere on the East coast to tell me that she was lecturing and "spitting through the open embrasure spaces!" She demanded to see me the next day when she got off the airplane to have me "fix" the issue for her. Long story short, I fixed the embrasure spaces by closing them down slightly. I subsequently called the laboratory and told them to give me the smallest open embrasure space I could have without closing it in on the gingiva. I placed the veneers a few days later and they were beautiful, in occlusion, the perfect shade and had a slight open embrasure space keeping the veneer off the tissue. She was unhappy and threatened to sue me unless I gave her a "suggested donation of $9000 to her Foundation", which I immediately refused. I am getting to the point here...

She next took out an ad in the local newspaper asking people who had cosmetic procedures performed by me to contact her for a Class Action suit against me. She also filed a complaint with the State Dental Board, who asked me for a copy of my records. The result was that her claims were frivolous, and we underlined in the copies of her chart that we sent to the Board what we had discussed with her about her disease process at every cleaning she had, noted by the hygienist in writing. There were 22 separate notes by my treatment coordinator about discussions she had with the patient about following through with suggested treatment, which the patient stated to the Board that we never discussed and just went ahead and did the work without her permission! And there were at least 20 entries in the records of my consultations and examinations over the years that she came to my office about the suggested treatment, which she finally elected to have. All of which was documented. The Board threw the case out...

One last thing to mention was what she said to me when coming into the office for me to close the embrasure spaces after her lecture on a Saturday, when no patients were in the office. Immediately, she came at me and put me in a hard headlock strangle hold, choking me and stating she was going to "kill me" if I did not put her teeth back the way they were when she first came to see me!

She was a large woman and towered over me, as well as "powered" over me. I should have called the police, but I felt that it would not help the situation or the dentist-patient relationship we had; however, soured it became. My point in telling this story is that you can never write enough documentation about what you do for the patient, what both of you say and what your treatment is or what and how the patient responded to all of it. Do not forget your informed consent forms, as it can come back to haunt you if you do forget. We made them in our office because in those days, it was not in fashion to have one, but we did. I never saw her again, except I had "peeked" at the 60 Minutes show on television to see her briefly and her smile was as big as life, looking great, despite the "sour puss" that she was. She has since passed away from cancer.

When someone is nasty or treats you poorly, do not take it personally. It says nothing about you, but a lot about them.

2.5.3 Forms Precede Function

There are many kinds of forms used for examinations of all kinds. Most dentists tend to combine many forms into a single form that suits their practice, and their forms are noticeably short and succinct. Others buy stock forms to make it easy. Many make their own forms, like myself, which I color-coded so we could easily find the different ones we used for different procedures. Forms are always changing based upon your knowledge level and base. If you tend to learn something useful and wish to put it in one of your forms then so be it, consider it done. The more one learns, the more one has at his/her disposal to meet their needs.

Forms are legal documents and should be dated and signed each time an entry is made. They are also good for use in medical and dental referrals as needed. Either way, they are used as an information base about the human "puzzles" that patients bring you and they are legal records that can be used in court, should the need arise to protect your interest, as well as that of the patient. There is no set Geriatric Dental Patient Form that I know of; as is, it behooves each of us practicing with geriatric patients to customize a form for this cohort of patient in our practices. The Geriatric History form should cover a lot of information, including an extensive and up-to-date medical history. My patient history form is designed for geriatric patients.

My forms consisted of a Dental history form; a Medical history form; a Head and Neck Screening Exam form; a Clinical Examination form; a TMJ History and Screening form; a Periodic Oral Examination form; a Schematic Tooth Chart form; a Social History form; an Appointment Plan form; Specialist referral forms; X-ray Laboratory forms, including CBCT (Cone Beam Computerized Tomography) laboratories; Dental laboratory forms and Consent forms for every procedure that I perform. I can modify my consent forms as needed by filling in the blanks. Depending upon the kind of patient I have, what their intentions were and are, as well as treatment needs of the patient and an assessment by me, the forms I use could be all the above, some of the above or one or two of the above. I was and still am modifying my forms to meet my needs, much of which is based upon my improved knowledge base over time. All the above forms are legal records and necessary to have.

It is a good idea to list the Geriatric Dental procedures that you do in your practice. Do not be afraid to cover the gamut of what you are capable of doing dental-wise and make a Consent form for each of the procedures in advance, instead of using a generic form and filling in the blanks. Each form should cover the procedure to be done, the risks of what is being done and the post-operative sequelae that may occur. These are important so that patients can acknowledge what you have informed them about. There should be a signature line at the bottom or the end of the Consent form for each of you to sign and date. Again, these are legal records, and it is important to "Inform Before your Perform". There should also be a form the patient must sign in lieu of rejecting what is recommended treatment. This is important for legal concerns and the record.

The following two-page form (Fig. 2.15) is an example of a standard Dental/Medical History form produced by the American Dental Association. It can be used for all types of patients, but it is particularly good for use with an older, possibly medically/mentally compromised patient.

ADA American Dental Association®

America's leading advocate for oral health

Today's Date: ______________________

Patient Dental & Medical Health History Information

To our patients: Please know that we may ask follow-up questions to make sure we have all of the information we need in order to treat you.

PATIENT INFORMATION

Last Name: | First Name: | Middle Name:

Home Phone: | Cell Phone: | Work Phone:

Email Address:

Mailing Address: | City: | State: | Zip:

Date of Birth: / / | Gender:

Occupation:

Emergency Contact: Name: | Relationship: | Phone:

If you are completing this form for another person, what is your name and relationship to that person? Name: ______________________ Relationship: __________

If executing this form as the patient's personal representative, I represent and warrant that I have full legal right and authority to consent to the performance of any procedure(s) on this patient. If for any reason I no longer have such legal right and authority, I will immediately notify the practice in writing.

DENTAL HISTORY & SYMPTOMS

What is the reason for your visit today?

Are you currently experiencing any dental pain or discomfort? ☐ Yes ☐ No If yes, where?

When was your last dental exam? / / What was done at that appointment?

When was the last time you had dental x-rays taken?

Please mark an "X" in the box ONLY if this applies to you.

Is it hard to open your mouth? ☐

Does it hurt to chew, bite or swallow? ☐

Do your gums bleed when you brush or floss your teeth? ☐

Have you ever had periodontal (gum) treatments like scaling and root planing? ☐

Do you have, or have you ever had, any sores or growths in your mouth? ☐

Do you clench or grind your teeth? ☐

Does your jaw click, pop or hurt? ☐

Do you have earaches or neck pains? ☐

Does dental treatment make you nervous? ☐

Have you ever experienced any of these sleep-related breathing disorders? ☐

☐ Mouth breathing ☐ Snoring ☐ Trouble breathing during sleep

Have you ever had a serious injury to your head or mouth? ☐

If yes, please describe what happened and when it happened: ______________________

Have you ever had problems with dental treatment in the past? ☐

If yes, please describe what happened: ______________________

Have you ever had a reaction to, or problem with, dental anesthesia? ☐

If yes, please describe what happened: ______________________

Are you unhappy with your smile? ☐

If yes, why? Please mark all that apply:

☐ The color of your teeth ☐ The shape of your teeth ☐ The position of your teeth

☐ Other. Please describe: ______________________

MEDICATIONS & OTHER PRODUCTS/SUBSTANCES

Please use an "X" to mark your answers to the following questions. Yes No ?

Are you taking any **blood thinners** (such as Coumadin, Warfarin, rivaroxaban (Xarelto®), dabigatran (Pradaxa®), clopidogrel (Plavix®), heparin or aspirin)? ☐ ☐ ☐

If yes, what medication are you taking? ______________________

Are you taking any medication to treat **osteoporosis** or Paget's disease? ☐ ☐ ☐

Some commonly-prescribed drugs include alendronate (Fosamax®), risedronate (Actonel®), ibandronate (Boniva®), zolendronate (Reclast®), and denosumab (Prolia®).

If yes, what medication are you taking? ______________________

Are you taking, or scheduled to take, an **IV medication** to treat bone pain, hypercalcemia or skeletal complications resulting from Paget's disease, multiple myeloma or metastatic cancer? ☐ ☐ ☐

Some commonly-prescribed drugs include denosumab (Xgeva®), pamidronate (Aredia®) or zolendronate (Zometa®).

If yes, what medication are you taking? ______________ How many years have you been taking it? ______________

Are you taking **hormonal replacements**? ☐ ☐ ☐

Do you use any form of **tobacco or nicotine products** (cigarettes, cigars, snuff, chew, bidis)? ☐ ☐ ☐

Do you use **vaping products**? ☐ ☐ ☐

How many **alcoholic beverages** do you have per week? __________

Do you use **controlled substances** (drugs), including marijuana, for either medicinal or recreational reasons? ☐ ☐ ☐

If yes, what substances? ______________ If yes, how often is your use? ☐ Daily ☐ Several times per week ☐ Weekly ☐ Occasionally

Was the substance prescribed by a doctor? ☐ Yes ☐ No If yes, for what reason(s)? ______________

Do you take any other **prescriptions and/or over-the-counter medicine(s), vitamins, herbs and/or supplements?** ☐ ☐ ☐

If yes, please list them here and include information about how much and how often you use each one. ______________

WOMEN ONLY: Are you:

Taking **birth control pills**? ☐ ☐ ☐

Pregnant? If yes, number of weeks: __________ ☐ ☐ ☐

Nursing? If yes, number of weeks: __________ ☐ ☐ ☐

Form S50021 To reorder call 800.947.4746 or go to ADAcatalog.org.

Fig. 2.15 Page 1 - ADA History form.

ALLERGIES
Please use an "X" to mark your answers to the following questions.

Are you allergic to or have you had an allergic reaction to:	Yes	No	?
Aspirin	☐	☐	☐
Barbiturates, sedatives or sleeping pills	☐	☐	☐
Codeine or other narcotics	☐	☐	☐
Hay fever/seasonal allergies	☐	☐	☐
Iodine	☐	☐	☐
Latex (rubber)	☐	☐	☐
Local anesthetics	☐	☐	☐
Metals	☐	☐	☐
Penicillin or other antibiotics	☐	☐	☐
Sulfa drugs such as sulfamethoxazole-trimethoprim (Septra, Bactrim), erythromycin-sulfisoxazole, sulfasala-zine (Azulfidine), erythromycin-sulfisoxazole (Eryzole, Pediazole) glyburide (Diabeta, Glynase PresTabs), dapsone, sumatriptan (Imitrex), celecoxib (Celebrex), hydrochlorothiazide (Microzide) and furosemide (Lasix)	☐	☐	☐
Other	☐	☐	☐

Please describe any "Yes" answers and include information about your experience. ______

MEDICAL & SURGICAL HISTORY

Date of last physical exam: / / What is your normal blood pressure (systolic, diastolic)?

Doctor's Name: Phone:

Please use an "X" to mark your answers to the following questions.	Yes	No	?
Are you in good physical health?	☐	☐	☐
Are you currently being seen or treated by a physician?	☐	☐	☐
Has a physician or previous dentist recommended that you take **antibiotics** before having dental work done?	☐	☐	☐
Have you had a **serious illness, operation or been hospitalized** in the past 5 years?	☐	☐	☐
Have you had any type (either total or partial) of **joint replacement** surgery (such as for a hip, knee, shoulder, elbow, finger, etc.)?	☐	☐	☐
Have you had a **heart valve replacement or heart surgery**?	☐	☐	☐
Have you had an **organ or bone marrow/stem cell transplant**?	☐	☐	☐
Have you traveled internationally within the last 30 days	☐	☐	☐
Have you had a fever (100.4°F or above) in the last 72 hours?	☐	☐	☐

If you answered yes to any of the above, please explain: ______

MEDICAL HISTORY SPECIFIC
Please use an "X" to mark your answers to the following questions.

Do you have, or have you been diagnosed with, any of the following conditions?

	Yes	No	?
Heart (Cardiac) Health			
Pacemaker/implanted defibrillator	☐	☐	☐
Artificial (prosthetic) heart valve	☐	☐	☐
Previous infective endocarditis	☐	☐	☐
Congenital heart disease (CHD)	☐	☐	☐
Unrepaired, cyanotic CHD	☐	☐	☐
Repaired (completely) in last 6 months	☐	☐	☐
Repaired CHD with residual defects	☐	☐	☐
Arteriosclerosis	☐	☐	☐
Coronary artery disease	☐	☐	☐
Congestive heart failure	☐	☐	☐
Damaged heart valves	☐	☐	☐
Heart attack	☐	☐	☐
Heart murmur/rhythm disorder	☐	☐	☐
Rheumatic heart disease	☐	☐	☐
Stroke	☐	☐	☐
Breathing (Respiratory) Health			
Asthma (COPD)	☐	☐	☐
Bronchitis	☐	☐	☐
Emphysema	☐	☐	☐
Sinus trouble	☐	☐	☐
Tuberculosis	☐	☐	☐
Cancer	☐	☐	☐
Type: ______			
Date of diagnosis: ______			
Chemotherapy: ______			
Radiation treatment: ______			
Blood (Circulatory) Health			
Anemia	☐	☐	☐
Blood transfusion	☐	☐	☐
If yes, date: ______			
Hemophilia	☐	☐	☐
High or low blood pressure	☐	☐	☐
Brain (Neurological)/Mental Health			
Anxiety	☐	☐	☐
Depression	☐	☐	☐
Epilepsy	☐	☐	☐
Mental health disorders	☐	☐	☐
Neurological disorders	☐	☐	☐
Post-traumatic stress disorder	☐	☐	☐
Traumatic brain injury or concussion	☐	☐	☐
Autoimmune Disease			
AIDS or HIV Infection	☐	☐	☐
Lupus	☐	☐	☐
Digestive Health			
Gastrointestinal disease	☐	☐	☐
G.E. reflux/persistent heartburn (GERD)	☐	☐	☐
Stomach ulcers	☐	☐	☐
Eye (Vision) Health			
Glaucoma	☐	☐	☐
Other			
Arthritis	☐	☐	☐
Chronic pain	☐	☐	☐
Diabetes (type I or II)	☐	☐	☐
Eating disorder	☐	☐	☐
Frequent infections	☐	☐	☐
Type of infection: ______			
Hepatitis, jaundice or liver disease	☐	☐	☐
Immune deficiency	☐	☐	☐
Kidney problems	☐	☐	☐
Malnutrition	☐	☐	☐
Osteoporosis	☐	☐	☐
Rheumatoid arthritis	☐	☐	☐
Sexually transmitted infection (STI)	☐	☐	☐
Thyroid problems	☐	☐	☐

Do you have any disease, condition, or problem that's not listed here? If so, please explain. ______

MEDICAL SYMPTOMS/GENERAL
Please use an "X" to mark your answers to the following questions.

In the past 30 days, have you:	Yes	No	?
had pain or tightness in the chest?	☐	☐	☐
coughed up blood or had a cough that lasted longer than 3 weeks?	☐	☐	☐
been exposed to anyone with tuberculosis?	☐	☐	☐
had a rapid or irregular heart beat?	☐	☐	☐
found it hard to catch your breath?	☐	☐	☐
had a high fever (greater than 101.5°F) for no reason?	☐	☐	☐
noticed a change in your vision?	☐	☐	☐
fainted for no reason?	☐	☐	☐
experienced vomiting, diarrhea, chills, night sweats or bleeding?	☐	☐	☐
had migraines or severe headaches?	☐	☐	☐

NOTE: It's important for both the doctor and patient to talk honestly about the patient's health before dental treatment starts.
I have answered the above questions completely, accurately and to the best of my ability.

Signature of Patient/Legal Guardian: ______ Date: ______

FOR COMPLETION BY DENTIST

Comments: ______

Office Use Only: ☐ Medical Alert ☐ Premedication ☐ Allergies ☐ Anesthesia

Reviewed by: ______ Date: ______

Form S50021 To reorder call 800.947.4746 or go to ADAcatalog.org.

Fig. 2.15 Page 2 - ADA History form.

2.6 The Evaluation Process

It is incumbent upon all practitioners to be skilled at evaluating what lies in front of us when a patient presents for treatment. In order to be effective at the process, one must be organized both mentally and physically to be able to ascertain information that will bring about a new light with respect to what the patients' concerns may be. Working systematically can be amazingly effective and keeping these systems in check during the examination process will help the practitioner to organize his/her thoughts and information that will eventually lead to a proper diagnosis. Looking at the areas that need to be inspected thoroughly is particularly important and necessary, especially when examining an older patient with multiple issues, both dentally and medically. Table 2.1 is a list in mnemonic form that will help the practitioner to stay aware and organized in the process of the *Geriatric Oral Cavity and Head and Neck* examination.

Table 2.1 Examination chart designed for screening

1	H = HEARING
2	E = EYES (movement, perla, nevi, sclera, color)
3	A = ALIGNMENT (occlusion, excursive movements, e.g., thyroid gland)
4	D = DILUENT (saliva - consistency/flow)
5	A = ANATOMY (intraoral/extraoral landmarks, e.g., thyroid gland)
6	N = NODES (auricular, cervical, occipital, submandibular)
7	D = DEXTERITY (opening/closing, excursive movement)
8	N = NERVOUS SYSTEM (swallowing, tongue movement)
9	E = ENAMEL (wear, caries, erosion, abfraction, restore)
10	C = CERVICAL GINGIVAL HEALTH/PERIODONTAL DISEASE
11	K = KICK OR GAIT (body language, movements)
12	E = EVALUATE
13	X = RADIOGRAPH
14	A = ASSESSMENT
15	M = MANAGEMENT

Mnemonic. Developed by Dr. Eric Z. Shapira

The mnemonic is written vertically in the form of **HEAD AND NECK EXAM**. Each letter stands for a specific system to look at or be aware of while examining the patient. If we look at the **H** for example, it stands for **Hearing**. Many times, older patients will wear some form of assisted hearing device that may not be written on the history form. We need to look for them and chart whether it is inside or outside the ear or a hearing assisted necklace worn on the neck as jewelry. We also need to ask if there is a device in one or both ears if the patient has a hearing disability. Most of the time, patients who are hearing impaired, that do not wear an assisted device, do not inform the dentist that this is a problem. Then the practitioner and staff find themselves raising their voices at the patient. This is a good sign of impairment of the patients hearing. Raising your voice is not a good idea, especially if there are other patients adjacent to where one is working.

E would be for the **Eyes**. I have never seen a dental history form that asked if patients wear contact lenses or glasses. It is always a good idea to find out and regardless of whether the patient is wearing either of those items, we need to protect the patient's eyes while working on them. We need to observe the function of the eyes. Have the patient follow your finger in an upward and lateral movement. This will tell you about the eye muscles, finding an astigmatism: whether they can track an object in good form and whether they can see our finger move. It also tells us if the patient can follow commands and pay attention. We want to look for pupils that are equal and reactive to light (PERLA), which may give us an idea about drugs someone may be taking or systemic eye issues and the subsequent functions of the eye. **A** is for the **Alignment** of the jaws and teeth. Our occlusion is important, and we should have the patient move in excursive movements to determine the lateral movement of the jaw, the opening and closing of the jaw and taking measurements of the protrusive, opening and centric positions including overbite and overjet. Of course, if the patient is edentulous, it is a moot point. **D** is for **Diluent** or liquid (saliva) in the mouth. We should look at each duct of the parotid, sublingual and submandibular glands and the accessory salivary glands on the roof of the mouth and the lips to make sure they are functional. One can do this by "milking" the gland and looking at the duct for secretion. **A** is for **Anatomy** of all the extraoral and intraoral landmarks. Making sure that there is symmetry is important. Charting the skin, the largest organ in our bodies, is important. We need to look for scars and nevi as well as charting their relative positions, color, size and measurements.

Many years ago, when I was an Assistant Clinical Professor at the University of the Pacific Dental School in San Francisco, a middle-aged woman came into the clinic for a student to examine her. I was supervising the student. I noticed a vertical scar on this patient's lip over the vermillion border from the mucosa to the outer skin of the lip. The student had overlooked the scar in his examination, so I called his attention to it and asked that he chart it. I signed off on his examination when he completed it. A year later, this patient was seen in the clinic again with a different student, having some restorative work done. She subsequently complained that a previous student, who went unnamed, had cut her lip with a dental handpiece and that she was in the process of filing a suit against the school. The clinical instructor saw that I had signed off on this patient's initial examination and that the student had charted it as part of his initial examination with the patient. In short, the woman in question backed down from her lawsuit as it was a lie and frivolous at the same time and could come back to bite her for perjuring herself. She was immediately dismissed from the clinic practice and told not to return. Therefore, a lesson in the importance of charting this information in the patient chart.

N is for **Nodes**. Checking lymph nodes is easy and will give the practitioner a chance to see if they are soft, tender and moveable or firm, fixed and asymptomatic. It will also allow us to check the thyroid gland in the neck at the same time. I have picked up countless tumors in the thyroid gland over the years and saved lives in doing so. Should this have happened to you already, you already know that when you find a tumor in its early stages, further investigation and referral are in order. You also know that you will have a patient for life in gratitude for saving their life. **D** is somewhat of a repeat of **Alignment**, already discussed. **N** stands for **Nervous System**. Checking the swallowing mechanism, the tongue and the gag reflex as well as movement, the feeling involved in these structures is particularly important. Feeling the tongue, lips, mucosa and such doing "bimanual palpation" is important to rule out tumors and improper function for one reason or another. Testing the 12 cranial nerves in and around the oral cavity is a good exercise as well. **E** is for **Enamel** and basically the condition of all the remaining teeth in one's mouth. **C** is for **Cervical Health** of the gingival tissues. We need to periodontal probe, chart recession, mobility and the presence of existing periodontal disease. **K** is for **Kick or Gait** of the patient. We want to look at body language, how a patient moves, sits, stands and walks. All these entities give us an idea of who we may be working with and their ability to function physically. Getting to the dental chair and sitting in it may be a chore for an elderly, compromised or special needs patient. It is for this reason that the K step in diagnosis starts when the patient comes into the office and again when they mobilize themselves towards the examination room, as well as leaving your operatory and office. **EXAM, E** is to **Evaluate** the patient. Utilizing all the modalities I have discussed here. **X** is for taking **X-rays** or other kinds of films on the patient as needed and warranted. **A** is for **Assessment** of all the information at hand that might affect subsequent treatment and then **M** is for **Managing** everything by placing it into a manageable, organized treatment plan and/or providing an alternate treatment plan(s) as well. Having all of this in place coupled with the medical, dental, economic and social histories, should give the practitioner a good base from which to start treatment of any kind.

Doing this *Diagnostic Mantra* will leave one well protected legally and reassured that future treatment will be organized and flow smoothly for the patient and the practitioner.

Older, more compromised patients of one type or another will need repetition, for the most part, in explaining what is going on dentally at the onset of treatment, due to possible short-term memory issues, which are much more common than far memory issues in cognitively impaired individuals. It is not just an issue about "Where did I put my car keys?" It is about continued treatment towards the long-term goal of a healthy individual.

Remember the **5 P**'s when getting ready to treatment plan your geriatric patients:

Poor
Prior
Planning
Promotes
Phailure

Should the older, more "set-in-their ways" patient resist the practitioner from doing any of the exams or filling out forms, then it is up to a caregiver or relative to do this for that person. If this is not possible, then there is no recourse, but to not treat this patient. Should the relative, guardian, Power of Attorney representative assure the practitioner that they will take care of the history in the best possible way, even though there may be limited information, and then sign the forms; the liability of care will be on their hands. The practitioner still needs to decide how to go about making the decision to treat or not to treat and decide what will be done.

Many times, in my practice in treating the older, medically and mentally challenged patients, I have had to have the next of kin or person with the Power of Attorney give permission for full sedation utilizing a dental anesthesiologist, in order to meet the needs of the patient. After attempting a cursory exam, should the patient allow it, one can ascertain the necessary treatment that is needed for the most part. It is not until the patient is totally under general anesthesia, that the complete examination and treatment is rendered. Because these are exceptional circumstances, some of the previous protocol, such as a complete head and neck examination, may be limited, in lieu of doing a more thorough intraoral examination to ascertain the extent of treatment to be done that day under general anesthesia and possibly another visit or two in the future to complete the necessary treatment. It is difficult treatment, to say the least, but knowing that treating all of what can be done to bring a compromised person with a compromised dentition, as well as diseased gingiva into a state of health, is worth the effort. Not all older compromised patients need sedation. It is an option to consider when there is an older, compromised patient who presents in an unmanageable way for care.

> **Note:** *Personal treatment forms mentioned in this section of Chapter 2 will be placed in the Appendix of this text for reference.*

References

1. *Oxford American Desk Dictionary and Thesaurus.* 2nd Edition, 2001. Oxford University Press: 355.
2. Shear MK. *Grief and mourning gone awry: pathway and course of complicated grief.* Dialogues Clin Neurosci. 2012 Jun;14(2):119-28.
3. Conejero I, Olié E, Courtet P, Calati R. *Suicide in older adults: current perspectives.* Clin Interv Aging. 2018 Apr 20;13:691-699.
4. Sinyor M, Tan LP, Schaffer A, Gallagher D, Shulman K. *Suicide in the oldest old: an observational study and cluster analysis.* Int J Geriatr Psychiatry. 2016 Jan;31(1):33-40.
5. American Psychiatric Association, *Diagnostic and Statistical Manual of Mental Disorders*, 4th Edition, 2002. American Psychiatric Association, Washington, D.C.
6. Shear MK. *Complicated grief treatment: the theory, practice and outcomes.* Bereave Care. 2010 Jan 1;29(3):10-14.
7. Mayo Clinic. Mayo Foundation for Medical Education and Research. *Post-traumatic stress disorder (PTSD).* Online: https://www.mayoclinic.org/diseases-conditions/post-traumatic-stress-disorder/symptoms-causes/Oyc-20355967?p=1;2021
8. *Oxford American Dictionary and Thesaurus.* 2nd Edition, 2001 Oxford University Press.
9. www.Edmesa.edu.outcomes-assessmentguide.12/20.

Chapter 3

The Preservation of Spit (Saliva) in a Drug Happy and Aging Society

"Kissing is good for teeth.
The anticipation of a kiss increases
the flow of saliva to the mouth,
giving the teeth a plaque dispersing bath..."
Unknown Author

3.1 Introduction

Saliva, or "spit", as some call it, is one our most valued human commodities. It is something we do not really think about, until we do not have any in our mouth and then the unconscious brain "kick's in" telling us that our mouths are dry and need lubricated. OK, where is the water? I am thirsty just thinking about this! However, as we age, the need for thirst is enhanced by a specific hormonal stimulus called **Angiotensin II** (Ang II), which is generated when the rate-limiting enzyme **renin** is secreted by the kidneys in response to hypovolemia or hypotension, whose action takes place within the pituitary gland. Thirst, as a desire and a specific signal, is the catalyst for us to replenish the wetness in our mouth. It is the alarm sounded regarding the lack of saliva, which tells us that we need to drink more fluids. It is the aging process that spawns this phenomenon, in part due to the lack of the hormone within the pituitary gland. Dehydration, on the other hand, is caused by the antidiuretic hormone or vasopressin. Excessive heat, overwork in such heat producing sweat; hence, the lack of a proper chemical balance in sodium can exacerbate serious dehydration allowing for an increase in thirst, asiallorhea or xerostomia of the mouth, as well as within the dysfunctional salivary glands and associated mucosal tissues.

3.2 What is Saliva?

Saliva is a viscous, clear, watery fluid secreted by the parotid, submandibular, sublingual and smaller, secondary accessory salivary mucous glands of the mouth; found on the lips and palatal tissues. Normal salivary secretions amount to approximately 1500 mL/day. It has been stated that a person's lifetime accumulation of saliva is enough liquid to fill a standard swimming pool! Saliva contains two major protein secretions, a serous secretion containing the digestive enzyme **ptyalin** and a mucous secretion containing a lubricating aid, **mucin**. Saliva also contains an enzyme called salivary **amylase**, which assists in the digestion of food, as well as destroying harmful bacteria and substances that can be deleterious to one's health. The pH of saliva is between 6 and 7.4 (basically neutral). Saliva contains large amounts of potassium and bicarbonate ions and, to a lesser extent, sodium and chloride ions. Saliva contains several antimicrobial constituents such as thiocyanate, lysozyme (a digestive enzyme) and the immunoglobulins **lactoferrin** and **transferrin**.

These salivary elements function in antimicrobial activity; mechanical cleansing action; control of pH; removal of food debris from the oral cavity; lubrication of the oral cavity; remineralization and maintaining the integrity of the oral mucosa, as well as digestion of food that we eat.

As an aside, when this Author was a child, he saw his grandfather make a bet or a business agreement with a friend by *spitting* in the palm of his own hand and then shaking hands with the other man, with whom he had made that agreement. I thought that this was the way people did business with each other back then, but I soon found out that it was unsanitary and forbidden for me to do the same by the number of "whacks" to my *derrière,* after telling my mom what I had seen! Such is life and the learning process...

The lack of saliva can be most detrimental to the health of the oral cavity, resulting in caries, gingivitis and periodontal disease, as well as problems with the mucosal tissue, lips and throat. Secondary inflammation from a build-up of *Candida albicans,* a common fungus in the oral cavity, can create associated issues of pain, redness, cracking and secondary bacterial and viral infections. The lack of moisture and the inefficiency in digesting the food that one chooses to eat can cause more involved issues within the stomach and intestines as well. So, it is all cause and effect when it comes to xerostomia, or the lack of saliva in the mouth.

Aging, in conjunction with the acquired inefficiency of an older person in cleaning one's mouth or lack thereof in cleaning altogether, can increase the potential for disease. Dementias and other diseases like Parkinson's disease, Multiple Sclerosis and being a mentally challenged individual add to the mix and can exacerbate oral disease.

Arthritis in one form or another has been discovered in 91 million U.S. adults. It is found in approximately 58% of men and 69% of women over the age of 65 years and older.[1] This disease can and does impede one's ability to hold a toothbrush effectively and to clean their mouth thoroughly in order to resist oral disease (Fig. 3.1).

3.3 Salivary Anatomy

The salivary complex of glands (Fig. 3.2) and associated ducts are found in the posterior part of the cheeks in front of the ears (the parotid glands); under the tongue in the anterior floor of the mouth (submandibular glands bilaterally) and the posterior floor of the mouth (sublingual glands bilaterally). These glands function 24/7 and are what keep our mouths moist and somewhat disease free.

With aging, the risk of **xerostomia** or dry mouth is increased greatly. It is the subjective sensation of "dry mouth", which is often (but not always) associated with hypofunction of the salivary glands leading to the absence of saliva.

3.3.1 Xerostomia

Xerostomia can be caused by certain health conditions seen at any age, but increased in older individuals with such issues as diabetes; stroke; thrush (yeast infections) in the mouth; Alzheimer's disease; dehydrating disease such as hypo- or hyperfunction of the kidneys; autoimmune disease; Sjörgren's syndrome; HIV/AIDS; lymphomas; medication and neurologic dysfunction. With any of these elements one can have xerostomia as a

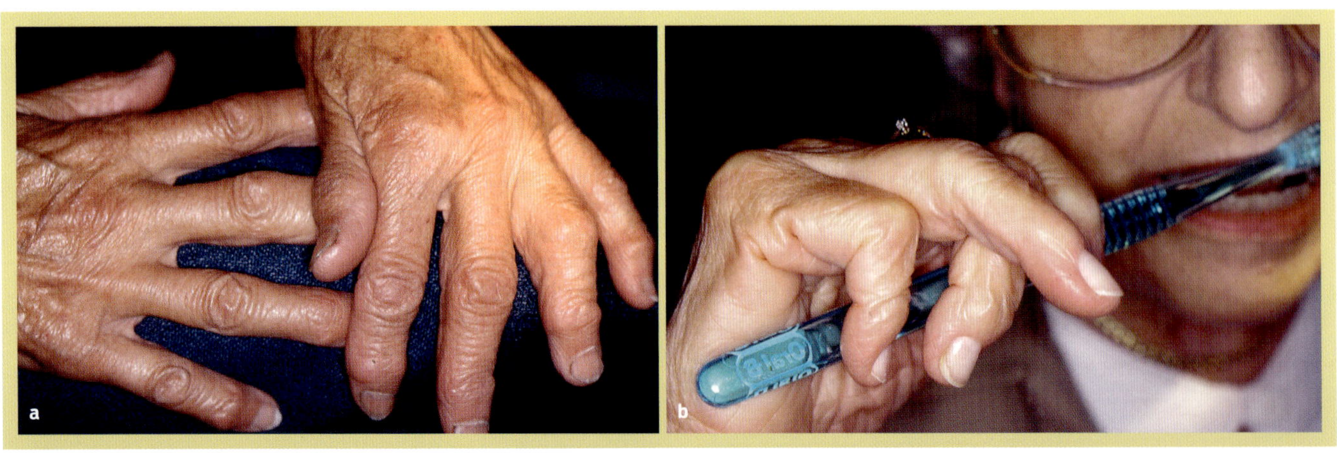

Fig. 3.1 Deceased 95-year-old patient with advanced arthritis (**a**), showing difficulty holding a common toothbrush (**b**).

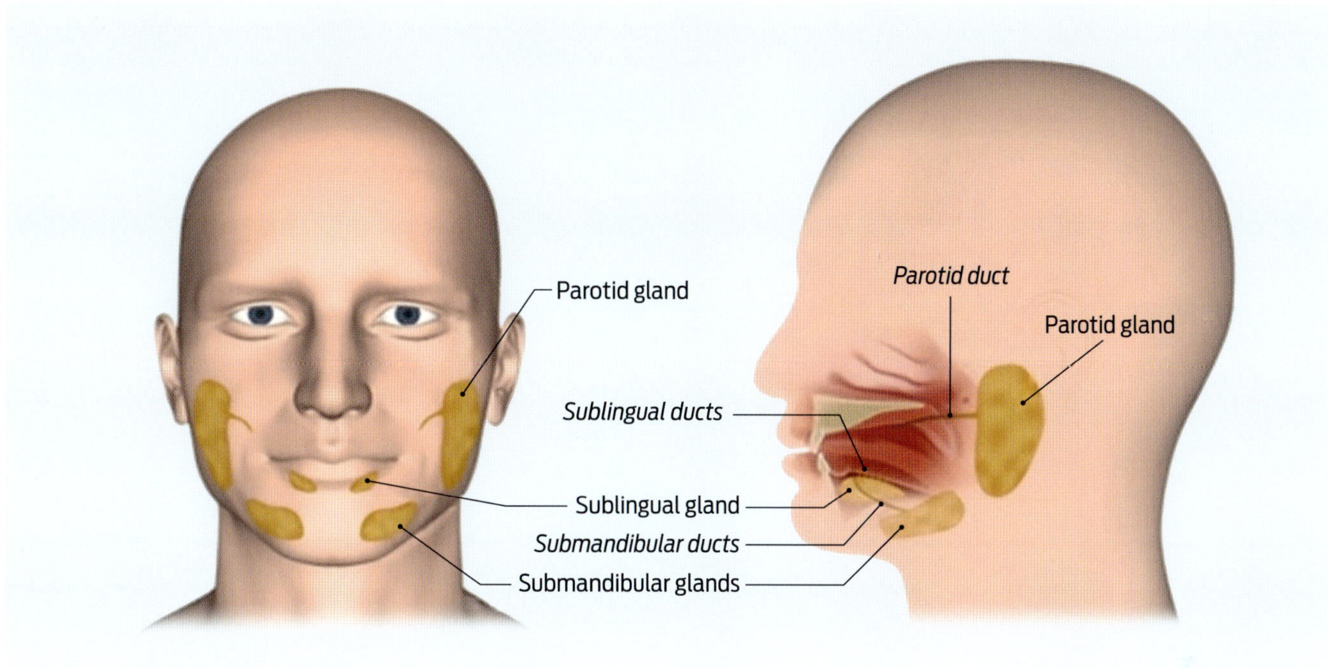

Fig. 3.2 Position of the major salivary glands.

by-product of their disease or malfunction issues. Common overlooked clinical issues can include snoring and mouth-breathing with the mouth open; tobacco and alcohol (ethanol) use; head and neck radiation; medications, especially antihistamines; vitamin D deficiency, which can cause Burning Mouth Syndrome (BMS) accompanied by a metallic or bitter taste in the mouth, as well as dry mouth from stress, anxiety, dehydration, and depression.

3.4 Baseline and Function

When examining an elderly person who complains, or not, about having a dry mouth, it is not enough just to peer into the mouth. The practitioner, besides looking, must touch the tissues in an intraoral examination, feel for the glands and milk the ducts to determine if there is function and saliva. It would even behoove the practitioner to take a sample of saliva to determine the rate of flow, if any, per minute. This procedural act helps give one a baseline for your oral examination of the tongue, mucosa, gingiva, salivary glands and associated ducts. Many times, an elderly person will exhibit a calcification in the duct or at the orifice of the duct that is palpable by the dentist, if he/she looks for this type of thing. Blocked ducts can be painful due to the inability of the patient to secrete saliva. Visually, one can see a dry tongue or a red shiny tongue, as well as gross stain and caries or incisal caries. All these things can be indicative of xerostomia, as seen in the accompanying photographs (Figs. 3.3, 3.4).

Dementia can lead to both xerostomia and the lack of self-efficacy in care. Older persons who have limited assistance at home or in an assisted living or memory community are at the mercy of

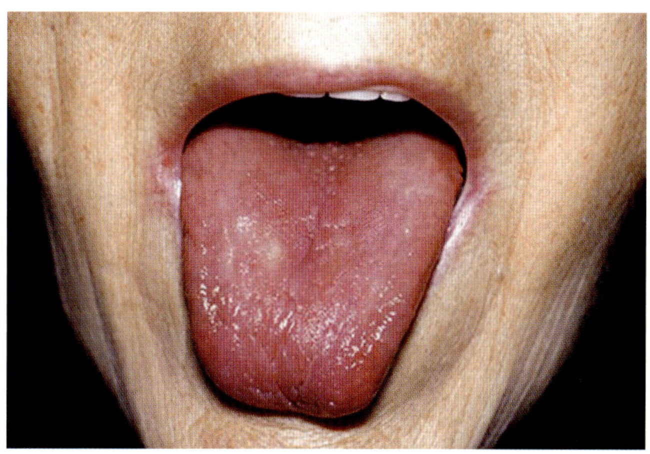

Fig. 3.3 Atrophic tongue with angular cheilosis and little to no saliva.[2]

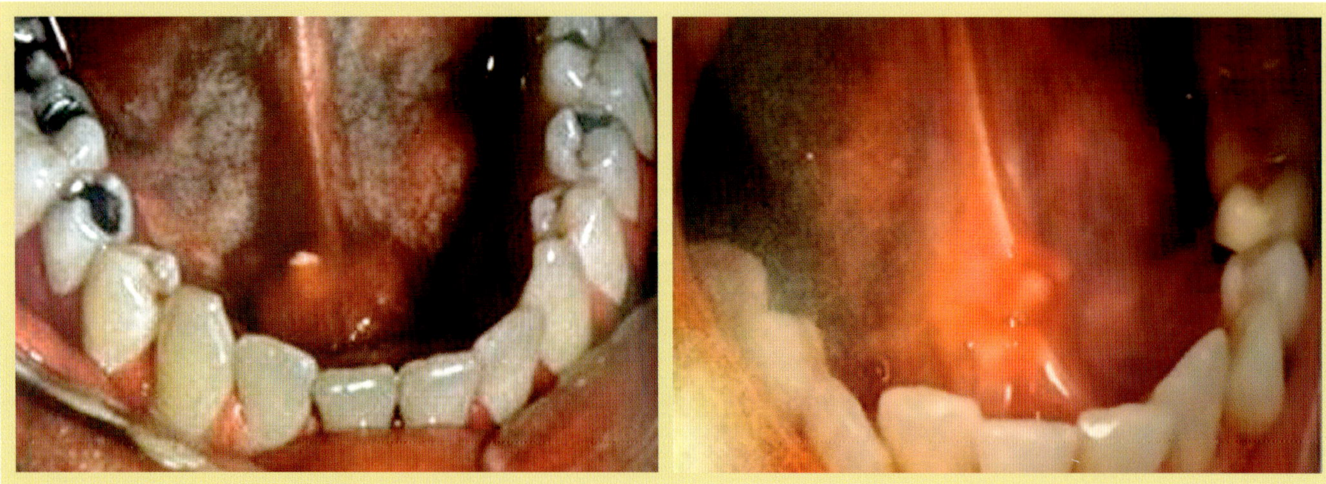

Fig. 3.4 Sialoliths (calcifications or stones) in Wharton's duct of the submandibular glands.[3]

the nursing aids for care. Many of these facilities and many of their employees do not know very much about oral homecare or oral disease. It is important for us as practitioners to assist them in learning about how to maintain a healthy mouth and dentition. This Figure 3.5 was of one of my long-term care facility patients showing the lack of care; hence, this person's disease as a result of the lack of self-efficacy over a long period of time. Advanced periodontal disease coupled with the loss of teeth, extrusion of remaining posterior teeth, heavy plaque and calculus present do not make for a total oral and systemically healthy person. Chronic disease in this case, along with her dementia, probably contributed to her untimely and anticipated death.

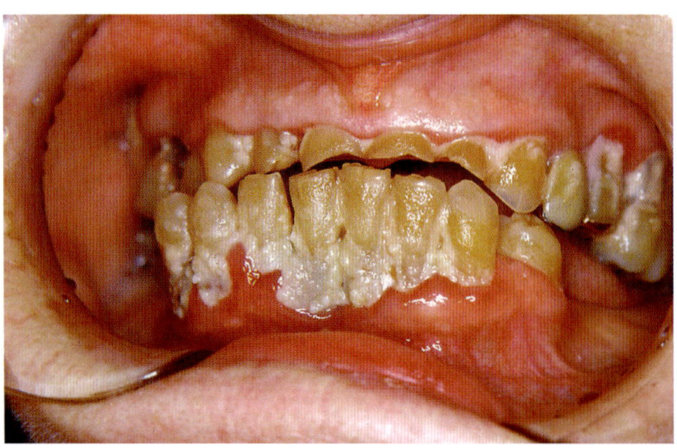

Fig. 3.5 Deceased 89-year-old patient with dementia, advanced geriatric periodontal disease and xerostomia.

3.4.1 Xerostomia in Depth: Cause and Effect

Many times there are common, overlooked clinical findings, with respect to the onset of xerostomia in the geriatric patient, that are caused by snoring and mouth-breathing with the mouth open; tobacco use; vaping; alcohol (ethanol); head and neck radiation; medications, such as antihistamines; antidepressants; antihypertensives; vitamin D deficiency, causing a dry, burning mouth syndrome, as well as a metallic or bitter taste in the mouth; antiulcer medication; SSRIs (Serotonin Reuptake Inhibitors); benzodiazepines; ACE inhibitors (Blood Pressure medication); decongestants; muscle relaxants; anticholinergics; anticonvulsants; antineoplastics; antiparkinsonian; antipsychotics; antispasmodics; CNS stimulants; diuretics; gastrointestinal medications; narcotics; HIV protease inhibitors; sympathomimetics and systemic bronchodilators, to name a few.[3] These clinical findings should be followed up on so that the salivary function can be regenerated to at least a minimal flow, which would be better than no flow at all.

The elderly patient, those with dementias and other psychological issues, take a myriad of medication type cocktails to assist them with maintaining some kind of "normalcy" in their lives or to sedate them into a more manageable person. Most of these medications that are dispensed can and do cause xerostomia.

Xerostomia is found in approximately 20-30% of the elderly, with a higher prevalence in aged wom-

BOX 3.1

Treatment Modalities of Salivary Issues

Associated treatment for **angular cheilitis** or **cheilosis** is the use corticosteroids coupled with an antifungal agent. A prescription drug such as *Lotrisone*® works very well in most of these situations. It is also possible that scarring may occur from these conditions over time, especially if left untreated. In these cases, a product called *Mederma*® can be used to reduce the effects of the scarring after treatment with *Lotrisone*®.

In cases of **asiallorhea** or **xerostomia**, one can sip on water throughout the day; use sugarless candy or gum with xylitol, which is anticariogenic; use an alcohol free and lubricating mouthwash and avoid mouth-breathing when possible. Oral lubricants such as *Xerolube*®, *Oral Balance*® gel and the like can be used all day long with no side-effects. *Xylamelts*® are small "dry tabs" that are placed over the parotid duct area at night to help secrete saliva. And then there is the "Old Wives" remedy of sucking on a lemon. But one needs to be careful of creating an acidic environment in the mouth due to the possible caries effect that could result. I advocate just thinking about eating or sucking on a lemon and your brain should do the rest...

For **sialorrhea**, or **hypersalivation**, one can take the prescriptions (atropine and pilocarpine), to help dry the mouth, but should be checked by a medical doctor first due to their possible cardiac side-effects.

Salivary issues of all kinds tend to complicate restorative procedures in the elderly, where caution should be a priority in treatment as well as planning. A mouth that is very dry makes dental treatment uncomfortable and sometimes intolerable. This has caused many cancelled appointments in my office until I learned how to cope with the issue of xerostomia.

Lubrication is a "key" to the success of your treatment. Constant lubrication of the lips is necessary. Stopping periodically, maybe every three to five minutes, for an oral rinse and a drink for the patient is necessary to keep the tissues moist, as well as using oral lubricants such as *Oral Balance*® gel placed on the tongue and allowed to be "swished" onto all the mucosal tissue, gingiva, and the tongue itself helps immensely. Moist cotton rolls tucked up under the cheeks are also helpful, so that the mucosa is kept moist; keeping the dry tissue from burning or tearing if retracted too much or with too much force. A prescription for pilocarpine can be used to stimulate saliva as well. Care must be taken with the use of the dental handpiece or other bulky, large equipment, by not rubbing it against the tissue while working, for fear of tearing the tissue just from the rubbing action itself. Lubricants such as *Aquaphor*® and *Cera Vie*® can be a home remedy and for use during treatment.

With the onset of hypersalivation, one must isolate teeth with a rubber dam for all restorative procedures that require dryness. When the dam is removed, a dry tab can be placed over the parotid gland duct, as well as cotton rolls under the tongue for moisture control. Of course, in some instances, I have pre-medicated patients with antihistamines or atropine as needed and as screened for in the patients' medical histories, to make sure there are no contraindications to treatment. It is best to be safe rather than sorry. As my father used to tell me when I was a young boy working in construction with him: "It is best to study the situation first, before you act upon trying to do it because if you don't do it right the first time, you always have to find the time, the energy and the money to do it over again and this is not good business". I have never forgotten that adage and it makes a lot of sense when treatment planning patients with these issues of xerostomia and siallorhea or hypersalivation. Always remember to: "Do No Harm".

en.[4] Dry mouth is a major issue with increasing age and should be investigated by the dental clinician. In older individuals, amongst the geriatric population, xerostomia not only affects the oral tissues, but has an influence on our ability to digest food properly in the digestive system, causing further systemic issues as well. Angiotensin I and II, enzymes that cause thirst, can affect the kidneys in the form of increased urination, which in turn, causes dehydration. The dental practitioner needs to investigate the older patient's general health making sure that his or her patients have good kidney health. True idiopathic xerostomia can and does cause an irreversible and physiologic degradation of the glandular tissue. This can be seen in sialographic examination; whereby one can see sclerosis and atrophy of the interlobar spaces and intralobular glandular tissue. Radiographic and sialographic testing shows no change if the condition is one of symptomatic or temporary xerostomia.

In other instances of having a dry mouth, salivary hypofunction or hyposalivation is the condition of having reduced saliva production which is different from xerostomia. One can diagnose hyposalivation by measuring salivary flow. There have been large scale studies on this effort that have demonstrated this issue through flow rates of saliva. The average unstimulated whole salivary flow rate is 0.3-0.4 mL/minute during waking hours. An unstimulated rate of 0.1 mL/minute or less indicates hyposalivation. People with hyposalivation experience inadequate bicarbonate and urea buffering, remineralization, and sugar and acid clearance, and may result in an increased caries rate. In a recent salivary function test, adults over 65 years of age with hyposalivation issues were more likely to lose at least one tooth more than those that did not have this condition.[5]

Symptoms such as the increase in dental caries, periodontal disease, sore throat (chronic), burning sensation of the mucosa, tongue and palatal tissues; difficulty speaking and swallowing, hoarseness and/or dry nasal passages and lips are all common issues with a chronic dry mouth. Subsequently, the entire aforementioned list of issues makes eating more difficult, followed by the results which may affect the individual's quality of life and bodily functions in many ways, including shortening of their overall lifespans.

Xerostomia is an original hidden cause of gum diseases and tooth loss in eight out of every 10 individuals. If left untreated it decreases the oral pH to an acidic environment, increases the development of plaque and dental caries. Oral candidiasis is one of the most common oral infections seen in the mouth in association with xerostomia. It is important for us as practitioners to continuously examine and re-examine our older, more frail patients for these entities.

3.5 Hypersalivation and the Elderly

Another physiological oral condition, that is not examined too often by dental practitioners, is hypersalivation or excessive saliva in the mouth. Again, this may be a function of the pituitary gland malfunctioning as it controls thirst. Vasopressin, produced in the pituitary gland, may act on receptors in the brain to create the effects of dehydration, which in turn may be manifested by an excess flow of saliva due to increased urination by the kidneys, causing the dehydration. Other causes of hypersalivation may include acid reflux, with the onset of a bitter taste and accompanying heartburn; cerebral palsy, due to muscle rigidity and a stasis in salivary flow without stopping; Parkinson's disease, with dystonia; severe dental caries and resulting discomfort from tooth aches; tonsillitis and associated pain as a trigger mechanism for hypersalivation; allergies; tumors and above the neck infections; sinusitis with pressure and pain; IBS (Interstitial Bowel Syndrome) with induced stomach ulcers; major tranquilizers; epilepsy medication such as *Dilantin*®; dementia medication such as *Aricept*® or donepezil; TIA's with loss of neurologic control of the salivary glands, and especially prevalent within the geriatric population, loss of vertical dimension creating angular cheilitis or chronic angular cheilosis (long-standing irritation) (**Figs. 3.6, 3.7**).

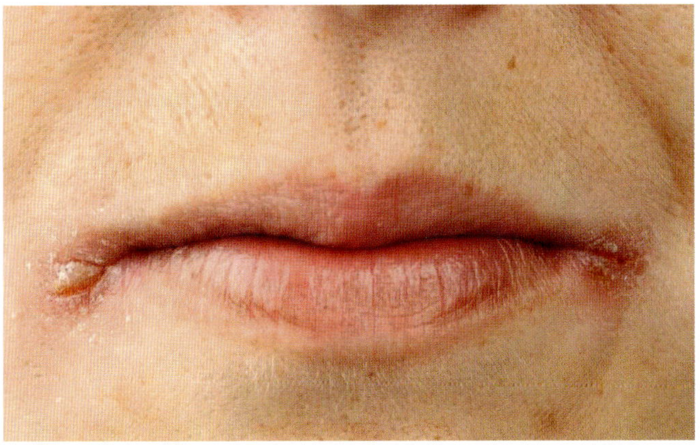

Fig. 3.6 Angular cheilitis due to loss of vertical dimension with a secondary fungal infection at the corners of the mouth and around the nares. The continuous leakage of saliva at the corners of the mouth is the result of hypersalivation. Also seen are the typical "thin" lip lines due to a collapsed vertical dimension and worn dentures.

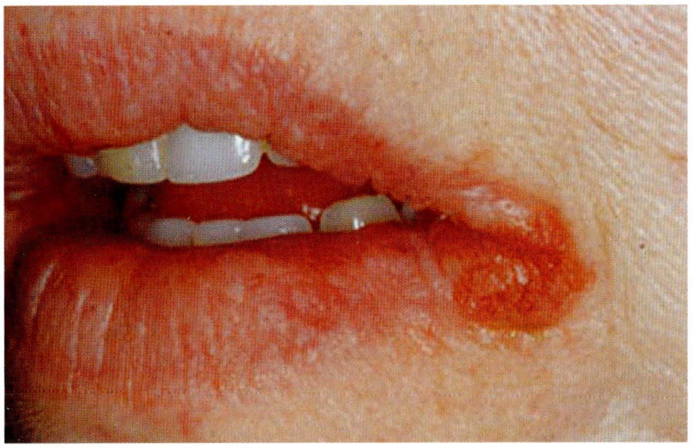

Fig. 3.7 Deceased 90-year-old patient with angular cheilosis (long-standing) with scarring and associated candidiasis at the corners of the mouth. This patient was edentulous, wore a full upper and lower denture and had poor hygiene habits.

References

1. Torgan, Carol, Ph.D. *Updated Estimates Suggest a Higher Number of U.S. Adults with Arthritis.* June 25, 2018. From: https://www.niams.nih.gov.
2. WebMD.com/oral-health/ss/slideshow-tongue-your health.
3. Kahn, Michael, A., DDS; Hall, J. Michael, DDS. *The ADA Practical Guide to Soft Tissue Oral Diseases.* Wiley-Blackwell, 2014: 1st Edition, p 102; fig. 3.77.
4. Wiener Constance R, Wu B, Crout R, Wiener M, Plassman B, Kao E, McNeil D. *Hyposalivation and xerostomia in dentate older adults.* J Am Dent Assoc. 2010 Mar;141(3):279-84.
5. Caplan DJ, Hunt RJ. *Salivary flow and risk of tooth loss in an elderly population.* Community Dent Oral Epidemiol. 1996 Feb;24(1):68-71.

Chapter **4**

Geriatric Periodontal Disease or Why Aren't Your Teeth in a Jar?

"Bid them wash their faces and keep their teeth clean."
King Henry IV, Part II – Coriolanus – Shakespeare

4.1 Periodontal Disease

4.1.1 Definition

Perio, from the Greek, means "around" and *odont* means "teeth"; therefore, periodontal disease is a disease entity that affects the tissues surrounding the teeth. This includes the bone; the ligaments attached to the bone that are also attached to the teeth (the periodontal ligament); the gingiva and the mucosal tissue attached to the gingiva. It is a disease that is pandemic in the world found in all species that have teeth, especially in humans. It is a disease that starts as inflammation in the space around the tooth, the gingival sulcus, called gingivitis. This initial disease state moves to the surrounding gingival cuff, attached gingiva and mucosa. It subsequently causes tissue redness, swelling and bleeding: the first signs of inflammation and disease. It progresses to a loss of gingival support and recession as well as loss of supporting bone with the possibility of eventual tooth loss caused by periodontal disease itself. Gingivitis is a precursor of periodontal disease.

4.1.2 Statistics

Approximately 47.2% of adults aged 30 years and older have some form of periodontal disease. Periodontal disease increases with age. 70.1% of adults 65 years and older have periodontal disease. This condition is more common in men than women (56.4% versus 38.4%), those living below the federal poverty level (65.4%), those with less than a high school education (66.9%), and current smokers (64.2%). Ethnically, the highest incidence of periodontal disease is found in the Mexican American sector of our society (63.5% versus 40.8%) compared to other races.[1]

I think it is safe to say that within the geriatric cohort of patients I have treated over the age of 65 years, over the past 45+ years of practice, I have found more periodontal disease in the elderly as compared to the younger generations I have treated. Almost 90% of the older women I have seen over the years have some form of periodontal disease. I say this because I have probably seen more older women patients over the years than men, and statistics show that men statistically do not live as long as women do. That is not to say that older men are devoid of this disease, because they are not. No one, at any age, is immune to this disease process.

4.1.3 Risk Factors

Risk factors in periodontal disease are varied and many (Table 4.1). Certain factors increase the risk for periodontal disease.

Risk factors present the initial nidus for periodontal diseases of all kinds. Varying stages of gingivitis include incipient, acute and chronic phases of this disease. It becomes a more advanced disease, namely periodontal disease, when there is distinct bone loss on any or all four sides of a tooth; not dependent on the fact that there is active inflammation present or not. It is the bone loss that distinguishes this disease from gingivitis.

Table 4.1 Risk factors in periodontal disease

• Smoking, vaping, chewing tobacco
• Diabetes
• Increased aging (mentally and physiologically)
• Poor oral hygiene
• Stress
• Heredity
• Mal-aligned and crooked teeth
• Underlying immune deficiencies (e.g., HIV/AIDS); leukemias; lymphomas; blood dyscrasia, to name a few
• Restorations that have become defective, broken and unrestored
• Medication use that creates xerostomia
• Bridges and crowns that are defective and no longer fit properly
• Female hormonal changes, such as with pregnancy or the use of oral contraceptives, or menopausal changes
• Addiction to drugs and/or alcohol
• Depression
• Loss of self-esteem
• Lack of self-efficacy
• Specific disease states such as dementia; arthritis; osteoarthritis; Parkinson's disease; multiple sclerosis; Down's syndrome and mental retardation, to name a few

4.1.4 Classification

Periodontal disease can be incipient, acute and chronic or advanced with specific levels, such as Class I periodontal disease, Class II periodontal disease, Class III periodontal disease and Class IV periodontal disease. Each number of the Class pertains to the level of the disease; whereby, Class I being incipient and Class IV being advanced and probably chronic. Everything in the middle range is also going from acute to more chronic in terms of the longevity of the disease and whether it was treated previously and returned for another round. Bone loss is the common denominator for all the Classes presented.

At the end of 2020, the American Academy of Periodontology (AAP) announced new information about reclassifying periodontal diseases, which were facilitated by emphasis on the basic ground rules, the clarification of ambiguities and the identification of "gray zones".[2]

Highlights of this discussion were the following ground rules: 1. Stage is a patient-based, not a tooth-based concept, therefore a single Stage is assigned per patient; 2. Stage can shift upward over time, if the periodontal status deteriorates, but the initially assigned Stage is retained even after improvement post-therapy; 3. the complexity factors that determine Stage must be evaluated collectively, not in isolation, to arrive at a clinically meaningful assessment; 4. a single Grade is assigned to a patient based on a deliberate evaluation of the "biologic fabric" of the case, in terms of history of risk for further progression, interplay of risk actors, and the two-way effects of periodontitis or its treatment on general health; 5. shift of Grade over time is possible towards either direction, after thorough, collective, evaluation of changes in the above parameters. Exemplified "gray zones" include a radiographically intact patient with minimal attachment loss in older age; presence of "frank" periodontitis affecting a single tooth; assessment of factors that do/do not lead to increased complexity of therapy.[2]

My reasons for discussing the "new classification of periodontal diseases" here at this juncture is that there are no references to systemic or other etiological evidence, as previously mentioned in this text, which confounds the diagnosis of periodontal disease itself in the new classification system. It is all based upon "Stages" that over time include the deterioration of a person's periodontal status based upon a "clinically meaningful assessment and clinical evaluation of an "interplay of risk factors", which I feel are not totally defined.

The photos of patients from my patient files, that I am exhibiting in this section of the book, are all periodontal disease patients that have either a systemic or etiological influence or a combined set of systemic symptomologies that contribute significantly to the periodontal disease each patient exhibited. The periodontal disease is not just a simple lack of care but is a conglomeration of factors which, when added to the mix of oral findings, adds another dimension to the diagnosis of periodontal disease and can be distinctively labeled *Geriatric Periodontal disease* with an accompanying Stage or degree of advancement to categorize it. All too often we, as practitioners, diagnose periodontal disease based upon the supporting tissues of the teeth that we see in our examination process and do not place much importance on the contributory effects of other factors, such as systemic or etiological entities that can and do exacerbate the oral disease process itself. One must study the medical aspects of disease to understand its ability to affect the entire system of the human body, and in this case the mouth of an older individual who may be severely compromised in many ways: hence, the label I have given this phenomenon of **Geriatric Periodontal Disease**.

The patient of Figure 4.1 was very recalcitrant about brushing or flossing her teeth and refused regular recall appointments for cleanings and examinations. She claimed that brushing and flossing caused her to lose her memory. She had an underlying dementia, unbeknownst to her. I found out from her daughter, who came with her to this appointment. There was no way that I would be able to convince this person that she needed dental care. It was a no-win situation for the both of us. She refused to allow me to fully examine her mouth, clean her teeth, probe her teeth or go anywhere near them, other than take these memorable two photos. Note that before I knew that this patient had a genetic disease, Alzheimer's disease, I labelled her condition by sight only as Advanced, Chronic Class II Periodontal Disease. One can see by the signs of red, swollen gingiva, heavy calculus (long-standing), heavy plaque and recession that this disease has been here for a while. The fact that this patient's daughter admitted to me that her mother had Alzheimer's disease, proves to be a confounding factor in her disease process. She also had some kind of heart issues as well. Geriatric individuals that are resistant to treatment or self-efficacy need treatment with general anesthesia. The daughter did not want to "harm" her mother or go against her wishes by giving us permission to schedule her mother for general anesthesia. Guilt is a factor in geriatric patient care, especially by their children. Many times, they will feel guilty, not wanting to go against their parents will, even when the parent is cognitively impaired and not rational. Our main weapon against this sort of response is education of the responsible party and documenting everything we told them. That relieves us, as practitioners, from the burden of neglect and possible litigation. It is unfortunate that we must think this way, but we live in a litigious society where people think nothing about bringing a lawsuit against a dentist for lack of informing them that there is an *unmet need* either in their treatment or that of a loved one who states they were not informed about the need for treatment. We need to practice defensively, but rationally. There is no excuse for ignorance and ignoring what your findings tell you should be discussed with those who are able to assist in their loved-one's care.

4.2 Geriatric Periodontal Disease (GPD): Assessment, Diagnosis and Care

I have "coined" a new classification of Periodontal Disease with the addition of one or more systemic or

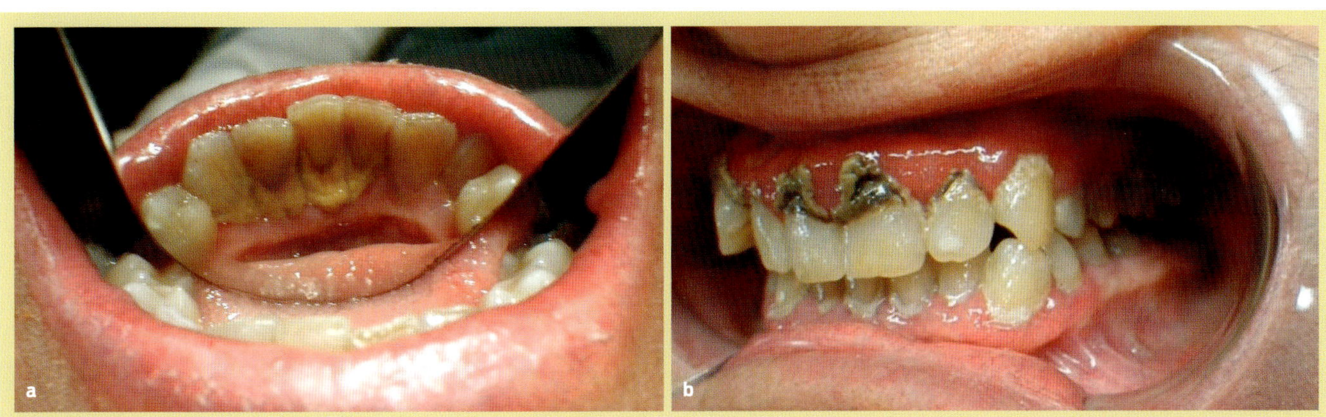

Fig. 4.1 Deceased 80-year-old female patient with advanced, chronic Class II periodontal disease (**a**) and advanced geriatric periodontal disease (**b**). Note the large sublingual defect with partial root exposure of all the lower anterior teeth. Present: heavy calculus, stain and red marginal tissue with moderate generalized bone loss (**a**).

deleterious etiological disease modalities, essentially one of the categories previously mentioned with the age distinction of being an older individual: **Geriatric Periodontal Disease** (GPD). It carries with it the same classification as periodontal disease in general, with the difference being the addition of either a systemic disease or acquired systemic disease, as well as one that involves the total body health of the individual. People who are immunosuppressed and are subject to one form of periodontal disease or another, tend to do more poorly than those who are not in the treatment of periodontal disease. Those persons who are fighting a systemic or localized disease or etiological issue are at a disadvantage when healing or in the resolution of periodontal disease as expected after treatment. For example, it is very risky, at the least, to treat a "special need" patient, such as an older Down's syndrome patient, and then expect their disease to go into remission when they may not comprehend how to help themselves or be able to care for themselves or allow anyone else to care for them in the process. The same is true for dementia patients, who may not know how to maintain self-efficacy anymore and need help from a caregiver, who may not be able to assist them when the patient either "acts-out", fighting and biting them in the process, or will not open their mouth for any reason. Who would want to continually try and help this level of patient? One can only beat their head against the wall so many times before it starts to hurt. But there is hope and direction. One must search for it in working with this type of patient while they are sedated or intubated.

Evaluating periodontal conditions in older, more compromised individuals takes knowledge, expertise, experience working with this cohort of people and the ability to be flexible in how one cares for such patients. If the general practitioner refers this patient for treatment to a specialist, he/she needs to know that the specialist has those necessary qualifications to care for the patient, as both the referring dentist and specialist are responsible for the care of the person being referred for treatment. The patient is still a patient of record of the referee practitioner and one that will have their follow-up care done by this practitioner as well.

Figure 4.2 shows this patient's issues: gingiva with red marginal tissue; gingival recession; broken teeth with retained roots; generalized calculus; generalized heavy plaque; root caries and generalized poor homecare as well as a patient who was suffering from advanced dementia. She would not open her mouth under any circumstances. If I placed my fingers too close to her teeth and tried to open her mouth to retrieve more information, she would snap at me like an alligator and try to bite me! She could not or would not talk, suffered from a previous stroke and had heart disease. She was medically compromised overall, which places her into this category of Geriatric Periodontal Disease.

She is what I call a "Silent Sufferer". Mainly, because she could not tell me what bothered her, or what she wanted to do with her concerns, if she had any to speak to us about? This makes this scenario mostly impossible to treat, unless her family would opt for an examination under general anesthesia, which they did not. They also did not want any teeth extracted... just a cleaning, which was impossible without sleep dentistry. It was a no-win situation. But it is a good example of Geriatric Periodontal Disease, as well as other forms of dental disease, as well as a lesson in futility. We cannot assist everyone, as "we cannot undo what our patients will not let us do". Hopefully, you may have learned this already in your practice working or treating people with this category of disease, as well as not beating yourself up over not being able to help your patient(s). We need to know that this type of patient is the most difficult to treat. I am sure her advanced periodontal disease exacerbated her systemic issues and was at the root of her demise in the end.

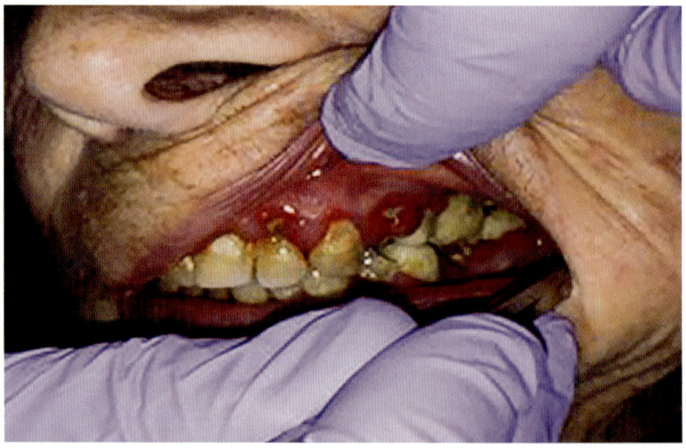

Fig. 4.2 Deceased 88-year-old patient with Class III-IV Geriatric Periodontal Disease (GPD) coupled with systemic disease.

Case Study 1

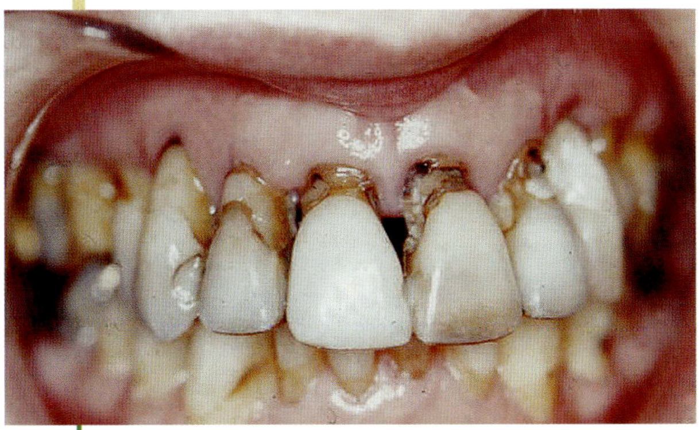

Fig. 4.3 Deceased 65-year-old patient with rampant root caries and Geriatric Periodontal Disease (GPD).

When the patient in Figure 4.3 took out her acrylic maxillary "gingival" denture, this is what I saw underneath. This woman was embarrassed about her appearance as she was an actress and always in the limelight, especially in live theater. She had the gingival denture made to cover her interproximal spaces in order to improve her appearance (apologies for not having a picture of this appliance). She had an active periodontal disease with severe bone loss, accompanied by gross root caries, heavy plaque and calculus, as well as mobile teeth that were stabilized by her acrylic gingival dental appliance.

What I did not know at the time I took this photo was that she had an underlying systemic disease, cancer. Take note of the "blanched" color of the maxillary and mandibular gingiva. She had a blood dyscrasia that created an anemic condition, which, within two years of the time I treated her, took her life. She was not one for going to the dentist or to a medical doctor for regular check-ups and care. She was not one for caring for herself and was only motivated by the way she looked. She was in denial about her oral disease. This denial coupled with her systemic issues eventually created the ultimate price for only being concerned about her esthetics, going to parties nightly and drinking alcohol and not her overall health and well-being.

The over-riding factor seen in most of these cases is the lack of homecare leading to periodontal disease. When coupled with a systemic disease or etiologic disease that affects the entire body, it manifests itself in an almost non-resolvable periodontal situation. There is always the exception: when both periodontal treatment and continuing care is initiated and followed through to the end with the proposed dental and medical treatment. But this is not always the case. In fact, what brought the patient to this situation in the first place was lack of their own self-efficacy and denial. These psychological factors are contributory in nature to the presence of this disease state in general. Having an underlying serious, life-threatening disease simultaneously makes the situation less successful in the long run. As practitioners, we need to look for these things in order to be able to determine whether what we intend to do to assist the patient is a viable treatment and whether there will be good odds of it being successful in the end.

Case Study 2

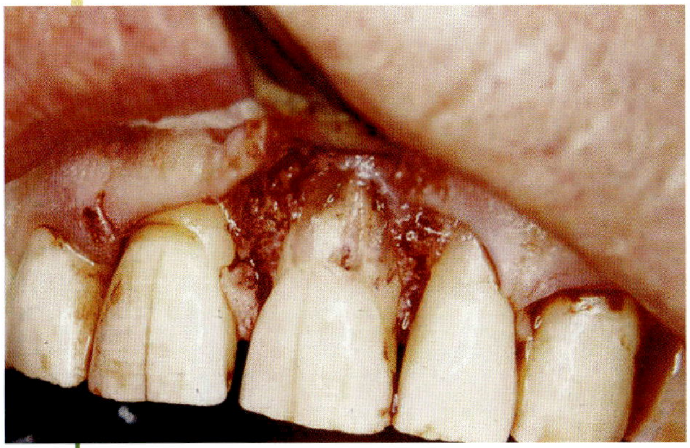

Fig. 4.4 Deceased 70-year-old patient with a deep periodontal pocket on tooth #9 with crazing.

The patient in Figure 4.4 had a fluctuant swelling above tooth #9. There was a deep periodontal pocket on the labial aspect with no mobility or discomfort, but which exhibited suppuration and bleeding on probing. Both entities are signs of active and chronic disease. The patient did regular homecare and had regular periodontal recall; however, this pocket was not evident until the swelling occurred, and it was not cleansable by the patient.

A full flap was lifted showing facial resorption of the root with crazing and severe bone loss (Fig. 4.5). The patient did not want to extract the tooth and opted for a "rescue" procedure, which involved a root repair and labial frenectomy to prevent further

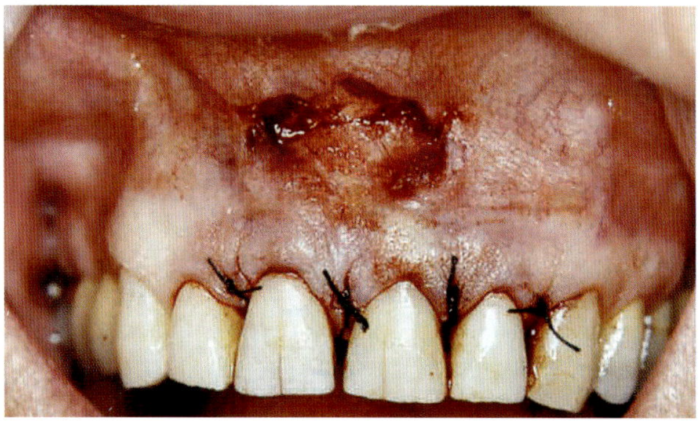

Fig. 4.5 Post-surgical repair and maxillary frenectomy.

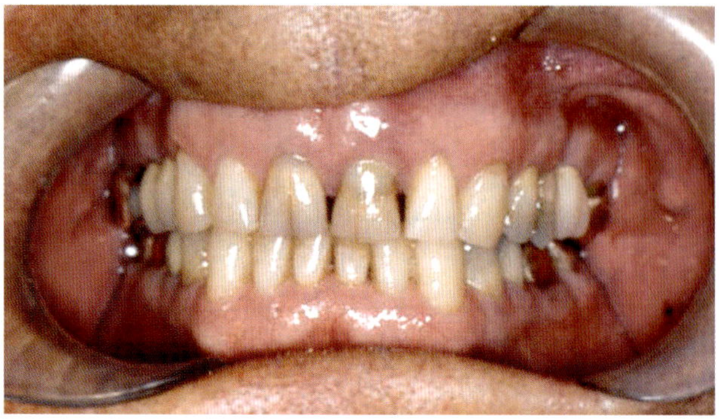

Fig. 4.6 Restored "Internal resorption" on tooth #9. Material is a glass ionomer that secretes fluoride. It is durable, hard, non-porous and light curable.

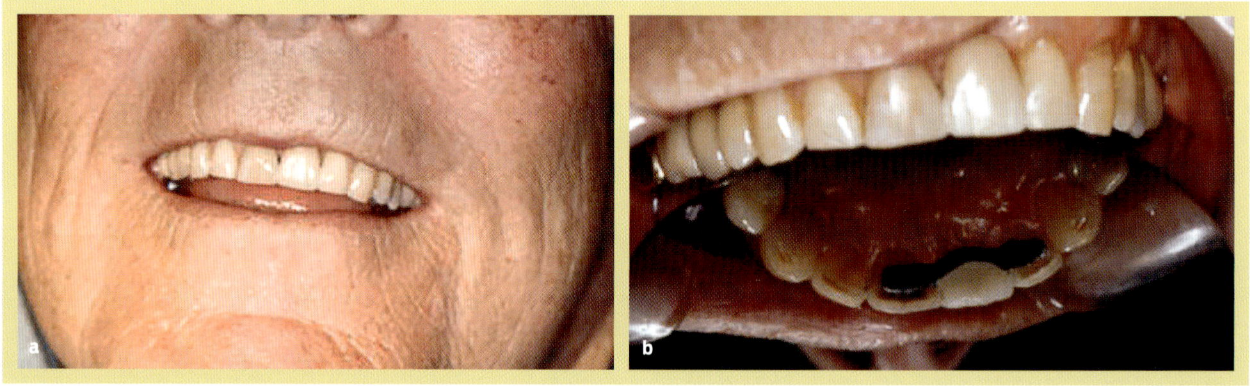

Fig. 4.7 (**a**) Maryland Bridge replacing tooth #9 as it was eventually lost due to non-healing. (**b**) Maryland Bridge from the underside or lingual surface.

"pull" of the mucosa, which might cause continued recession of the marginal gingiva in that area in the future, compromising his esthetics (**Figs. 4.6, 4.7**).

As an aside, sometimes life gets in the way of one's best intentions. As it turned out, this patient returned for a routine cleaning and in doing his examination I found a hard mass in his thyroid gland, which turned out to be malignant. I referred him to his MD for further testing and care. He had just lost his wife and refused to have anything done. This reaction and subsequent lack of treatment cost him his life within 6 months of finding his metastatic disease. I am sure this tumor was there for some time before I found it. Denial played a part in his decision not to see his medical doctor or dentist regularly, as well as wanting to be with his wife again. His periodontal condition worsened in the process and was classified as Geriatric Periodontal Disease (GPD).

4.2.1 Etiology of GPD Outside of Systemic Disease

Case Study 3

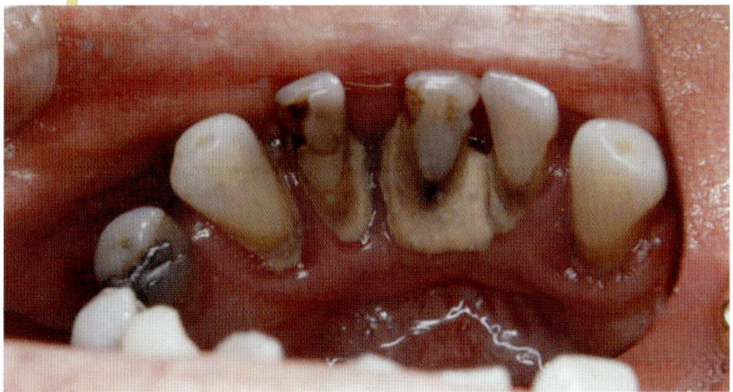

Fig. 4.8 Deceased 65-year-old patient with Class III-IV Geriatric Periodontal Disease (GPD).

The patient in **Figure 4.8** was both a long-term smoker and alcoholic. As evidenced by this photo, one can see the clinical results of abuse with chronic alcohol and smoking, which in this case went hand in hand. The patient had been smoking since his teen years and drinking alcohol since then as well. He grew up on a farm, was not well educated or cared for by his parents and left home at an early age to find his way in the world. This person's continuous lack of care, both by himself and not having gone to a dentist for routine maintenance for years, created the periodontal condition that can be seen in **Figure 4.8**. He had gross calculus, recession, plaque, missing teeth, mobility, caries, stain and inflamed and bleeding gingiva. His addictions to alcohol and smoking have added a systemic aspect to his Geriatric Periodontal Disease, that being liver and lung diseases. Newton's law: for every action there is an opposite and equal reaction plays out here in the example I am posing with this patient.

He came in for an examination because of the issues I mentioned, but could not afford treatment per se. Even my reducing the fees did not persuade him to help himself. Again, denial is a factor here in his decision-making process. After all he had been abusing his body for over 40 years with alcohol and tobacco addictions. I am sure depression was a factor here and I referred him to a counselor with the County Department of Mental Health, which offered free care to underserved and indigent people.

This patient never returned to my practice, and I could only hope that he found some care for his issues.

Case Study 4

The patient in **Figure 4.9** presented for treatment after not being able to eat well for some time. Her chief complaint was not only the inability to chew her food properly forcing her to eat starchier, soft foods, but also causing her digestive issues. She suffered from missing teeth; broken teeth; decay; periodontal disease; root caries; extrusion of her posterior maxillary teeth; xerostomia; bleeding gingiva and generalized pain in her mouth. She was also a

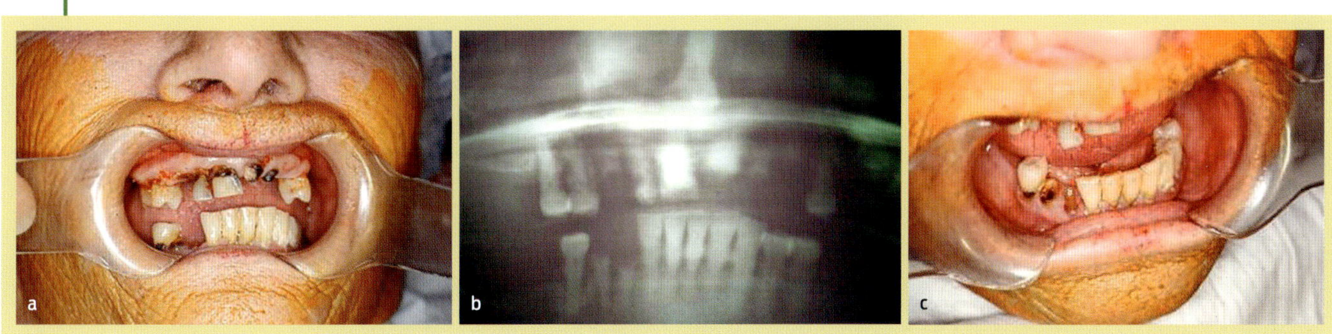

Fig. 4.9 (**a-c**) Deceased 80-year-old woman with geriatric periodontal disease and general dental disease.

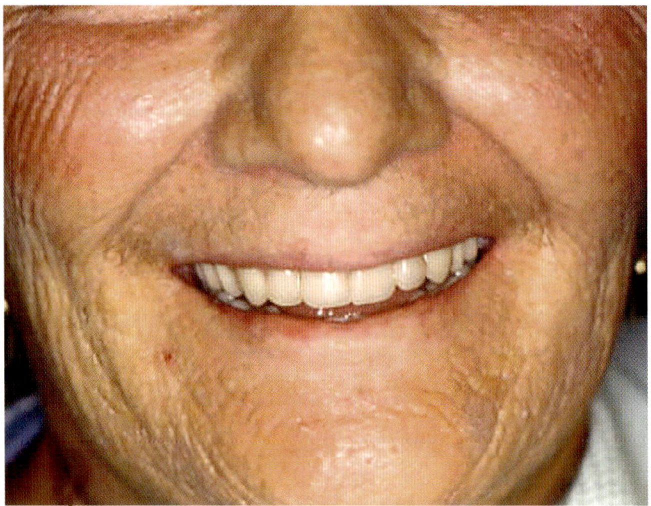

Fig. 4.10 Deceased 80-year-old woman with previous geriatric periodontal disease and general dental disease wearing her full new dentures.

long-time smoker and user of alcohol. Her request was for me to remove all her remaining teeth and make her a set of dentures. She also suffered from cognitive decline.

Medically, this person had a gastric ulcer and Irritable Bowel Syndrome (IBS). These medical issues were probably a result of the combination of the kind of food she was forced to eat and the amounts of her daily apportionments of Bourbon. After a medical consultation and clearance for treatment, I followed through with her request, under local anesthesia, but not before going over the treatment plan, discussing my findings and her oral disease findings with her and explaining the relationship between what I found and her medical condition. I also explained how important it was to come back at least twice a year for an oral examination and to limit or stop her smoking and drinking habits (**Fig. 4.10**).

The etiology of periodontal disease outside the systemic system of the body is overly complex and can and does cause secondary disease entities within the human system. Inherently, it is important for us, as dental practitioners, to learn medicine and those facets of diseases caused by outside vectors that can invade our systems and manifest themselves in the oral cavity. This not only includes our habits that develop over time, but bacterial and viral infections, aberrant systemic infections and tumors from malfunctioning organ systems, genetics (which play out at a 70% influence on how our ancestral history can affect our overall continued health) as well as our diets, the water we drink, the vitamins we may take, all of which can cause oral disease by manifesting symptoms in our mouths.

We know from studies and experience that "we are what we eat". I am not sure who came up with that slogan, but it is relatively true. In discussing this aspect of our lives, I will get intimate by telling you a true story about what happened to me that demonstrates this issue. Some 40 years ago, I was working in a lab and donated some needed blood. About an hour after I donated, a technician came to see me and showed me my centrifuged blood in a test tube. The packed cells were at the bottom and the plasma/serum was at the top of the tube. The plasma was supposed to be clear, but it was not... it was snow white! I asked what was going on and was told that my triglycerides, normally seen in adults at 150 milligrams per deciliter (mg/dL or less than 1.7 millimoles per liter), were 3000 mg/dL! My results were 20 times the normal reading and extremely dangerous. With some additional testing, it showed that I did not have a specific lipase (enzyme) to break down fats. I immediately saw my primary care doctor and was placed on a low-fat diet and given some medication to help control this condition. I then took blood from my immediate family members (mom, dad, brother and sister) and found out that my father, my younger sister and I had this condition, and my younger brother and mother did not. Heredity was playing a major factor here in my family's future health concerns. For the next 25 years I became a guinea pig for different labs throughout dental school and beyond, donating my blood for experiments to try and see how this condition could be rectified. In one such experiment not too long ago, the participants were involved in taking vitamin B_3 or niacin. There were 12 doctors participating in the experiment, including myself, and we started with taking 50 mg of niacin a day until after three years we were taking 5000 mg a day. This proved very deleterious to our overall health after this time. The researchers were watching our lipids go down in the process, but they were not watching anything else. Apparently, while this was making our lipids normal, it was making our blood sugar abnormal, by causing our cells to become insulin resistant. Yes, that is right; we all became Type II diabetics from this experiment. I was angry, as were the other doctors, but at this point all we could do was diet, exercise and take medication. Unfortunately, it was not reversible...

This experiment has shown me how a simple vitamin can change your life while taking it in excess. It has changed my life forever, for which I had been angry about for many years; but now, I have become more subdued because I have the knowledge gained from this experience to evaluate my family and patients who tell me their respective histories. I can counsel them and show them from my own example what might be healthy and what might not be good for them.

Many years later I had a patient come into my practice. She was attractive, around 45 years of age, but looked stressed and distressed, as well as unhappy and in visual discomfort and aged. Taking her history was interesting because she told me that she was vying for a job in her company that would mean a huge increase in salary and stature, but she had a lot of competition for the position. Because of her mindset and the advertising in our society about various things, she heard of *Gingko biloba*, an herb that is "supposed" to increase one's mental acuity and memory. It had been plastered all over the TV and directed at senior citizens, in general, because of the assumed thinking that seniors tend to lose their memories as they age. *Gingko*, as people called it, was supposed to enhance your memory and make you "sharp as a tack".

My patient had several teeth that were causing her discomfort as well as bleeding gingiva. She was taking mega aspirin, acetaminophen, and hydrocodone meds as well for her tooth pain. She asked me to do some root canal therapy on the teeth that were bothering her. In my head and neck exam I noted exceptionally large masseter muscles, worn teeth from bruxing and clenching and fractured teeth, especially some of her lower molars. I made an appointment for her, and she returned a few days later. I noted when she got into the dental chair that she had multiple bruises on her legs and arms. Being a "mandated reporter", I asked her if someone had abused her lately. She became truly angry and said "No!" emphatically. I then asked her how much *Gingko* she was taking? She answered, "About a bottle a day". I asked why? She told me about wanting to be smarter and more astute than her competition at work vying for the new job. She felt that the more of this herb she took, the more improved her memory and actions would be. She was convinced that this action would get her the new position she longed for. The stress involved during this process, as well as her habits, were literally causing her demise instead.

I tell this story again, to prove a point: taking vitamins, herbs and pharmaceuticals in excess can lead to side-effects that are unknown, sometimes dangerous and life-threatening; but most life-changing in the immediate sense. *Gingko*, in excess diminishes one's platelets and can make one bleed internally. The fact that this patient was taking this herb, that was not regulated by the FDA, in excess, while coupling it with other medication that virtually did the same thing, made her susceptible to a bleeding disorder endangering her life. I referred her back to her MD and to a counselor to help assuage her stress. I do not know if she ever had those root canals...

4.2.2 Bruising

This patient was not a senior, but I have seen many older people do similar things without knowing what it will do to their bodies and minds. We must take adequate histories when working with all our patients, but especially our elderly, who may not remember what they are taking or even how much. I always ask for a written list and verify it with a caregiver or family member and their physician as well. Then I can counsel the patient after I have all the facts before I treat them.

Bruises can last for up to two weeks or more depending upon the type of injury. A subcutaneous bruise, such as that of my patient was somewhere between Stage 1 and 2. I did not see the bruises on her legs the first visit because she was wearing slacks and a long-sleeved shirt. The second visit, a week later, she was wearing a short dress with short sleeves, making her bruises more visible. I am placing this Bruise Color graph (Fig. 4.11) in this text for your interest and use when assessing bruises on your patients. Most of the time when seeing red bruises, they are recent and Stage 2 bluish to purple bruising in older people especially, may lead one to infer that they are taking blood thinners of some kind or baby aspirin or the like. Something for you to ask questions about before your dental treatment begins.

I am posting *The Stages of Bruise Colors* chart for your use. You may find that geriatric patients have bruises on their forearms, hands and possibly legs, if you can see them. Knowing medicine, pharmacy and the like will reassure you that these may possibly be from anticoagulant therapy. Elders are also subjected to abuse, especially physical abuse. It is a common finding among older people who either have a caregiver or a nurse that may be abusive to them. It is always prudent to ask questions about bruising and your right as a mandated reporter to do so.

Rashes, hives and irritations can be from etiology outside or inside the body. Emotions play a role in this as well. Allergies to foods, medicines, virus infections, fungal infections and bacterial infections can all mimic these symptoms, and they can be seen in the oral cavity on mucosal surfaces as well as the gingiva.

Our older elders usually have a suppressed immune system and are susceptible to these findings. We also need to look for these things in areas that are visible to us, especially the mouth. Figure 4.12 is an example of the symptomatic response of the body to produce an oral "marker" for a systemic disease. In this case, it is the measles virus, which shows Koplik spots on the posterior soft palate of a patient. Other systemic diseases where oral symptoms can erupt are Herpes Simplex virus, *Candida*, yeast of fungal infections, venereal disease, such as syphilitic lesions and chancres, as well as cancerous lesions that may be metastatic or localized.

I have compiled a list of common medications that are used for geriatric patients and an accompanying list of oral sequelae (Table 4.2). This list is an especially important adjunct to your dental armamentarium. I hope that you find it useful and a good reference.

4.3 Periodontal Disease and its Effects on Dental Caries

Dental caries go hand in hand with being one of the most pandemic of all human diseases.[4]

In most instances, caries was born from the same nidus of bacteria as is periodontal disease. The difference being that there are different forms of periodontal disease, and caries as well. I believe that dental caries is more diet related and specific for tooth structure and not the destruction of the periodontium.

As we age, our teeth are subjected to many stressors such as wear; fracture; restorations; injury; extraction and movement. There is no formula for which or what comes first and, in fact, many elders who have most all their teeth find them in pretty much in "unscathed" condition. My own mother-in-law (Fig. 4.13) had all her teeth until she was 100 years young, and they were in very good condition. There was some incipient wear and light

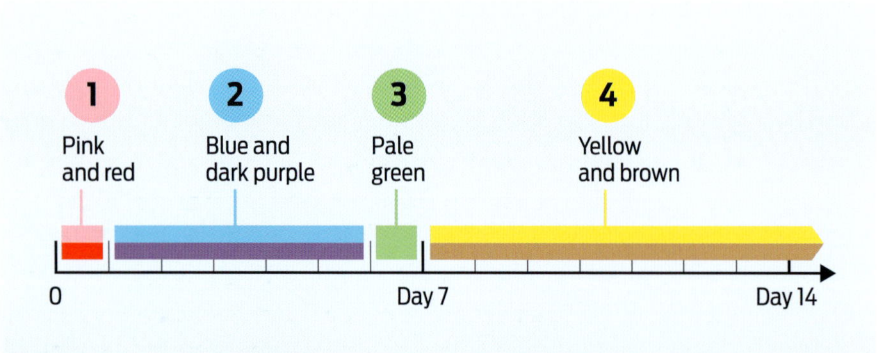

Fig. 4.11 The stages of bruise colors.

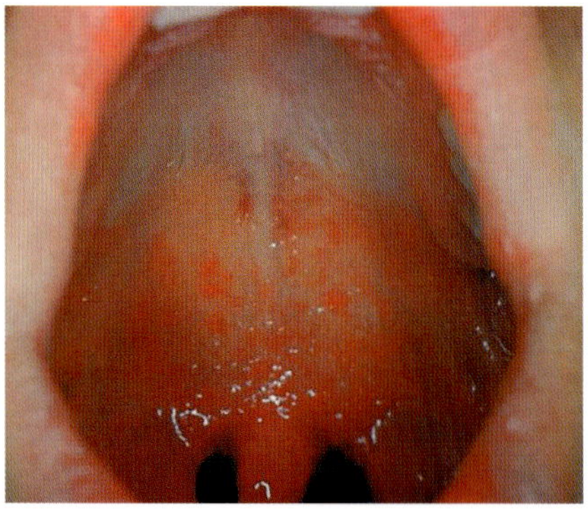

Fig. 4.12 Koplik spots on the soft palate 2-3 days after the onset of the measles virus.[3]

Table 4.2 Summary of oral sequelae of commonly used geriatric medications*

Drug category	Drug	Oral problem
Analgesics	• Aspirin	• Hemorrhage, erythema multiforme
	• NSAIDs	• Hemorrhage
	• Barbiturates, codeine	• Erythema multiforme, xerostomia or ropey saliva
Anesthetics (local)	• Benzocaine, crocaine hydrochloride, lidocaine	• Taste disorders
Antiarrhythmics	• Procainamide	• Lupus-like reaction
	• Quinidine	• Lichenoid mucosal reaction
Antiarthritic	• Allopurinol, auranofin, colchicine	• Taste disorders
Antipyretic	• Dexamethasone, hydrocortisone	• Taste disorders
Anti-asthmatic	• Advair (inhalers)	• Xerostomia, altered sense of taste
Anti-inflammatory	• Levamisole, D-penicillamine, phenylbutazone, salicylates, 5-thiopyridoxine	• Taste disorders
	• Gold salts	• Taste disorders, lichenoid reaction, oral pigmentation, vesiculo-ulcerative stomatitis
Antibiotics	• All	• Oral candidiasis
	• Erythromycin	• Hypersensitivity reaction, erythema multiforme, vesiculo-ulcerative, stomatitis
	• Penicillin	• Hypersensitivity reaction, erythema multiforme, vesiculo-ulcerative stomatitis
	• Chloramphenicol, Ciprofloxacin, Clindamycin, Dapsone, Isoniazid, Sulfa antibiotics, Tetracyclines	• Erythema multiforme
	• Minocycline	• Melanosis
	• Chlorhexidine	• Brown pigmentation of teeth and tongue
	• Ampicillin, cefamandole, ethambutol hydrochloride, griseofulvin, lincomycin, metronidazole, niridazole, sulfasalazine, tetracyclines	• Taste disorders
Anticoagulants	• All	• Hemorrhage, ecchymosis
Anticonvulsants	• Carbamazepine	• Erythema multiforme, taste disorders
	• Phenytoin	• Erythema multiforme, gingival enlargement, taste disorder
Anticholinesterases (Memory Enhancing Drugs)	• All-Aricept (Donepezil) • Reminyl (Galantamine) • Exelon (Rivastigmine) • Cognex (Tacrine) • Memantine (Namenda), NMDA-Receptor antagonist	• Bad/Acidic taste in mouth, facial edema, gastric reflux
Antidiarrhea	• Bismuth	• Dark pigmentation of the tongue and gingiva
Antihistamines	• All	• Salivary dysfunction, xerostomia
	• Chlorpheniramine maleate	• Taste disorders
Antihypertensives	• Calcium channel blockers	• Gingival enlargement

(continued)

(continued)

Drug category	Drug	Oral problem
ACE Inhibitors		• Vesiculo-ulcerative stomatitis, pemphigus vulgaris
	• Chloramphenicol	• Vesiculo-ulcerative stomatitis
	• Hydralazine	• Lupus-like reaction and erythema multiforme
	• Methyldopa	• Lupus-like and lichenoid mucosal reaction
	• Thiazide diuretics	• Lichenoid mucosal reaction
	• Minoxidil, Verapamil	• Erythema multiforme
	• Acetazolamide, Amiloride, Captopril	• Taste disorders
	• Diazoxide, Diltiazem, Enalapril maleate	• Headache, dizziness, constipation
	• Ethacrynic acid, Nifedipine	• Headache, dizziness, constipation
Antilipidemic	• Cholestyramine, Clofibrate	• Taste disorders
Antimycotics	• Griseofulvin	• Erythema multiforme, black pigment/tongue
	• Amphotericin B	• Taste disorders
Antineoplastics	• All	• Oral candidiasis, hemorrhage, viral infection, aphthous stomatitis, vesiculo-ulcerative stomatitis
Antiparkinsonian	• All	• Salivary dysfunction
	• Levodopa	• Taste disorders
Anti-reflux agents	• All	• Salivary dysfunction
	• Cimetidine	• Erythema multiforme
Anti-thyroid	• Carbimazole, Methimazole, Methylthiouracil, propylthiouracil, Thiouracil	• Taste disorders
Antioxidants	• Octyl gallate	• Allergic ulcerations
Anxiolytics	• Benzodiazepines	• Salivary dysfunction
Chelating agents	• Penicillamine	• Ulcers and *Pemphigus vulgaris*
Corticosteroids	• All	• Oral candidiasis, recurrent oral viral infections
Immuno-suppressants	• Azathioprine, Bleomycin, 5-FU, Methotrexate	• Vesiculo-ulcerative stomatitis, taste issue
	• Cyclosporine	• Gingival enlargement
Hypoglycemics	• Sulfonylurea agents	• Erythema multiforme
	• Glipizide, Metformin and derivatives	• Taste disorders
Muscle relaxants	• All	• Salivary dysfunction
	• Baclofen, Chlorzoxazone	• Taste disorders
Others	• Etidronate, Germine monoacetate	• Taste disorders
	• Idoxuridine, Iron sorbitex, vitamin D	• Taste disorders
Psychotropics	• All	• Salivary dysfunction
	• Glutethimide, meprobamate	• Erythema multiforme
Phenothiazines		• Oral pigmentation, tardive dyskinesia
	• Lithium carbonate	• Erythema multiforme
	• Trifluoperazine hydrochloride	• Taste disorders
Sympathomimetics	• Amphetamines, Amrinone	• Taste disorders
Vasodilators	• Bamafyline hydrochloride, Dipyridamole, Nitroglycerin patch, Oxyfedrine	• Taste disorders

* (Compiled by Eric Z. Shapira, DDS, MAGD, MA, MHA. 2011, updated 2021©.)

crazing, but her gingiva was normal and healthy as well as her teeth. She went for regular dental care and practiced good self-efficacy. It was not until the age of 100.5 years that her dentist talked her into removing a lower wisdom tooth; the only adult tooth of her life she would lose. I begged her to keep it, but her dentist, whom she trusted deeply, informed her that she had a deep caries interproximally and that it would be costly ($) to keep the tooth. Her tooth was in position, stable and the gingiva was healthy around it. The caries had been arrested and a temporary restoration had been placed previously. The choices he gave her were "a gold crown or extraction". However, despite my pleading with her to save it, she believed that he was right and took it out.

I was more conservative with her in my thinking because at her age, close to 101 years, I did not want to see her have any added stressors put on her, as she suffered from hypertension, had several TIAs (Transient Ischemic Attacks) in the past and was on blood thinners. Her dentist never got a medical clearance and went into the extraction blind. Not a good idea.

I am a follower of the **KISS Method** of treatment with older, compromised patients: **Keep it simple stupid** method! As luck would have it, she survived the treatment to see another day.

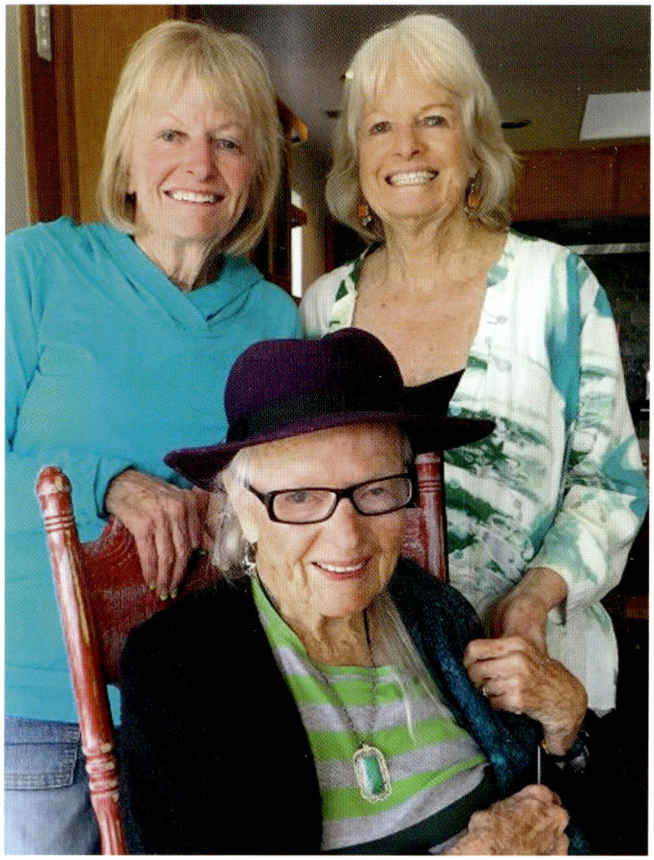

Fig. 4.13 My deceased mother-in-law at almost 101 years of age, with her two daughters, and all 32 of her teeth! (My wife facing us on the right-side, behind her mother.)

The more one invests time in the patients' history, the more understanding one has of the necessity for medical clearances prior to any invasive treatment. Luckily, my mother-in-law listened to me about getting a medical clearance from her physician and brought it with her to her dental appointment. I also recommended that she stop taking her blood thinner medication three to five days prior to extraction and to verify that with her MD, which she did. Even though her dentist did not do this, I had her covered and kept her safe from harm to the best of my ability.

The bacteria causing occlusal caries are *Streptococcus mutans* and those causing interproximal caries are *Lactobacillus acidophilus* as the main culprits. As we age, and as possibly expected over time, we find that the gingiva will recede exposing the roots of our teeth, essentially allowing us to see the dentin and/or cementum that the root is formed from. If there is a periodontal pocket around a tooth, the bacteria causing supragingival caries may not be the antagonist here that creates root caries. Anaerobic bacteria take precedence over the aerobic bacteria when it comes to gingival and subgingival root caries (Fig. 4.14) and bone loss as well.

Anaerobic bacteria are those that live in an oxygen deprived area, such as the gingival sulcus or inside a periodontal pocket or bony defect. *Bacteroides forsythus* is a fusiform anaerobe associated with active periodontal lesions. Other pathogenic anerobic bacteria are spirochetes, black-pigmented bacteroides species, such as *Porphyromonas gingivalis* and *Prevotella intermedia*. Spirochetes, *Treponema denticola* is the only species found in all periodontal lesions and produces such chemicals as collagenase, peptidases, hyaluronidase and keratinolytic enzyme, which in turn produce noxious end products that cause the inflammatory response in periodontal diseases.[5]

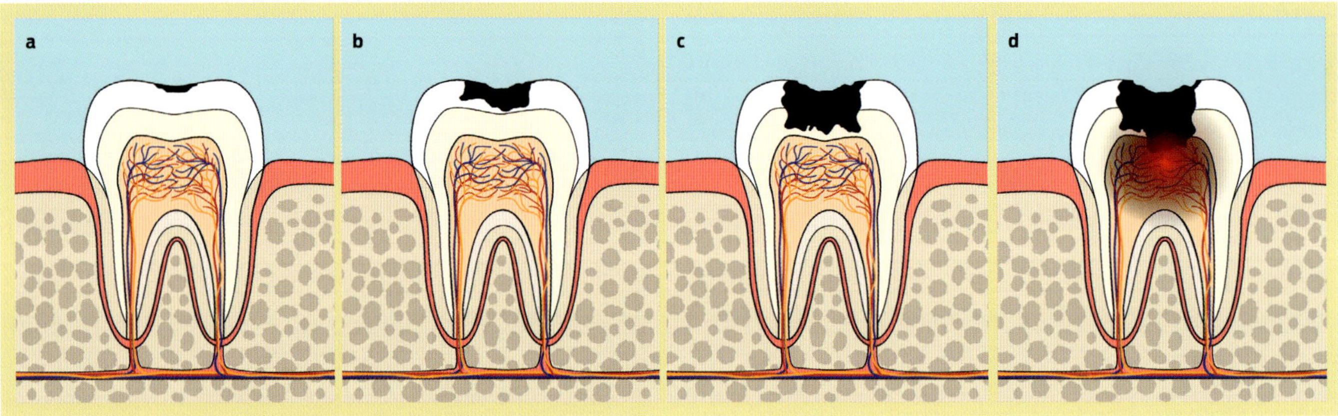

Fig. 4.14 (a-d) Stages of dental decay over time. *(CanStockPhoto.)*

When the gingiva is inflamed or swollen, as well as develops periodontal pockets that are larger than 5 mm in depth, it is difficult to clean these areas. The bacteria that live under the gum tissue, as well as above and around the sulcus, appreciate any kind of substrate that has some form of sugar (sucrose) in it as its prime source of metabolism. While digesting these carbohydrates, acid is produced as a by-product of this metabolic process, which, in turn, demineralizes the enamel of the tooth crown over time and the dentin of the tooth root surfaces as well. The root surfaces are softer and less able to resist the effects of the bacteria and, as a result, root caries (Fig. 4.14) develop much faster than those in the crowns of the teeth.

There are 200 to 300 bacterial species colonized within the mouth, but only a limited number of these species participate in dental decay (caries) or periodontal disease. The tooth surface normally loses some tooth mineral from the action of the acid formed by plaque, an accumulation of food debris, metabolic carbohydrate remnants, sticky mucous and bacteria, after ingestion of foods containing fermentable carbohydrates. This mineral is normally replenished by the neutralizing and rinsing action of saliva between meals. However, when fermentable foods are eaten frequently, the low pH (5.0 or less) in the plaque is sustained and a net loss of mineral from the tooth occurs.[5]

It is likely that in older age, the decrease or loss of salivary flow, especially serous saliva as opposed to the more viscous saliva, causes the plaque to continue producing acid for a greater period of time, which, in turn, produces more damage to the tooth. Again, xerostomia is a major problem for most people, but extremely dangerous in older people who lose their sense of thirst and become both dehydrated and caries prone simultaneously. Coupled with a decreased immune system as we age, an elder's inability to chew their food properly, due to lack of teeth or significant wear, means a resultant diet of softer foods that contain more carbohydrates and sugars. This type of diet leads to both the risk of diabetes, periodontal disease and rampant decay without continuous proper care.

Periodontal disease can establish itself when the gingiva detaches from the teeth as a result of an inflammatory response to plaque. Plaque, made up of sticky debris or biofilm and bacteria, in turn, produce compounds such as H_2S, NH_3, amines, toxins, enzymes, and antigens, to name a few that elicit an inflammatory response that is protective, but is also responsible for loss of periodontal tissue, pocket formation, and loosening and subsequent loss of teeth.[5]

In the many older persons I have examined and treated over the years, I have seen some form of generalized, periodontal disease, coupled with dental decay going hand in hand. Fewer elder patients have exhibited healthy mouths than those that have been infected. The reasons are many and I realize that everyone is different. Therefore, the practitioner must look at the histories of these people and the myriad of entities that could have and did affect them over their lifetimes, socially, medically and dentally. This will give one the needed answers on how to approach discussing the cause and effects of the past and their care in the future with the patient.

Figures 4.15 and 4.16 show both subgingival caries into the pulp of an upper bridge abutment coupled with advanced periodontal disease in the form of GPD. This patient is in her 80's and is immunosuppressed due to a blood dyscrasia and suffers from poor homecare as well. The bone graft was performed in Mexico at a clinic. This patient's care was dependent on where she could get the best price for whatever she needed. Her homecare was less than perfect. She declined my care when I told her the bridge and the decayed tooth should be removed for treatment and the fee was also an issue for this patient pursuing further treatment from me.

Daily tooth brushing by the patient and regular professional cleanings by the dentist appear to be adequate to prevent periodontal disease, for the most part. Rigorous debridement of tooth surfaces is the standard treatment usually, utilizing root planning. Often, some form of surgery using LANAP (Laser Assisted New Attachment Procedures) with a dental laser is used or traditional surgical procedures with a scalpel, etc., is used to improve access to root surfaces to diminish the pockets. Recent studies suggest that short-term use of antimicrobial agents, especially metronidazole and doxycycline, are beneficial both orally and placed locally into the periodontal pocket as an adjunctive treatment.

LANAP is an FDA approved laser procedure and will assist in regaining lost tissues and bone from periodontal disease. It is less painful than more traditional treatments, coupled with less post-surgical sensitivity, resulting in less recession and truly little, to no downtime after treatment. It is my treatment of choice when dealing with older, more compromised patients because it is conservative and effective in reversing periodontal disease. Since many older persons on multiple drug therapies have systemic or etiological issues that affect their ability to heal, this form of conservative gum treatment is my first choice with patients. It is also a great motivator to get patients on track again to do effective homecare and continue with regular recall.

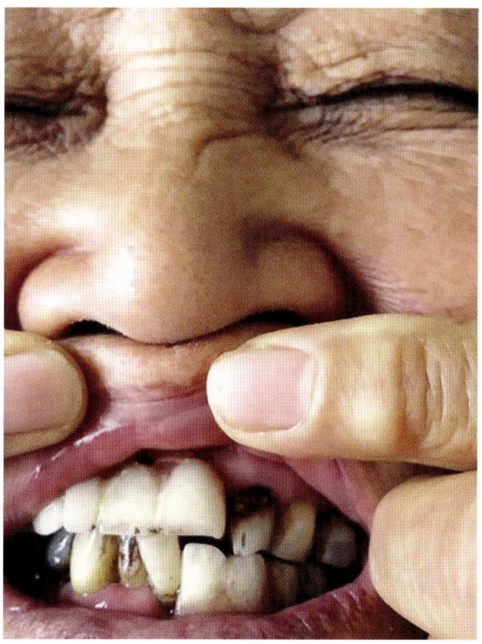

Fig. 4.15 70-year-old woman with both advanced periodontal disease in the form of GPD, coupled with chronic advanced caries. The crowded teeth did not help her in terms of her oral hygiene care. This patient suffered from heart disease and hypertension, as well as diabetes. Her medical care was not managed very well, and this photo was taken in the hospital, where she went for medical management of her conditions.

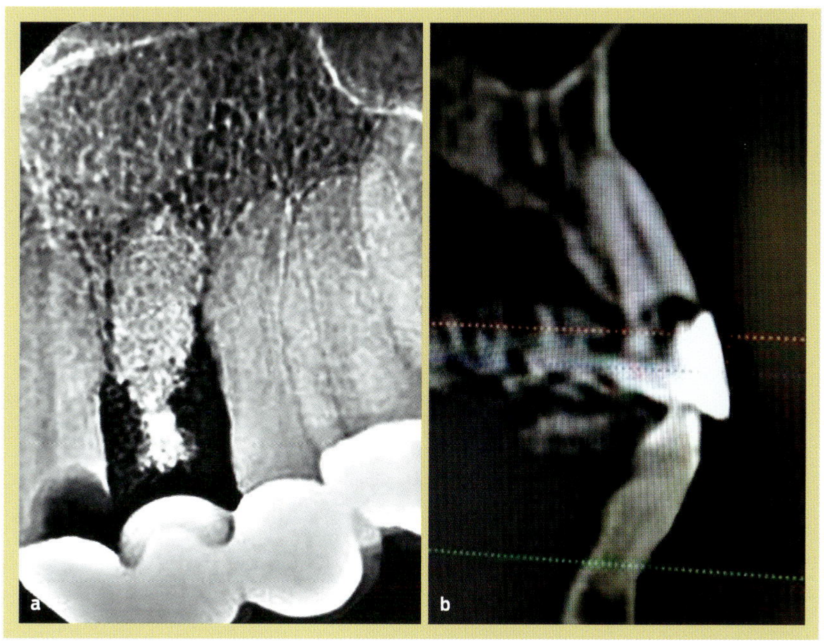

Fig. 4.16 80 year-old-woman with circumferential and subgingival root caries on her upper left cuspid. (**a**) The CBCT-3-Dimensional radiograph shows a face forward view of the decay, with a poorly done bone graft in the upper left first bicuspid area, and the lateral view CBCT (**b**) shows almost total separation of the tooth root from the crown portion of the tooth due to decay, as well as "no" labial bone on the tooth root at all.

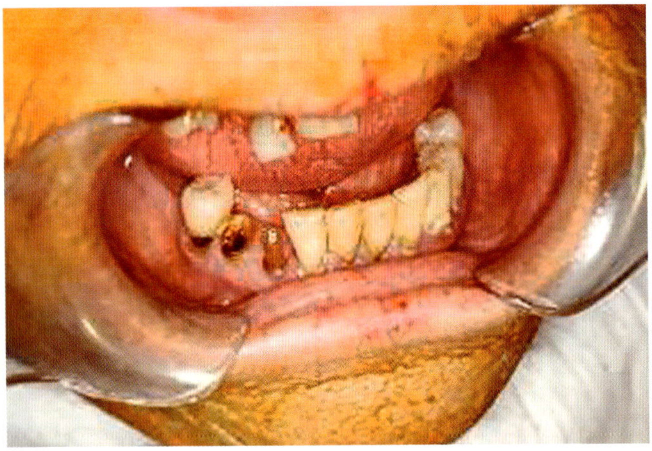

Fig. 4.17 75-year-old patient with chronic moderate periodontal disease, mobility, caries, and attrition of the anterior incisal surfaces of the lower teeth. Local etiology and lack of more frequent periodontal recall and homecare is the main cause of these issues.

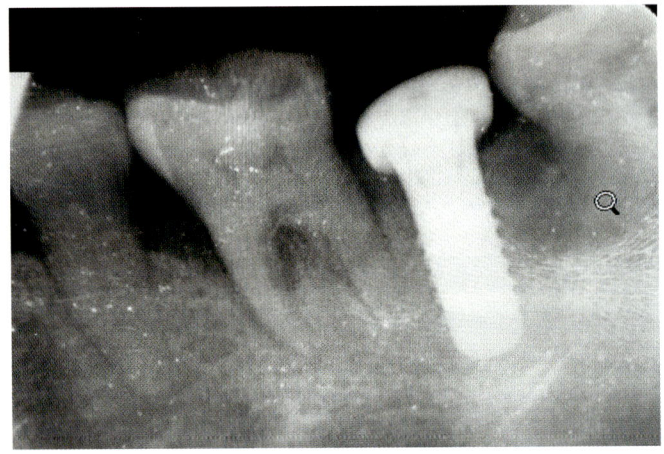

Fig. 4.18 75-year-old patient with advanced, generalized periodontal disease and GPD, coupled with dental root caries. Poor homecare, lack of recall and dementia were the cause of this disease process. Note: someone placed an implant into an extracted root socket of a lower second molar that had a bone graft previously; but the crown was never placed, and the bone graft was failing.

Periodontal disease is usually painless until late in the disease process, when the teeth are so loose that some discomfort may appear when chewing (Figs. 4.17, 4.18). Food that is retained within the periodontal pockets may instigate a sudden onset of microbial growth which could result in a painful abscess. Once the abscess breaks or drains from the periodontal pocket, the pain is lessened or gone. Unfortunately, when the gum heals over, the same etiology is there to create a "repeat performance" of the scenario. All the while, the bone is disintegrating around the tooth and the infection can become systemic in nature, exacerbating any pre-existing systemic issues, as well as causing teeth to be lost in the process. Patients can become severely ill from periodontal disease due to the lack of treatment and preventative care (Figs. 4.17, 4.18).

Clinical dentistry in my practice has been close to 85-98% effective in treating periodontal disease and arresting it, for the most part. Various surgical procedures can maintain the periodontium as well as replace the lost bone in some instances. Grafting of tissue and bone can improve the support of the tooth and the esthetics when the gum tissue and bone have receded, and the stability of the affected teeth is managed. The stopgap in the number of persons, who can be treated, in most cases, is the patient themselves. Cost is a major factor with older people who are low-income, have no dental insurance and whose choices of treatment reflect this kind of negative action. Both dental caries and periodontal disease are major factors in tooth loss and oral health. Educating our patients is a most important process in keeping them safe from harm and healthy overall. It takes time and effort to do this care; however, when you have an older, physically compromised, possibly cognitively impaired patient as well, these efforts may go unwanted, unheard and undone. Therefore, it is important to involve the caregivers, the family and those people who are there for the compromised older adults in our lives, in assisting them with prevention and manual care of their mouths and bodies.

4.4 Charts

4.4.1 American Academy of Periodontology New Guidelines

These recent guidelines in Table 4.3 are based on severity and complexity. Stages I-IV are listed in Table 4.3. The severity is based on probing depths, while the complexity is based upon the same, but also includes bony defects listed and other signs and symptoms related to chewing, pain, bite collapse and remaining teeth present.

In Table 4.4 grading is based on progression of disease and causative agents such as biofilm pres-

Table 4.3 1. Periodontitis: Staging.

Periodontitis	Stage I	Stage II	Stage III	Stage VI
Severity				
Interdental CAL (at site of greatest loss)	1-2 mm	3-4 mm	≥5 mm	≥5mm
RBL (radiographic bone loss)	Coronal third (<15%)	Coronal third (15%-33%)	Extending to middle third of root and beyond	Extending to middle third of root and beyond
Tooth loss (due to periodontitis)	No tooth loss	No tooth loss	≤4 teeth	≤5 teeth
Complexity				
Local	Maximum probing depths ≤4 mm Mostly horizontal bone loss	Maximum probing depths ≤5 mm Mostly horizontal bone loss	In addition to Stage II complexity: • Probing depths ≥6 mm • Vertical bone loss ≥3 mm • Furcation involvement Class II or III • Moderate ridge defects	In addition to Stage III complexity: • Need complex rehabilitation due to: • Masticatory dysfunction • Secondary occlusal trauma (tooth mobility degree ≥2) • Severe ridge defects • Bite collapse, drifting, flaring • ≤20 remaining teeth (10 opposing pairs)
Extent and Distribution				
Add to stage as descriptor	For each stage, describe extent as: • Localized (<30% of teeth involved); • Generalized; or • Molar/incisor pattern			

American Academy of Periodontology, 2018.

Table 4.4 2. Periodontitis: Grading.

	Progression		Grade A: Slow rate	Grade B: Moderate rate	Grade C: Rapid rate
Primary criteria Whenever available, direct evidence should be used.	Direct evidence of progression	Radiographic bone loss or CAL	No loss over 5 years	<2 mm over 5 years	≤2 mm over 5 years
	Indirect evidence of progression	% bone loss/age	<0.25	0.25 to 1.0	>1.0
		Case phenotype	Heavy biofilm deposits with low levels of destruction	Destruction commensurate with biofilm deposits	Destruction exceeds expectations given biofilm deposits; specific clinical patterns suggestive of periods of rapid progression and/or early onset disease
Grade modifiers	Risk factors	Smoking	Non-smoker	10 cigarettes/day	Early onset disease ≥10 cigarettes/day
		Diabetes	Normoglycemic/ no diagnosis of diabetes	HbAlc <7.0% in patients with diabetes	HbAlc ≤7.0% in patients with diabetes

American Academy of Periodontology, 2018.

ent, length of time present, the etiology of smoking and diabetes are also listed.

A note of interest with these two Charts is that the only reference made to systemic or etiological factors are smoking and diabetes, with respect to periodontal disease. A recent research paper published in July 2021, in *JAMDA*: "The Journal of Post-Acute and Long-Term Care Medicine" showed that tooth loss is a risk factor for cognitive impairment and dementia. With each successive tooth loss, the risk of cognitive decline grows. A growing body of evidence shows the connection to having untreated periodontal disease in later life to significant tooth loss and the onset of dementia. Almost 38,000 participants were in the study at NYU.

References

1. Eke PI, Dye BA, Wei L, Thornton-Evans GO, Genco RJ; CDC Periodontal Disease Surveillance workgroup: James Beck (University of North Carolina, Chapel Hill, USA), Gordon Douglass (Past President, American Academy of Periodontology), Roy Page (University of Washington). *Prevalence of periodontitis in adults in the United States: 2009 and 2010.* J Dent Res. 2012 Oct;91(10):914-20.
2. Kornman KS, Papapanou PN. *Clinical application of the new classification of periodontal diseases: Ground rules, clarifications and "gray zones".* J Periodontol. 2020 Mar;91(3):352-360.
3. CDC.gov/measles/symptoms/signs-symptoms.html. Measles: signs and Symptoms. Accessed March 2021.
4. U.S. Surgeon General Reports, Department of Health and Human Services, 2000.
5. Loesche, WJ. *Medical Microbiology.* 4th Edition, Galveston (TX): University of Texas Medical Branch at Galveston; 1996. Chapter 99: *Microbiology of Dental Decay and Periodontal Disease.* Accessed March 2021. www.ncbi.nlm.nih.gov: books-NBK8259.

Chapter **5**

Considerations in Treating the Older Compromised Patient: «*Who Am I and What Am I Doing Here?*»

"Be who you are and say what you feel because those who mind don't matter and those who matter don't mind."

Dr. Seuss

5.1 The Ability to Communicate Properly with a Compromised Patient

The first step on the ladder of the list of things to do is to know who your patient is **ahead of time**. If you find out that they are either an older "special needs" patient, an elderly compromised patient in some way or an older patient with medical issues, this might affect your treatment success. "***Know before you go***" has been a motto of mine for many years and it has helped me in many ways, both in understanding what I am basically going to be dealing with medically and possibly how to treat, cope and communicate with the patient about their dental needs.

Secondly, one must consider ***a change in the thinking process*** and not depend on how or what one has learned, if anything, about communicating in the past. In an informal survey I did while teaching at the University of the Pacific, Arthur A. Dugoni School of Dentistry in San Francisco and at the University of California School of Dentistry in San Francisco, where I also instructed, both senior classes at these two schools were polled and I found that the students had a minimum of one hour of communication taught to them in the four years of school they were just about to graduate! Not enough!

One must **consider a change in the thinking process of the compromised patient** as well. Being mentally, medically or physically compromised in some way may have changed the way a person communicates in general; therefore, a change in thinking on the practitioner's part and that of the patient should be considered. Changes in speech, ability to listen or hear and comprehend speech are all viable issues that do occur in people as they age normally, but more so with patients who suffer with disabilities. It is important to realize that no matter who you are confronting with information, that a person's perceptions are their reality, for the most part. It is up to us, as practitioners, to assist our patient's in understanding by educating them during this important consultation time and the time they spend with us as a patient. It is a never-ending process.

Communication is the basis of everything we do in life, and we must master this subject before we can hope to successfully achieve the heights of a great dental practice. I will go into this subject in depth in the coming chapter of this book, but for now realize this is the first step to getting to your proposed treatment on any patient that you see.

Discussions with this patient grouping of elderly, cognitively impaired, special needs, medically compromised, hard of hearing and mentally compromised individuals must be in simple straightforward and understandable terms. Therefore, this protocol should be addressed:

It must be in short sentences coupled with eye-to-eye contact, and in a friendly, caring tone of voice.

- Since we are in a visually oriented society, the use of photos, models, drawings or illustrations, radiographs, videos and even the assistance of our other patients, who are willing to talk to your consulting patient as an adjunct to your discussion, would be a favorable addition to the mix.*
- A time for questions and answers should be set aside for discussion after your presentation.
- Always check in with your patient and their caregiver or family members and ask if they understand what you are talking about and ask them to repeat what they have heard. This is the test as to whether they heard you and understand what you said to them.
- It is always good to have a caregiver or family member with the patient, who can take notes or record the conversation, as well as who can ask necessary questions.
- Ask permission to discuss finances for the scope of proposed treatment. All of this should be done before treatment is initiated.
- It is important to carry out these suggestions regularly and repetitively for the same treatment.
- Make sure that **The Consent to Treatment** is signed and dated, acknowledging that the patient and/or patient representative has heard, understood and given permission for the proposed treatment.
- Give copies to the patient and keep the master form for the office files.
- Make sure to have a sheet listing possible post-treatment sequelae for every type of treatment rendered and give that to the patient or caregiver prior to the procedure, keeping a signed copy for the office file.
- Give the patient or caregiver a post-treatment instruction sheet for the care that is, or will be rendered, keeping a copy for the office file.

Once you have practiced this exercise several times, or more, it will become a natural part of your armamentarium. You will be able to see an increase in your case acceptances and an increase in your referral base. This way you will be building a reservoir of trust with your patients and a referral base in the process, based on mutual respect, understanding and acceptance of your skills.

We must find ways to "unlock" the minds of our compromised patients, if possible, in order to provide them with the "keys" to successful treatment. We do this with an effort to communicate on every level to achieve mutual understanding as our goal.

5.2 Polypharmacy and Treatment Issues in the Compromised Patient

Polypharmacy or the mix of taking many medications at the same time is of great concern when treating the compromised, older patient. After the age of 65 years, a good number of aging adults are taking 5 or more medications a day. Various global studies have shown that on an average of 2-9 medications per day are taken by the elderly. At the same time, the prevalence of inappropriate medication used by the elderly was found to be from 11.5%-62.5%.[1]

My mother, who was medically compromised, just before she passed away at the age of 97, was taking about 14 pills a day to keep her alive. I suggested, in lieu of her impending death and poor health condition that she be taken off all her medicines. Some of my patients are taking double the number of pills that my mother took, essentially

Table 5.1 Symptoms caused by polypharmacy
• Tiredness
• Sleepiness
• Decreased alertness
• Constipation
• Diarrhea or incontinence
• Loss of appetite
• Confusion
• Falls
• Depression or lack of interest in one's usual activities
• Weakness
• Tremors
• Visual or auditory hallucinations
• Anxiety or excitability
• Dizziness

* Give the patient the drawings to study at home.

for the same reasons my mother took these medications. It is incumbent upon us to know what these medications are given for and to not give the patient something that will create an adverse drug reaction in our offices or their living facility, as well as compromise their health in any way.

There should be a heightened sense of awareness regarding polypharmacy when seeing the older, more compromised patients. There is a greater risk for adverse drug reactions (ADRs) because of the metabolic changes and reduced drug clearance associated with aging; thus, the risk is further exacerbated by the increasing number of drugs used in both medicine and dentistry alike. The symptoms caused by polypharmacy are usually not picked up by both the patient and the practitioner unless they are extreme and life-threatening. Symptoms can be as in Table 5.1. The most serious symptomology would be anaphylactic in nature and most likely seen in the dental setting at any time and under any circumstances.

The most consistent risk factor for ADRs is the number of drugs being taken, i.e., as the number of drugs taken increases, so does the risk of ADRs increase exponentially. Polypharmacy may also lead to decreased medication compliance, poor quality of life and unnecessary drug expenses. Older patients who find that their medication lists are expanding and who do not have the ability to afford these medications will have a higher risk rate of a reaction when they voluntarily stop taking a medication without realizing the consequences.[1]

Dentists who prescribe medication for pain, including narcotics, which can become addicting, or antibiotics, which patients can become sensitized to requiring either higher doses or a different type of antibiotic or combination thereof, can cause adverse reactions and possible life-threatening issues if taken to excess over time. To reduce the incidence and adverse effects of polypharmacy medication regimes of the elderly, their medications should be evaluated both by the dental practitioner and by the physician on a regular basis.

Looking at how one prescribes medication, it must be understood that less is more and the possibility of prescribing a lower dosage would be preferred over a higher number of pills being prescribed per day. For example, using a higher strength antibiotic two times a day rather than a lower strength antibiotic three to four times a day, especially when the patient is medically compromised and taking many other medications. Drug interactions and reactions need to be looked at when using injectable anesthetics and oral medications for discomfort and infections, which are used in the dental office for these kinds of treatment. These can interact with other medications being used for systemic issues of the patient and could be contraindicated for use. If you ask the patient about their medications and if they are susceptible to adverse reactions, will they know how to answer you?

Questions to ask the patient and oneself, as well as questioning the physician about the patient who cannot answer the questions are:

- Does each medication have an indication? What for?
- Are there any medications that are duplicating therapeutic indications that you are aware of?
- Are the dose, route and frequency appropriate for each medication?
- Has the patient experienced any adverse effects secondary to the medications received?
- What is the risk versus benefit of each medication?
- Are there any drug-drug, drug-disease, or drug-allergy interactions?
- Does the patient use more than one pharmacy?
- Does the patient have multiple prescribers?
- Are there any concerns with adherence to the prescribed medications?
- Is the patient taking any over the counter medications, vitamins or herbal products?
- Considering the identified health conditions, is the patient receiving therapy in accordance with the latest guideline recommendations?
- Is the patient responding to therapy in accordance with the patient-specific goals?
- Are there physiologic changes that would affect the patient's response to therapy?
- Does the patient have adequate support, e.g., insurance and family/caregiver?
- Does the patient understand why they are taking the prescribed drug and what the side-effects might be as well as how to take the medication?
- Does the patient know what to do if something irregular or unexpected happens to them while taking the prescribed medication?

Case Study 1

I am reminded of a chronic pain patient I had many years ago. The patient was in his mid-60s, a smoker, diabetic, overweight and a closet drinker who would come into my practice on a regular basis, about every other week, saying he had a severe toothache. He asked for radiographs and then indicated that he needed a root canal on whatever tooth he stated was bothering him, due to his intolerance not to the pain. If I obliged him by completing an endodontic procedure that was perfectly done, he still complained of severe pain and demanded a narcotic medication. I would give him an antibiotic because he did have some broken down teeth and decay near or into the pulp, but he always said it did not help and went back to asking me for a "pain killer". I tried to give him NSAIDs (Non-Steroidal Anti-Inflammatory Drugs), but he would always come back for something stronger. One day he came into my office when I was not there and saw my young associate dentist. She gave him an exam and ended up giving him a prescription for more narcotics, as he convinced her that whatever I had done was not working.

I later found out about what care she rendered to him and called the pharmacy, finding that he had received up to 10 other prescriptions from other practitioners in the Community over a month's time for the same drug and issues! The pharmacist also told me that this patient was a "chronic" pain patient with severe back pain and his MD (Medical Doctor) prescribed over 300 hydrocodone pills a month for him!! The patient had become addicted. About six months later, this patient had a heart attack and died. He was taking at least eight or nine other medications at the same time for his medical conditions. I believe the narcotics hastened his demise and were a cause of an adverse drug reaction ultimately affecting his heart.

I knew this person well, as he was my office alarm specialist. Prior to his death, I called his MD and told him about my concerns with the patient. I informed him that I found out how much medication he was dispensing for the patient and that I thought he was overdosing. He told me a story about a cancer patient that had been in a newspaper article awhile back that was dying and in severe pain. The patient requested an extraordinarily strong narcotic, *Dilaudid®*; however, the MD he had refused to give it to him for fear of addiction. He was dying... did I say that? This MD stated that after the patient died, his family sued the doctor for neglect winning a $14 million dollar judgment. It did not do the patient any good as he was not there anymore.

My patients' MD, dealing with our patient, was practicing his prescribing out of fear. A big mistake for him because he was harming the patient, who was now creating issues outside of his back pain in order to get more drugs. As licensed practitioners, we need to be prudent about the way we prescribe, not just what we are giving the medication for but answering the list of questions I addressed, calling the pharmacy and being aware of what other medications the patient is taking, as well as considering saying the word **NO** to our patients. This, more than anything else, would be a prudent thing to do if we realized that we were being used or played by a patient to do more than what is called for in treating them and something that is not ethical as well.

As an aside, the patient's medical doctor was reported to the State Medical Board and the Federal Drug Administration, who eventually took away his license to practice and his license to prescribe drugs and medication.

Medications are proven useful to manage the comorbidities of diseases and extend life. Improper overuse of medications often results in toxicity, morbidity and a plethora of problems. We associate aging, for the most part, with an accumulation of comorbidities for which multiple medications predictably will be prescribed. Taking multiple medications is within guidelines for treatment of hypertension, diabetes and heart failure for the achievement of treatment goals. Additional patient comorbidities translate to concomitant medications, which may result in a "prescribing cascade".[2] This can occur with medications being added to treat or prevent the effects of other medications or with the addition of drugs being taken for different reasons which can cause life-threatening scenarios. With respect to the elderly and more compromised patients and the amount of medication they take, it is important to always do baseline measurements of:

1. Blood pressure;
2. O_2 saturation with a pulse oximeter (they are very inexpensive and can be bought online or in a local drugstore) and
3. Respirations per minute. These test results become your legal record, a gage for you to couple with the amount and kind of drugs your patient is taking and your vehicle for reporting to the patient's medical practitioner or to EMS (Emergency Medical Services).

Case Study 2

I am reminded of a time when an 80-year-old woman came into my office for care. She sat in the dental chair and chatted away with gossip and questions and whatever else she could squeeze into the conversation. I noted that she was having trouble breathing and I was not sure whether this was from talking so fast and for so long, or some other entity. I immediately took her blood pressure, which was high, and her O_2 saturation, which was low, around 81. It should not have been below 97 on a good day. She was taking lots of medication, most of which I cannot remember as I am writing this paragraph, but I knew she was hypertensive, diabetic and had a history of asthma and COPD (Chronic Obstructive Pulmonary Disease).

I started to delve into her medical condition when she slurred a few sentences at me and passed out. I immediately called 911. She was having a TIA (Transient Ischemic Attack). The office staff had called her son, who was an Emergency Room physician. He got to my office at the same time the EMS people did and the first thing he said to me was, "**What did you do to her!?**". He yelled this blaming statement into my face in a loud and angry voice. I told him in a quiet voice that I did not do anything to her and that I believe she had a small stroke in the dental chair. People, and physicians are not exceptions, are quick to blame and sue. This was what was behind his words. I acknowledged his feelings of anxiety and agreed with him that I was anxious too. He later called me to apologize after he realized that I had not even started treatment on her at that time. Thank goodness I was not in the middle of some involved procedure and have my patient have a stroke right in front of me. It was not the first time, nor will it be the last. It is important to be prepared for the unknown.

Having this patient's vitals for the paramedics and upcoming hospital staff and symptoms as well, gave them an edge up on treating her. She ended up being alright after several days in the hospital for observation and was given some blood thinners. Apparently, she stopped taking some of her medication on her own accord several days before, but had not reported it to anyone, including me. Having a current list of medication is important and germane to a patient's overall health. Checking each time, they come in for a visit should be routine by going over the list and asking if there are any changes, additions or deletions of medication. Record the information and sign it in your chart. I have worked in many offices, other than my own, whereby the primary dentist literally writes three of four unintelligible words in the chart. "NO" information about the changes in health history, medications or issues. No recording of the kind of local anesthetic or amounts used, or information other than something like #29 DO Comp. This is a terrible mistake.

If I were in the middle of a procedure and had injected the previous patient with local anesthetic when her stroke hit, I can assure everyone that this would have come back to "bite" me if I had only written "Carbocaine 3%" and nothing else. I did tell the patient's son that I saved her life by what I did and made it easier for the paramedics because of the information I gave them. I think it took a while for this to sink in and could have been the reason for spawning his apology for blaming me for her issues that day.

5.3 Systemic Disease Effects on the Oral Cavity in Older Individuals

Systemic disease is an extremely broad topic, and I will cover what I can with respect to our aging population, who are subjected to more diseases because of their age and because of their declining immune system and ability to fight disease.

Looking at the Table 5.2 of chronic conditions, one can see the overall increase in systemic disease states over several years.

Table 5.2 Percent of middle-aged adults and seniors having common conditions

Chronic Conditions	Ages 45-64	Ages 65+
Arthritis	30%	58%
Hypertension	30%	50%
Hearing loss	15%	45%
Visual impairment	20%	300%
Diabetes	23%	35%
Dementia	100%	46.9%
Parkinson's	15%	30-50%
MS	1 in 750 increased over 65	

Centers for Disease Control, 2021.

5.3.1 Arthritis

Arthritis is a major concern among aging adults because it is so debilitating, especially when it comes to the hands and oral care (Fig. 5.1). Utilizing an electric brush makes the patients grasp much easier. Some people with this malady use a small racquetball or the like, on the end of a hand brush, in order to assist them in holding it properly. There are bicycle grips available that a toothbrush can be placed onto in order to help hold the brush with compromised hands and fingers, which make it useable, less painful and more efficient for the patient.

5.3.2 Diabetes

Diabetes in our society is rampant and has been labelled a "new" coined word: "Diabesity", because the disease is both genetically inherited as well as diet related. Diets high in carbohydrates can cause diabetes over time. Either way, this disease affects our immune systems and breaks down our defenses against bacterial and viral predators. Diabetic gingivitis is seen as a precursor to periodontal disease (Fig. 5.2), which is associated with the breakdown of the supporting tissues of the teeth. Yes, it can happen at any age; however, older people are more prone to the effects of this disease because of their lowered immune response to infection and their slow response to healing. Treating a diabetic patient can be difficult, to say the least, because one must work with their medical doctor to make sure the patient is on the proper medication, as well as checking with the patient on a regular basis that they are compliant with their medications. It might even behoove the dental practitioner to keep a glucose testing kit in the office for use prior to surgical or interventional procedures such as surgery, use of deep scaling and curettage and laser treatment of any kind. This way, the dentist will know whether

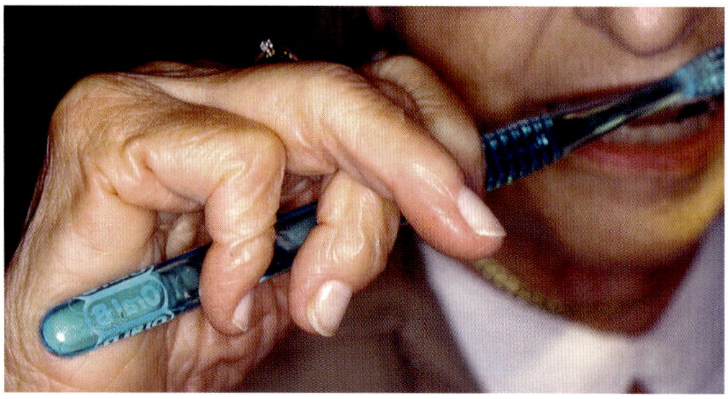

Fig. 5.1 Osteoarthritis in a deceased 95-year-old female patient, making brushing and homecare most difficult.

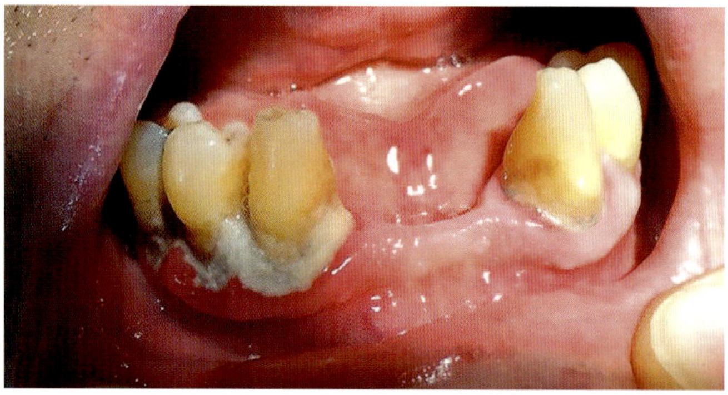

Fig. 5.2 Diabetic periodontitis in a deceased 80+ year-old man who was cognitively impaired as well. Seen here are red gingiva, swelling, recession, poor homecare with mega plaque and calculus, all signs of an inflammatory condition due, in part, to his disease status and lack of proper homecare.

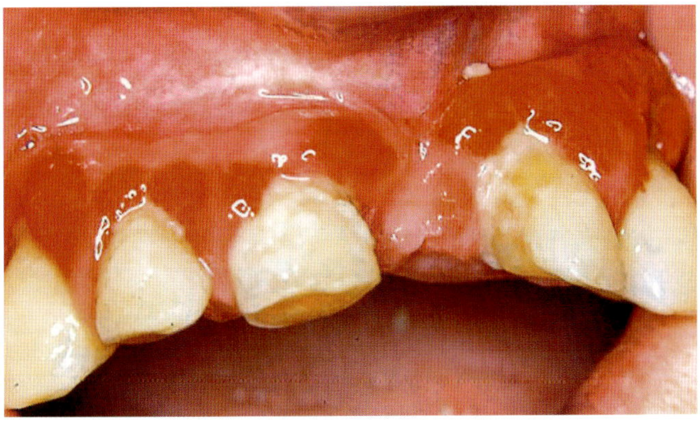

Fig. 5.3 Deceased 60-year-old female with multiple sclerosis showing chronic inflammation and advanced periodontal disease (GPD).

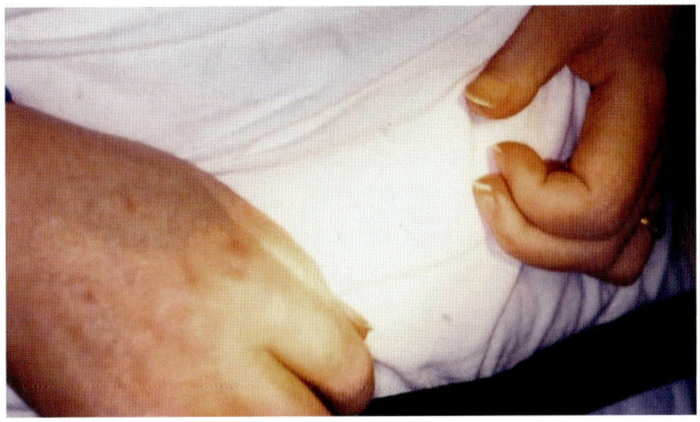

Fig. 5.4 Deceased 60-year-old female with multiple sclerosis, showing stricture of the hand muscles and loss of control in the use of the patient's arms, hands and fingers, making homecare impossible.

to treat the patient with antibiotics and pain meds in the face of a blood sugar that is not normal and/ or not treat at all. ***The Testing Kit*** should be a normal part of the office emergency kit. It is relatively inexpensive and an adjunct to proper care of your patients with diabetes. Nutritional counseling should also be considered by the practitioner or the hygienist in the office. Because most patients see their dentist more times in a year, than a physician, they feel more comfortable discussing their personal issues with the office staff, assistants, hygienist and dentist. This in turn is a good starting point to discuss dietary concerns with the patient who may be obese as well as diabetic. I have had great luck with this and my patients.

5.3.3 Multiple Disease Types

In Parkinson's disease, Multiple Sclerosis, Down's syndrome and Alzheimer's disease there is a point in time, usually in an advanced state, whereby the recipients of these diseases lose their cognition and ability to continue their homecare regimen by themselves. Besides this aspect of not being able to care for oneself, Parkinson's disease with its tremors, confusion, weakness and generalized decreased immune response allows for the inability to do just about anything. Multiple Sclerosis (MS) causes a stricture of the muscles and patients have a difficult time being able to control how they hold things, suffer from loss of strength and vision and breathing impairment (Figs. 5.3, 5.4). Down's syndrome patients tend to acquire Alzheimer's disease and subsequent dementia around 40 years of age and do not generally live much longer than this age. If they do, it is an anomaly. In all these instances, it is exceedingly difficult for the patient to have self-efficacy. Recommending shorter dental hygiene visits, periodontal scaling, laser treatment and general anesthesia may also be prudent with these types of patients for achieving more thorough results.

My Down's syndrome patients, as well as the other types of patients I mentioned here, were all slated to return for recall every two to three months. In some cases, it took general anesthesia to be able to provide dental care for them, especially the Down's syndrome patients, because of the difficult nature of the disease itself and the lack of cooperation of the patients. Older patients with blood dyscrasia, such as lymphoma, leukemia, various forms of anemia and the like, tend to manifest some of their symptoms in the gingival tissue; blanched tissue may be indicative of anemia, as well as blanching in the lower eyelids. I always roll down the lower lid of the eyes to see the color of the eye mucosa during my head and neck exams. If the inner lid tissue is white or blanched, the person is usually anemic, and I send them for testing. If the gingival tissues are swollen, red and bleeding, even with good homecare, it is a sure bet that a blood dyscrasia, such as leukemia or lymphoma, may be an underlaying cause. I also question the patient and send them for testing as well.

Treatment on these kinds of patients is a bit tricky and one should have a diode laser handy for hemostasis, should the gingival tissue bleed extensively during a routine cleaning or other treatment that might cause bleeding within the gingival tissues.

Case Study 3

Complicated Treatment of a Medically Compromised Individual

Many years ago, I had an older woman in her early 70's as a patient, with end-stage leukemia (**Fig. 5.5**). She requested me to rehabilitate her entire mouth! I was flabbergasted for the most part at her request. I questioned her about it and asked her for her rationale to do so at this time in her life. She was wearing a wig due to the loss of her hair, having just finishing a second round of chemotherapy. She told me that she did not feel good about the way she looked or smiled and wanted to look good at her funeral. Her appearance affected her self-esteem, and so she felt that it was important to feel good in the context of her eminent death, as well as remaining attractive for her husband of over 50 years while she was alive. Far be it from me to deny her last wishes, so I agreed to rehabilitate her mouth. However, I asked her if we could have a meeting with her husband and herself. He was a retired medical doctor and I wanted him to know what was going on prior to initiating treatment. She agreed to have him by her side.

The consultation with the two of them was surprisingly illuminating and beneficial for them as well as for me. There was so much love between them that there was no question about the fact that he wanted her to be happy at any cost. After speaking with the couple for some time about how long the treatment should take approximately, and the probability that it may not get finished before her death, as well as the possible discomfort she might feel during the procedures, I felt uncomfortable discussing this necessary aspect of care with her, but it needed to be done. However, she made it easy for me by acknowledging my concerns and my ability to do what she asked, telling me how appreciative she was of my willingness to make her feel "whole" again. To her, her teeth were one of the most important possessions in her life and she wanted her smile to show her gratitude for a life well lived, as well as her inherent beauty, even in death. I was so very humbled, to say the least, that I cried in front of her and her husband.

In the process of treating this patient with her systemic disease, I was confronted with a lot of bleeding from her gingiva and used mega amounts of *Astringedent*®, by Ultradent, to acquire hemostasis around the teeth in order to take adequate impressions. I did not have a laser back then, unfortunately, only an electrosurgery unit. Her teeth were worn and yellowed and scattered gray coloring as well (**Fig. 5.5**). She had some recession and old metal crowns. Her gingiva was blanched. Her vertical dimension was collapsed, and her anterior guidance was in group function with all her teeth, with no independent anterior guidance.

After treating my medically compromised patient for several months, one arch at a time, with not only the "normal" trials and tribulations of full mouth reconstruction, but coping with and handling the oral issues during prepping and taking impressions in a blood free environment, bonding in a dry environment, and allowing the patient rest periods in between each impression, it was most difficult for both of us. In today's world an iTero® type scanner would make the treatment much less of a hassle in terms of taking electronic impressions and a lot less uncomfortable for the

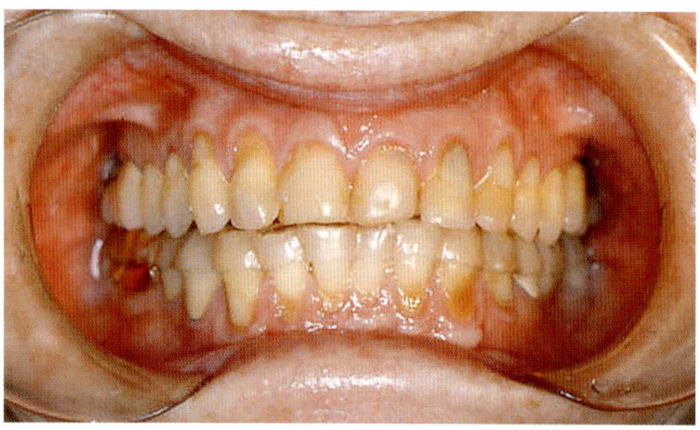

Fig. 5.5 Pre-treatment photo of now deceased 70-year-old woman with lymphoma.

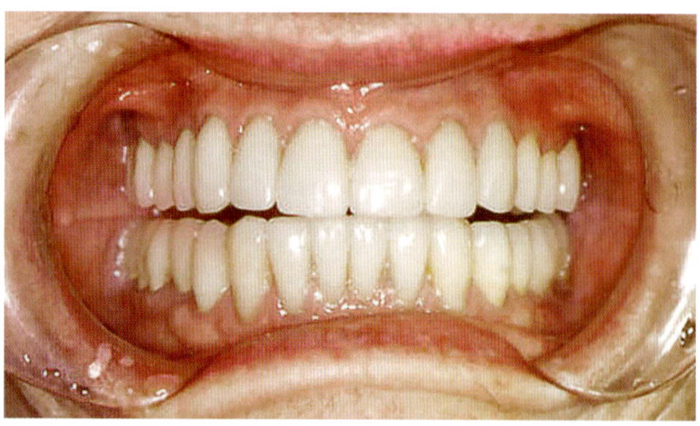

Fig. 5.6 Post-treatment of full mouth porcelain rehabilitation showing anterior guidance.

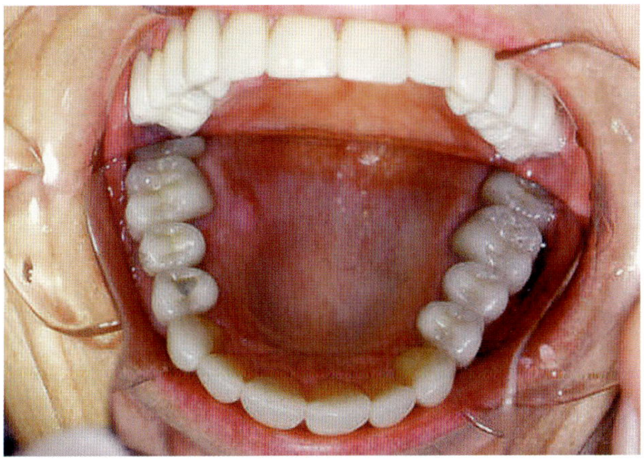

Fig. 5.7 Finished all porcelain case of now deceased lymphoma patient.

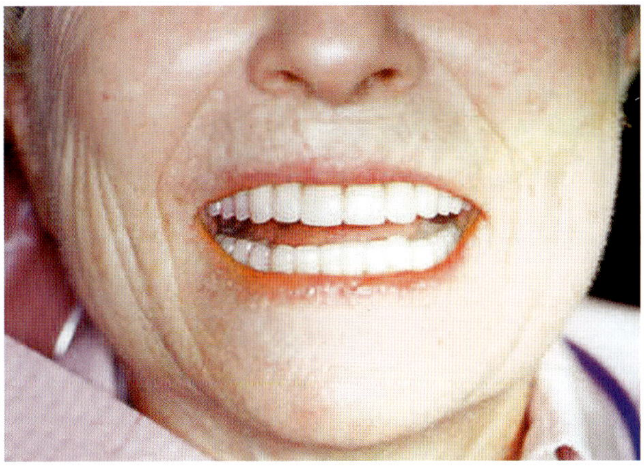

Fig. 5.8 Post-treatment photo of now deceased lymphoma patient with her new smile and wig.

patient. The electronic scanner would save time, energy and exhaustion on both our parts had we had it back when I did this case (Figs. 5.6, 5.7).

Overall, the main goal was to give my patient a better smile, overall appearance and a feeling of happiness and self-worth, which we did. It was worth it in the end to see her smile (Fig. 5.8).

5.3.4 Conservative Restorative Treatment on a Medically Compromised Patient

Case Study 4

Another medically compromised older patient, with a blood dyscrasia, presented with a missing tooth and inflamed gingiva. The patient had limited finances and it was up to me how I wanted to present this case. I felt that being conservative was an important facet of treating older and medically compromised individuals, so I suggested we bond in a bridge. There was some slight gum inflammation and recession with minimal to limited bone loss. The patient liked the idea of staying conservative and agreed to a bonded porcelain bridge. A "wing" preparation was placed on the lingual aspect of the lower left cuspid, #22. A porcelain only, minimal preparation onlay was produced for the lower left second bicuspid, #20, and a pontic for the edentulous area where tooth number #21 had been (Fig. 5.9). Due to bleeding issues, the preparations were kept above the gingiva. The pontic was completely flossable and cleansable. The patient had no discomfort the entire time and it only took two visits (Fig. 5.10). The cost and procedure were doable and appreciated.

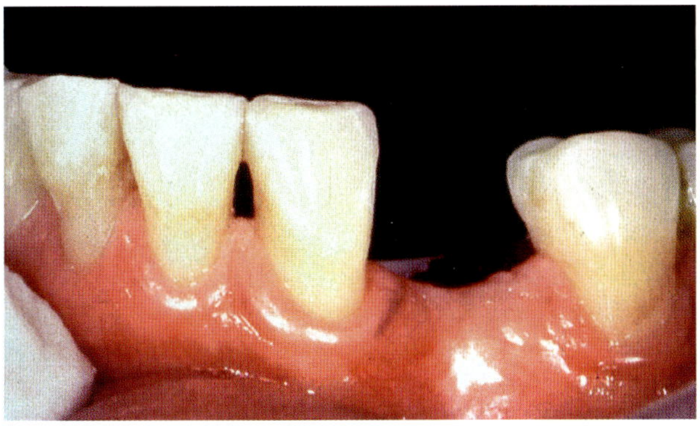

Fig. 5.9 Deceased 65-year-old patient with a blood dyscrasia, missing #21.

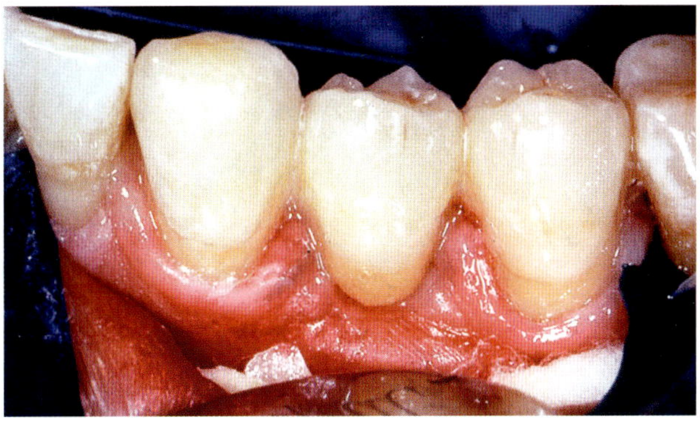

Fig. 5.10 Deceased 65-year-old patient with a blood dyscrasia, with a bonded porcelain bridge #21.

Other diseases, such as diabetes mellitus (DM) in an advanced state, can be responsible for a breakdown of the gingival tissues with a resultant advanced periodontal disease or geriatric periodontal disease, as well as a decreased immune response. These types of periodontal disease associated with advancing systemic disease are deleterious to the systemic aspects of one's body. The inflammation triggers an immune response that can spread the bacteria into the system and increase the irritation and reaction of the tissues to a decreased ability to heal themselves, if overwhelmed. In turn, according to recently published articles in multiple dental journals, chronic advanced periodontal disease was found related to both breast cancer, pancreatic cancer, oral, esophageal, head and neck, lung cancer, melanoma, heart disease and stroke.[3,4]

In a recent study, the Women's Health Initiative Observational Study monitored 73,737 postmenopausal women who had never been diagnosed with breast cancer. About 26% of the women indicated they had "gum" disease. After 6.5 years, 2,124 women were diagnosed with breast cancer. These results indicated that the risk of breast cancer was 14% higher in women who had gum disease compared to women who did not. The average risk of breast cancer is about 12%; therefore, an older woman with gum disease had a 13.5% risk of breast cancer, as well as contracting other cancers and heart disease.[3] These research studies show the relationship between oral disease and systemic disease and vice versa, especially in the older cohort of our Society.

5.4 Cognitive Aspects of Treating the Older and More Compromised Patient

In treating the older compromised patient, the practitioner must learn to assess the patient both through their medical and dental histories, which hopefully they have read prior to the appointment time, and with the conditions that they bring with them. Whatever they bring with them to the dental office, the dentist and the staff need to address their concerns by having an organized discussion with them after the clinical examination takes place in a quiet, uninterrupted space away from the dental operatory. I have done this for years and it proves highly effective in getting to "Yes" with the patient and/or with their respective representatives.

Another discussion one should have that will prove prudent and rewarding is with all ancillary dental personnel who will have contact with the patient(s), in one way or another, so that everyone will be on the "same page". It is important to know how to speak to an older person, especially a medically or mentally compromised one. Showing a patient a brochure on a treatment, or giving them a choice of watching a video, inherently will not answer all their questions. So, it is important that someone with dental knowledge sit with them while this is happening to be able to do this task. Conversations can be recorded in writing and then typed into the record. They can be used to send to the patient about what was discussed and getting their approvals, as well as a legal record of treatment options. One cannot go wrong in this direction and more than one consultation is usually needed for more understanding, both with the patient and family members or caregivers who can relay the message to family.

It is not enough to assume that our patients understand everything we tell them or explain to them. Even the assistance of visual clues, such as models, videos or the use of a mouth mirror, does not always get the point across. We, the practitioners, need to hear the patient out, repeat the information if necessary and confirm that they, the patient and/or their family member, understand what they saw or/ and what they heard. Then and only then can we get some consensus on what lays ahead and what the treatment choices and acceptance will be.

For all compromised patients, but especially those with Mild Cognitive Impairment (MCI), a precursor of dementia, Dementias, in the general category of mental impairment and Alzheimer's disease, it will be more difficult to reach a mutual understanding of the proposed treatment through any means, the ability to understand and agree to an Informed Consent and be aware of what it is that they are doing in the dental office. Mind you, this is all dependent upon the level of their disease; however, it is essentially important that a responsible relative who has Power of Attorney is there to assist in making the decisions for the patient with respect to present and future care and acknowledgment of their advanced cognitive decline. It is a difficult scenario, to say the least, and a big challenge for the practitioner and the relatives.

In working with older, mentally challenged individuals who are basically "special needs" patients, I have found it satisfactory to even examine them under general anesthesia. Radiographs can be taken at that time and a treatment plan worked up as well, prior to presenting it to the family member who is financially responsible for the care of the patient. I spoke of the "**Silent Sufferer**" previously in this book and this is the best way to go forward in terms of treatment and treatment success with positive outcomes. One can have a dental anesthesiologist either come into your practice and deliver the anesthesia or everyone goes to the anesthesiology office, the local Surgicenter or to the local hospital for the treatment and care. The issue with this is that the General Practitioner, the Endodontist, the Oral Surgeon and the like, must bring their entire armamentarium to the place of treatment, other than their own offices, where everything is in place and with a more comfortable working environment for the practitioner and staff. It is much easier and more prudent to treat the compromised patient this way. I say this from personal experience!

In general, working with older adults requires mutual respect based on trust and the ability for two-way open communication. Working with mentally, acoustically or visually challenged individuals takes a little more effort to achieve this endpoint and requires assistance from one's staff and the attending family member in charge of the patients financial and care needs in order to get a positive consent for treatment.

5.5 The Necessary Training of Staff for Working with "Compromised" Patients

My father, a building contractor, used to tell me that "**if you don't do something right the first time, you will have to always spend a lot more time, effort and money to learn how to do it all over again**". This statement never failed to impress me and has been a mantra of mine through my entire professional career. He also told me to "**study the situation before I ever embark on doing anything about it**". This was another wise mantra given to me by my father to follow during both educating people about a particular treatment plan and the actual treatment itself. In his case it was building construction and in mine and yours it is oral rehabilitation, both similar ventures.

Newton's law of physics states that "for every action, there is an opposite and equal reaction". I use this in the context of reinforcing what we tell patients, their families and/or caregivers about prospective treatment and how it affects the outcome of said treatment. Firstly, in training staff, it is important to not just talk or tell them how to do things, but to show them as well. This will imprint far better in their minds than just telling them what they should know or do. Secondly, there should be a list of written questions that we go through with the older patient and/or their responsible family member to ascertain whether they understand what we are informing them about, in order to see how much they understand before signing a **Consent to Treatment** form. There should be an Informed Consent form for every kind of treatment one does in his or her practice. Each form should have a place for a patient or Guardian signature as well as the practitioner and a witness (usually a staff member) and the date.

The staff can be evaluated on this aspect of their responsibility in their job position every so often (set a time and date) in order to determine whether they are imparting what it is you want them to convey to the patient and family about the treatment and concerns you have, and any outcome concerns you may have as well. Assuring that the patient and family have an opportunity to ask questions in an open and honest fashion builds trust and allows for mutual understanding and respect for one another.

The **list of questions** to ask the patient and/or family and caregiver with regards to getting positive feedback about continuing with dental treatment options are in Box 5.1.

These questions will help all parties be on the same page. They are questions designed by me to get to a patient's feelings rather than just deal with

BOX 5.1

List of Questions to Continue with Dental Treatment

- Were you able to understand what was being discussed with you by the dentist about treatment?
- Will you please tell me what you thought you heard in your own words?
- Is there something you do not understand about your issues that brought you here for treatment or that may not have been discussed by the dentist?
- What do you think the unmet need is that you have about your care?
- Did the dentist explain what he or she wants to do to assist you with your oral concerns?
- Did a staff member speak with you to explain to you again, in different terms, what it is the dentist recommends we do to assist you?
- How better could we have served your needs? Is there anything else that would have helped you understand the situation better or something else you would have liked to have heard from the dentist or staff person who spoke with you?
- How do you feel about moving forward with your treatment care options?
- Is money an issue with you regarding your acceptance of future dental care?
- Do any of the side-effects of treatment that you learned about scare you, and if so, how do you feel about your choices?
- Will you come back to see us and if so, would you like to get started with making an appointment for your dental care?
- Would you consider referring friends and relatives to our office for dental care?

the information at hand. People's feelings are all too often not brought into play when discussing a major procedure(s) that may cost a lot of money. Most people usually make their decisions with their emotions or hearts and not their heads.

People, especially older individuals, are most sensitive about financial issues, especially if they do not have much income. Working on a feeling level lets one know that you care and have concerns for them regarding making the right choices. Also, most patients tend to communicate more with the staff members on their dental visits and not so much with the dentist. This makes for a situation whereby the patient-staff bond might be more than that of the patient-practitioner bond. So, the staff people in the office can help make the environment, the conditions of care and treatment much more meaningful for the patient, more so than the practitioner, whose main goal is to get the patient to accept treatment and then complete it in the long run.

The staff needs education on proper communication techniques, including active listening and giving feedback. I will discuss this in Chapter 7. The staff needs to learn from their practitioner what he or she expects of them when discussing treatment with the patient. They also need training about the techniques the dentist is going to be offering to all patients, so that they can discuss these things in depth, in an educated way with the patient as well. The use of models, slides, books, fact sheets, brochures about procedures and videos, all need to be part of the arsenal of the staff person(s) that will ultimately discuss treatment with the patient and family members. **We are in a visually oriented Society**. Understanding how things flow in the office with respect to educating the patient and family members is half the battle in getting consensus to do the recommended care plan. Seeing what needs to be done is much more effective than just hearing about it.

Talking about money with the patient and family is a sensitive issue. It is imperative that the office have various plans to accommodate the patients who have no dental insurance and those that do, who may need supplemental income to pay for recommended treatment. Having a list of credit unions to work with, Care Credit type plans and even In-House insurance plans that the dental office can offer, are all things that make it much easier for the patient, especially the older patients to accept and continue treatment options.

5.6 Understanding the Needs of the Compromised Patient

Working with the compromised patient requires special abilities on behalf of the staff. Recognizing when one has either a medical issue, a psychological issue or a combination of issues is the first step in understanding "who" it is you are working with. Secondly, familiarizing oneself with the issues at hand, in advance, will help the staff person become more understanding and empathic with the patient and the patient's well-being while in the office. Getting older brings with it an entire cadre of issues from hearing loss, eyesight impairment, cognitive decline, mobility issues and security issues. All these things need to be recognized and discussed, as well as nurturing and reassuring the older compromised patient that one understands their issues and concerns. This, in turn, will reassure the patient that the office cares about them and will certainly assist in helping the patient to make the right choices when deciding about their patient care. Older people will need periodic breaks to use the restroom more often while in the office, may need more water to drink as well as a snack to eat while in the office for a long procedure due to possible hypoglycemic episodes.

The staff needs to be aware of these things in order to assist the dentist as well as the patient in general. Those patients' "special needs" will need to be accommodated in order to make their dental experience comfortable, secure and successful.

An older patient I had for many years suffered from osteoarthritis, which was most debilitating and, in the end, caused the death of the patient. However, before his death occurred, he came to his dental appointments every three months as recommended because of several reasons. Firstly, he liked the way he was treated by the staff. He felt that everyone on the staff knew he had a disease that was constricting and life-changing, as well as frustrating for the patient. The staff was attentive to his needs and always reached out to make him feel welcome and comfortable. Secondly, we assisted his needs when he came in. He was moody at times and the staff learned to assess this moodiness and ask him questions. We took an interest in him as a person. He was a retired teacher and appreciated the questions we asked him as well as the interest we showed in him as an individual.

The patient drove himself to our office, even though he could not walk! He had a lift on his vehicle whereby he could use his motorized wheelchair to help himself in and out of his van. He had limited use of his hands as well. He used a joystick to drive with two fingers, and a brake with another two fingers on the opposite hand. It was a most difficult situation with respect to his survival and we knew it. I taught my staff to be prepared for people like him with disabilities. His wife could only do so much, especially with his homecare because he could not open his jaws very wide for her to clean his teeth due to his severe osteoarthritis. So, he came to see us more often and we reduced the fees he paid in order to keep him healthy. This meant a lot to him.

The patient was able to manipulate his wheelchair (Fig. 5.11) so our hygienist could readily clean his teeth in a comfortable manner for both she and the patient. We moved our dental chair to the side of the room, so he had more access for his wheelchair space and his needs. We gave him frequent breaks and had to take him to the restroom more often than the norm during his time in the office. His hands were distorted from the arthritis and could not do the job of efficient self-cleaning of his teeth and mouth. He could only use his fingertips and not his entire hand to function manually. It was most frustrating for him, and we recognized that. The staff was incredibly supportive and empathic

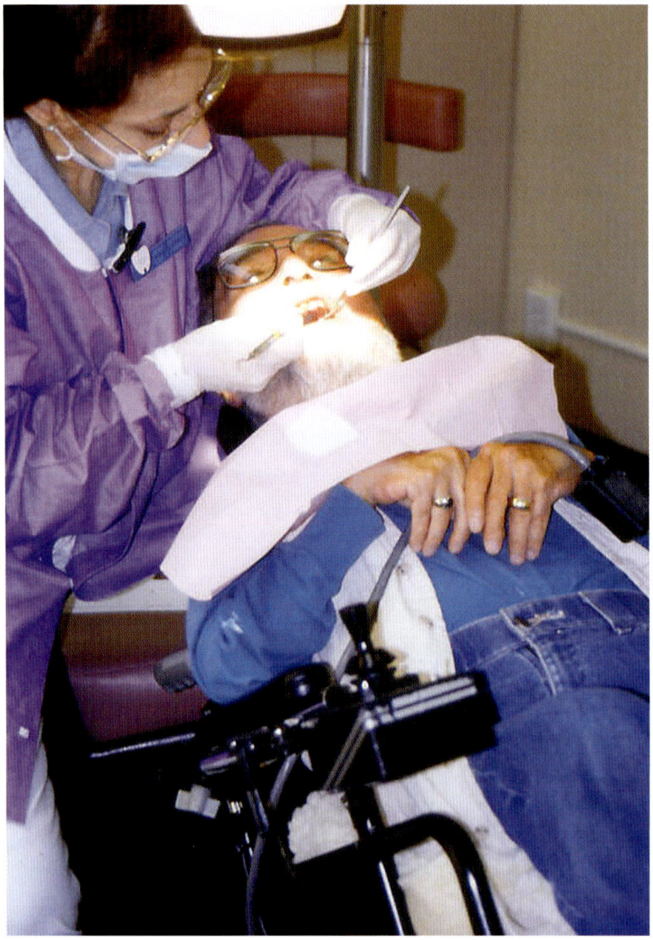

Fig. 5.11 Deceased 65-year-old patient with crippling osteoarthritis in an adjustable motorized wheelchair.

Table 5.3 Learn to adapt to the road with patients who need special assistance

• Discuss options with patient
• Make a room for treatment
• Utilize the wheelchair for the procedure, if possible
• Support yourself
• Have supports and pillows available for props
• Make sure there is an adequate airway
• Have a tonsillar suction for unexpected emergencies, such as dropping a crown down someone's throat
• Have emergency equipment on-hand and for training the staff

with him until he passed away about the age of 75 years young from his crippling disease and its "consequences".

Accommodating compromised patients is essential. Lastly, learn to "be a friend" and take not only an interest in these people but their families as well, who are trying to cope with almost impossible odds sometimes themselves. It is frustrating for them as well. So, we developed a call system with a "tickler file" alerting us every couple of weeks, to call these patients and their families to check in and see how they were and if they needed anything that we could assist them with. This unexpected courtesy and care did more for patient care and respect than one can imagine. Secondarily, it was a practice builder for us, but primarily, it was a bond we created with the patient that promoted their continued interest in their oral and systemic health and relationship with our office (Table 5.3).

I have stated before that "**no one cares how much you know, until they know how much you care**". Keep this saying close to your heart and read it to yourself often to remind yourself that you, as a dental practitioner, are a healer and a gift to your patients, not just a technician who makes them look beautiful or orally functional. Your patients are people and the people who are compromised need a lot of "TLC" (Tender Loving Care) because they may not get it anywhere else. Allowing your staff to participate in the specialized care of these patients spreads the joy and appreciation that your practice brings to all your patients (see Box 5.2). It also gives them the self-confidence and respect they may need or long for which they have not found anywhere else. One must look within, to promote our feelings, and actions from without.

5.7 Emergency Preparedness

The dental staff being prepared for a medical emergency in the dental office can be the only hope that the person having the emergency has, in order to have the emergency reversed, ultimately saving their life. Thinking that "***It Won't Happen Here!***" is a misnomer because emergencies happen everywhere and when one least expects it, especially in the dental office.

DEFINITION: *a **Medical Emergency** in the dental office may be an unexpected event that can include accidental or willfully bodily injury; central nervous system stimulation and depression; respiratory and circulatory disturbances, as well as allergic reactions that can and do impede life or the health and safety of the patient.*

Our roles in crisis should be a well thought out with a written plan that is practiced repeatedly so that you remember "**Practice Makes Permanence**". A motto I have practiced and advocated all my professional life.

Having each member of the dental team assigned to a specific duty during a medical emergency in the dental clinic or office will ultimately save lives and prevent wasted time, when time is of the essence. If you think that these things do not happen in a dental setting, you are mistaken... they do!

BOX 5.2

Some Rules of the Road with Patients Who Need Special Assistance

As a practitioner running an office and having ancillary professionals working with you on older individuals, some of whom may be compromised, here is what I think you need to do with your staff:

- **Ask your staff members what they would like to learn and why?**
- **What does each staff person feel is their strength?**
- **How does each of your staff members feel about working with older, compromised people?**
- **Is there something that scares them about working with people like this? What?**
- **What does each staff person know now about working with and treating older, more compromised patients? What would they like to learn?**
- **Is there any staff member who does not want to work with these types of individuals? (This is an important question because it illuminates this person's anxiety about whatever they are afraid of, in themselves.)**

You can incentivize your staff by paying them extra or rewarding them in some way for their time in learning new techniques and taking the time to improve on all aspects of their job specifications, especially when compromised patients are involved.

You can ask one of your older patients to be involved in educating your staff as well by setting up a scenario whereby your staff has to meet, greet and educate him or her about the office and the program planned for that day of treatment. The patient can be filled in beforehand about how they should act with the staff member, essentially role-playing someone they are not, just to make it a bit difficult for the staff person until they get what they are up against. Role-playing is a great teaching tool for your staff.

Think up some scenarios such as the patient being hard of hearing or vision impaired; the patient being short tempered or cognitively impaired to the point of him/her not being able to respond in kind to the actions of the staff person working with them, and possibly the inability of the patient to sign a consent form, etc. See how the staff person reacts. Instructions after the role-playing can be done in a group setting, so that everyone learns from everyone else. You can opt for a professional to come in and lead the discussion as well. Either way, the staff needs to know the expectations of the dental practitioner in working with his/her compromised older patients. This way everyone is on the same page, which, as I stated before, is the only way to have a unified staff, ready to promote an organized and caring practice.

Emergency→

Emergency Categories and Events

May include the following:

- Cerebral Vascular Accident (CVA-Stroke).
- Syncope (Fainting)! The most common emergency in a dental office.
- Seizure.
- Pseudo-seizure.
- Anaphylaxis (from any cause, i.e., anesthetic, oral or intraoral medication or materials and medicaments used in or around the mouth).
- Hematoma.
- Myocardial Infarction (MI) – Cardiac Arrest.
- Angina Pectoris – Chest pain above or around the heart.
- Cuts to the lip, mucosa, gingiva or tongue.
- Prolonged bleeding (from an extraction, an injection or wound).
- Asthma attack.
- Diabetic events (hypoglycemia or hyperglycemia).
- Hypertensive event or hypotensive event.
- Injuries and falls.
- Eye injuries (Foreign bodies, excessive light reaction).
- Sound (Excessive noise with hyper-reaction and Emotion).
- What is the code word for an office emergency? (Mine is "STAT" and I call it out very loudly!!)
- Nose or inhalation emergencies.
- Choking.
- Burns (from spills of any diluent, such as etchant or acid used in dental procedures onto the patient's skin, eyes or in the mouth; from warm or hot instruments or lasers, electrosurgery instruments or hot waxes or other flammable materials).

RESPONDING: *how we respond to preventing some or all these entities and how we react when one of them occurs is something that needs information, knowledge and proper protocol in place and the necessary emergency equipment in the office or clinic.*

Ask yourself:

- Where is my ammonia pellet?
- Where is the emergency kit?
- Where is the defibrillator?
- Where is the portable oxygen?
- Where is the pulse oximeter and blood pressure cuff?
- Do I need an adult, adolescent or child's cuff? (Some geriatric patients will need a child's cuff and others an extra-large adult cuff. Make sure you have all the sizes handy).
- Where is the phone?
- Where are my colored safety goggles, glasses or *Foamy*® patient eye protection wrap-around goggles?
- Where are my co-workers? Are they close enough to hear me call out? Are my co-workers prepared to act and to assist?
- Where is the eye-wash station?"
- Where is the printed map of where these things are in your office? Is it on the inside of a cabinet door in each operatory? Is it in a drawer in each room?
- What is the code word for an office emergency? (Mine is "STAT" and I call it out very loudly!!)

In your brain, where it will not help anyone but yourself, if that? Remember the Boy Scout motto: **BE PREPARED!** All these things are important in the scheme of things during a medical emergency and should be known prior to any dental treatment or care.

What to Look for and What to Do

- Look at the patient's when they arrive. Scan them quickly and thoroughly with your eyes, assessing them as a first impression.
- Are they awake, talkative and timely?
- Are they dressed appropriately?
- Are their pupils normal?
- Do they look at you or away from you?
- Is their speech normal?
- Do they react to your commands and suggestions?
- How is their gait-fast, slow and/or unsteady?
- How is their overall demeanor?

> **RESPONDING:** *All these observations will give you and your staff insight into whether you will need to be concerned that something is not right to begin with, as you ready yourself for doing dental treatment on an older, compromised person. Follow the Dick and Jane Rule of Functional Analysis:* ***Stop, Look and Listen. Then take Action, if needed.***

- Have you checked the condition and whereabouts of all the emergency equipment and supplies you may need prior to treatment?
- Look for any patient resistance or immediate challenges that face you about your intended treatment or combative efforts on the part of the patient, both verbally and physically before they enter the treatment room.
- Ask yourself "**Am I Capable** of responding properly to my observations and subsequent treatment?" If you feel uncomfortable at the first moment of meeting resistance or in your gut you know that this challenging patient will be too much for you to treat in the office then **stop!** and either refer to a specialist, dismiss the patient from treatment that day or entirely or call for assistance.

If you have a patient who presents with medical challenges, think ahead to what you might do, prior to treatment, if they had an emergency associated with their present medical condition. Role-play in your mind, the steps needed to attend to them and have what you might need close-by when you initiate treatment. This could save you a lot of headaches in the end, as well as a life, should a medical emergency arise on your watch.

- Do you have an **ammonia ampule** taped to an inside cabinet door or under the cabinet next to you in each working room?
- **Always** ask the patient for an update on their medical history prior to initiating treatment **every time** they come into see you for dental care. They might not tell you on their own about changes they have had medically since their last visit to see you. This could be a lifesaver.
- **Always** note in writing in the patient's chart both the *subjective information* the patient gives you and your *objective observations* about their attitude, physical and mental conditions before, during and after treatment. This material is a legal record and report that may save you lots of grief in the event something happens to them in the dental chair, walking out or even coming into the office, or sometime after treatment outside your office, which could come back to haunt you.

Notes on Conditions of Medical/ Dental Emergencies

Keep a notebook with you to take notes in the event of a medical or dental emergency. List the categories of the emergency noted below and write in the space accordingly in your book. Notes on conditions should follow the **SOAP Method** of reporting. That being a mnemonic for:

- **Subjective** (Anything the patient says of does from coming into the office until leaving the office);
- **Objective** (What you observe in the course of seeing your patient walk into the office until leaving your office after treatment);
- **Assessment** (A summary of the condition of the patient before, during and after care);
- **Prognosis or Plan** (That being: how the patient progressed, ended-up after treatment and how they felt before leaving your office and after treatment, as well as in their dismissal from your office and any return visit to come being noted).

A written "note" by the practitioner is a legal record and should be in the SOAP format. Example:

S "The patient stated they were nervous upon entering the office before they said anything else or responded to our greeting".

O *Noted*: "The patient was jittery, had a flushed face, was speaking rapidly without listening to what was being said to her and she was perspiring as well".

A "The patient was obviously nervous and was asked if she would like to use the restroom or sit down for a few minutes and have a glass of water before going to the dental operatory. The patient did not say much, except "thank you, I will have some water". "We told the patient to relax for a few minutes, catch her breath and then we would take her to the back of the office for treatment care".

P "The patient seemed calm and collected when we took her back for dental care. We took her blood pressure, pulse and respiration, as well as a pulse oximeter reading, all of which were normal (Note information with readings in the chart). Treatment was started after an informed consent and went as planned. The patient was dismissed in good stead and in good health and spirits. Post-treatment instructions were given to her to follow for the rest of the day, and she was asked if she was OK, to which she responded, "Just fine, thank you".

Post note: "The patient was called several hours after she left the office to see how she was and if her anesthetic had worn off and if she was comfortable. I thanked her for being a good patient and hoped that she enjoyed her experience here. I asked her if there was anything we could have improved upon in terms of her care or if she would have liked to have changed anything about her care". (These are especially important questions to ask because they show ownership in what you have done; they tell the patient that you respect their opinion; they show an interest in the patient and they show that you ultimately truly care about how she feels and thinks regarding her visit and care in your office. These create or enhance trust, mutual respect, admiration and a committed patient in the end, who may refer you many more of her friends and relatives for care as well.)

Headings of Possible Medical Emergencies to Log into Your Journal or Notebook

- Cerebral Vascular Accident (Stroke-CVA)
- Syncope (Fainting)
- Seizure
- Pseudo-seizure
- Anaphylaxis
- Hematoma
- Myocardial Infarction (MI) – Cardiac Arrest
- Angina Pectoris
- Cuts to lip, mucosa, gingiva or tongue
- Prolonged bleeding
- Asthma attack
- Diabetic events (hypoglycemia or hyperglycemia)
- Hypertensive event or hypotensive event
- Injuries or falls.
- Eye injuries (Foreign Bodies, Excessive light reaction)
- Sound (Excessive noise with hyper-reaction and emotion)
- Nose or inhalation emergency
- Choking
- Burns

RESPONDING: *Remember, emergencies and accidents in the dental office, whether it be outside the front door or within the confines of the office itself, are under the purview of the practitioner. It is ultimately the practitioner's responsibility to handle these situations with the help of his staff.*

Staff Assignments for Emergency Drills

- One person should be appointed to call 911 emergency after the doctor calls a "STAT". This means, I want it right now! It is an Emergency. I used STAT as a code word with my staff, to not alarm the other patients in the office.
- One person oversees getting the emergency kit and oxygen, pulse oximeter and defibrillator. If you have a large staff, then you can have another person get the oxygen tank (small with wheels on a carrier).
- One staff person should take copious notes about who said what from by-standers to staff to patient to family members, to the dentist and their actions. (Very important if one goes to court). It never hurts to write **too much**.
- One assistant should always stay with the practitioner to assist in CPR, or the patient or anything else the dentist needs.
- Another person should be the peacekeeper and try to keep the patients or family in other rooms calm and collected as well as out of the way of the treatment room and the emergency.
- Other staff members who were not assigned a specific job can be "floaters" and assist where needed or when requested.

5.7.1 Practicing Emergency Drills and Role-Playing

Once a month or more, I would take a staff person aside, inform them they would be the person having an emergency inside or outside the dental office and give them the type of emergency it was supposed to be and the role they would play as the "victim". Then, unexpectedly, I would give her a sign, such as my whistling "**Dixie**" and she would act out. The staff never knew who the emergency patient was or the nature of what it would be. They knew their jobs and positions to take when there was an emergency. I made sure everyone was doing their work. The other patients in the office were cued in and all was in place. Then I whistled "Dixie" and watched the exercise play-out. Most scenarios involved events with older patients who were medically compromised.

When it was all over, we sat and talked about how we could have made things better, or if there was anything else we could have done to make it better in the first place or at all. Again, I use the phrase, "**Practice Makes Permanence**". It is not so much perfection that is important, but the autonomic and automatic response of doing something you are trained to do without thinking too much about it. Perfection comes from years of experience; however, nothing is ever totally perfect until we know the patient survives in good stead, the staff did everything they were supposed to do and more and the practitioner who is in charge tells everyone it was a perfectly "good" job.

Case Study 5

As an example of an actual dental emergency in my office was a young-looking middle-aged patient who came into see me for a restoration on an upper right second molar. We were doing amalgams in those days, so there was noise from the triturator or mixer that was disturbing, as well as a lot of things we had to prepare for before we did the restoration. The patient was noticeably quiet and subdued and asked for nitrous oxide, which she had never asked for before from me. Her husband was a volunteer fireman and aircraft mechanic. She was attractive and demure. I had placed a topical anesthetic and then placed the nitrous oxide mask on her with 20% nitrous and about 80% oxygen. She had also requested music and a headphone, which we gave her. So here we have a sensory deprived patient both with hearing, some light sedation and goggles over her eyes to protect them but blocking her vision. The injection was given, which she did not feel. I waited a few minutes and then started drilling the preparation and removing the decay. It was a "run of the mill" technical procedure.

The pulse oximeter was on her finger as well showing 98% oxygen saturation. I saw her hand go up from the chair with her wrist still on the chair as she was doing what looked like directing a band. I asked the assistant to turn off the nitrous and crank up the oxygen, just because I thought something "fishy" was going on. Obviously, one would think she was keeping time to the music, but she apparently let loose with what seemed to be a seizure of some sort. I took off the nitrous mask immediately, placed a mouth prop in her mouth and a tongue depressor so she would not swallow her tongue. She seemed unconscious but awake and thrashing and making erratic arm movements. I called a STAT. The team went into action and in two seconds I had an IV into her arm administering 5 mg of Valium. It did nothing to stop this event. She just continued to thrash as we maintained her airway and tried to keep her safe. The fire department showed up with the police and her off-duty husband! His first words to me were "what the F-K did you do to her?! He immediately made a blaming statement and directed it at me. I told him I did nothing out of the ordinary and that she was having a seizure of some sort and that I was trying to keep her from harm. I then asked him politely to get out of my face. He was demanding to take her to a hospital some 30-45 minutes away, when we had one in our community, albeit small, about 3 minutes up the road, which is where I told him we were taking her first. The fire chief agreed with me.

Long story short, the husband made such a stink at the small community hospital that they told him to take her to the big hospital some 30-45 minutes away. The ER doctor was an Intern and gave the patient phenobarbital and *Dilantin®*, which further sedated the patient. I used an AMBU (Auxiliary Manual Breathing Unit) bag on her all the way over to the other hospital. They took her to their ER and gave her more sedating drugs, which I asked them not too. All they did was finally stop her from breathing. Talk about an emergency. She was whisked off after that and I did not see her for several days. Her husband came by to inform me he was going to sue me for neglect. Nice guy!! The lawsuit was frivolous but lasted 6 years. It created much stress for me and my wife and my staff. Finally, after years of testimony, and after claiming that the wife (patient of mine) had brain damage, the other party agreed that I did nothing wrong, could find nothing wrong and that the wife was fine... and would drop their suit against me if I agreed not to sue them for ***malicious prosecution***, which I said I had to think about. I did not want to drop this issue of bringing litigation against them but did so for the sake of my marriage and my own peace of mind. I tell this story because there are people out there who will do anything to sue anybody. Keeping proper records, having the right emergency equipment and supplies that are up to date, practicing emergency drills and perfecting them, and learning how to communicate in a good way with our patients will hopefully keep you from having an experience like the one I had. Then no one can take your integrity away from you, no matter what.

Older, more compromised patients are bound to have medical emergencies and I have had many to cope with in my career from stroke, heart attacks, seizures, syncope, vasovagal responses and elevated blood pressure episodes, allergic phenomena, angina, acute asthma and allergy attacks, choking and aspiration of a dislodged crown, a drug addict swinging a baseball bat asking for drugs and an irate, cognitively-impaired older man with a gun demanding that his wife bring his grandson out to him or he'll start shooting at the office and everyone in it. A scary situation, need I say more.

I was always prepared and knew what I had to do innately because I had practiced these techniques for handling emergencies repeatedly for years. I even had emergencies outside the door to my office, whereby no one could open the front door to get to the patient, who had passed out in front of the door before entering the office. We had to go out a back door with all our equipment and run around the building to the front, while my receptionist called 911!

So, emergencies do happen in the dental office and there are a higher percentage of them that happen with older adults and medically/mentally compromised individuals. One third of older adults fall each year, and falls are costly to both the patient in terms of morbidity and mortality and to the health system.[4] Between the years 2003 and 2010 the rate of falls and fall related injuries among people aged 65 years increased from 60.4% to 68.8% per 1,000 population. Older adults in the 75-84-year-old group increased from 67.4% to 81.3%, a significant finding.[5] Redesigning and retrofitting our offices, making them safe for our older patients is especially important. Falls in older individuals are listed as one of the top five causes of death in the U.S. according to the CDC.

Medical emergencies were most likely to occur in the dental office during and after local anesthesia, primarily during tooth extraction and endodontic procedures as well. Over 60% were attributed to syncope, with hyperventilation, the next most frequent at 7%.[6]

BOX 5.3

Essential Emergency Medication

Essential Emergency Medication for the dental office should include, but not limited to the following:

1.	Oxygen	for almost all medical emergencies	100% inhalation
2.	Epinephrine	for anaphylaxis, asthma and cardiac arrest and 1 mg i.v. for cardiac issues	0.1 mg i.v. or 0.3-0.5 mg i.m.
3.	Nitroglycerin	for pain from angina	0.3-0.4 mg sublingual
4.	Antihistamine	for allergic reactions	25-50 mg i.v. or i.m.
5.	Albuterol/ Salbutamol	for asthmatic bronchospasm	2 sprays inhalation
6.	Acetylsalicylic acid (ASA)	for myocardial infarction	160-325 mg orally

Additional Emergency Medication can include the following:

1.	Glucagon	for hypoglycemia in an unconscious patient	1 mg i.m.
2.	Atropine	for clinically significant bradycardia	0.5 mg i.v.
3.	Ephedrine	for clinically significant hypotension	5 mg i.v. or 10-25 mg i.m.
4.	Hydrocortisone	for adrenal insufficiency/recurrent anaphylaxis	100 mg i.v. or i.m.
5.	Morphine or nitrous oxide	for angina like pain non-responsive to nitroglycerin	2-5 mg i.v./35% N_2O
6.	Naloxone	for reversal of opioid overdose	0.1 mg i.v.
7.	Lorazepam or midazolam	for status epilepticus	4 mg i.m. or i.v.
8.	Flumazenil	for benzodiazepine overdose	0.1 mg i.v.

Essential Emergency Equipment should also include:

1.	Tonsillar suction	for recovering swallowed or inhaled foreign bodies and cleaning gross debris
2.	Long beaked forceps	for retrieval of swallowed foreign bodies
3.	Rubber hose	for tourniquet use
4.	Airway/mouth prop	to protect the tongue, lips and cheeks from damage during seizures
5.	Needle holder and sutures	for closing wounds on lips, cheeks, tongue and mucosa
6.	Antiseptic	for wounds outside the mouth
7.	Bandages of all kinds	for cuts, abrasions, open skin injuries
8.	Antibiotic ointments	for all skin wounds and lip injuries
9.	A paper bag	for panic attacks and pseudo-seizures*
10.	Eye drops for foreign bodies and chemical wash	
11.	Eyewash station in the office (more than one would be good; every operatory would be perfect) (It is the law to have at least one.)	

One can customize an emergency kit and have what he or she thinks is necessary to have on hand just in case you must wait some time for the paramedics to show up at your office door.

Do not be shy about using these entities.

* Having a walker, cane, wheelchair, and any portable O_2 tank, mask, or Ambu bag on hand as accessories to your emergency supplies would also be germane to treating the older, compromised patient, as well as anyone else who is in need that frequents one's office.

Case Study 6

I must mention a dental emergency patient that was brought into my office after a fall in the bathtub. She was close to 9 months pregnant and when she slipped and fell as she got into the tub, she placed her arms over her belly, to protect her baby, and then hit her face on the tub as she fell into it! She broke her upper front teeth, all four of them and was bleeding profusely. The roots were still embedded in the ridge. She kept making noises of having pain continuously. I got the bleeding stopped and the remaining teeth pulp capped; however, she still made sounds as if she were in pain, with her eyes closed and wincing, still clutching her belly all the while.

The woman, unbeknownst to me, was in labor! We immediately called 911 and went into "Emergency" mode. Everyone took their places and before we knew it, the patient was delivering in the dental chair! And guess who was the deliverer?

I do not think the patient was in that much dental pain because I had given her a local anesthetic, albeit short-acting, but enough to assist her while being treated for her dental needs. I think she went into labor the moment she fell in her tub. And by the time she was in our office, the delivery was taking place. So again, be appraised that any kind of emergency can take place in a dental office, and one should be prepared for them all. The older patient is more apt to fall victim to an emergency anywhere. That is why we always need to be aware of their histories and their overall health situation.

I have given you a cursory list that will help you get started (Box 5.3). It is less expensive to make your own kits, but there are commercially available ones on the market you can purchase. If you are unsure about handling an emergency or stabilizing a patient in an emergency in your office and waiting for the paramedics, then there are many classes available which are offered by The Red Cross, The Fire Department, The American Heart Association or various medical and dental schools, and dental societies who give courses in first aid and emergency medicine.

References

1. Dagli RJ, Sharma A. *Polypharmacy: a global risk factor for elderly people.* J Int Oral Health. 2014 Nov-Dec;6(6):i-ii.
2. Hoel RW, Giddings Connolly RM, Takahashi PY. *Polypharmacy Management in Older Patients.* Mayo Clin Proc. 2021 Jan;96(1):242-256.
3. Post-Menopausal Women with Gum Disease Seem to Have a higher Breast Cancer Risk. Accessed from BreastCancer.org. 3-21. https://www.breastcancer.org/research-news/gum-disease-may-be-linked-to-higher-risk.
4. Freudenheim JL, Genco RJ, LaMonte MJ, Millen AE, Hovey KM, Mai X, Nwizu N, Andrews CA, Wactawski-Wende J. *Periodontal Disease and Breast Cancer: Prospective Cohort Study of Postmenopausal Women.* Cancer Epidemiol Biomarkers Prev. 2016 Jan;25(1):43-50.
5. Shankar KN, Liu SW, Ganz DA. *Trends and Characteristics of Emergency Department Visits for Fall-Related Injuries in Older Adults, 2003-2010.* West J Emerg Med. 2017 Aug;18(5):785-793.
6. Haas DA. *Management of medical emergencies in the dental office: conditions in each country, the extent of treatment by the dentist.* Anesth Prog. 2006 Spring;53(1):20-4.

Chapter **6**

Just in Case You Want to Talk "Turkey..." Truth and Consequences

"Never let success get to your head; never let failure get to your heart."
Anonymous

6.1 Case Studies in Geriatric Dentistry-Dental Rehabilitation

Oral-dental rehabilitation can be a complicated, multi-vectored scenario with respect to the presenting dental issues of the patient, as well as the medical, dental, social, psychological and economic histories of the patient. Many times, you may be presented with a one tooth scenario that has been the bane of existence for the older patient, who, in turn, may want it extracted, when you know that it is an important tooth to save or salvage in the scheme of things. As I have stated previously in this text, my father's quote to me as a young man, "**study the situation**" before making any suggestions or taking any actions as to how you, as the practitioner, might treat the issue at hand.

One should not be the "Bull in the China shop", so to speak, and rush right into both telling the patient what you will do, let alone doing it without discussion. Even restoring one tooth can be a challenge and one of the most complex issues in an oral-dental rehabilitation. Why, you may ask? Because, for every action there is an opposite and equal reaction. For every fractured or broken tooth there is a reason. For fractured teeth repeatedly there is a reason. Let us **use all our senses** to diagnose a patient's unmet needs before we attempt to treat them.

For example, I had an older gentleman farmer, in his 70's, come into my office one day to complain about the fact that he just had a front lower incisor restored with composite and, within two days, it fractured again. Apparently, this was the fourth dentist who attempted to fix the problem and the impatient patient stated that he thought he should just take out this tooth. He wore a lower partial denture and only had his front six teeth present. To take out this tooth meant one of several things:

1. The patient had no more money to spend on his teeth (economic reason).
2. The patient did not want to bother fixing it and rebreaking it again (physical and time reasons).
3. The patient wanted me to fix it but had reservations about my skills (irrational and uneducated reasons).
4. The patient refused to have me examine him thoroughly to determine the root cause of the issue so this would not happen again (irrational, controlling, unreasonable and unfounded reasons).

I ended up explaining to him that I found it necessary to do an exam to see why this had happened to him at least four times before. I told him that I did not want to be the fifth dentist he went to that he blamed for it breaking again and then subsequently going to a sixth dentist to complain that I did poor work. I was surely studying the situation as it was. The patient obviously had a poor dental IQ and probably did not frequent a dental office unless he had an issue with something like this present need. So, after some coaxing, he let me do a full exam on him. In doing so, I noticed that he had a collapsed bite and flattened and worn denture teeth on the poster flanges of his lower partial and flattened opposing natural teeth on the maxillary arch. With a collapsed vertical dimension, he was bound to break his lower anterior teeth, which he abused by eating hard foods and substances on them, as well as having constant force placed on them by his upper natural teeth in an edge-to-edge arrangement. It was obvious to me that no other dentist discussed opening his bite up with him, or if they did, he had refused due to financial reasons. I received permission to take impressions of his mouth, so I could show him how they lined up and better explain the reasons why his lower front tooth or teeth were breaking as they did. **We are in a visually oriented society,** and this was a man who was so oriented, to a point.

In the meantime, during my intraoral examination, I observed a small, approximately 5×6 mm greenish in color, "grape-like" elevation at the junction of his hard and soft palate. I took photos of this lesion with a millimeter ruler for my record. I told him that I could place some bonded material on his remaining broken tooth, but that it might not hold up, depending upon how he treated it, and that I would make it just out of occlusion to minimize his force on it to help keep it from breaking. At the same time, I informed him about the lesion on his palate, which was non-painful and one that he did not know existed. I suggested a referral to an oral surgeon for biopsy, but he refused by saying "Just fix my tooth". Which I did, but I was not done with him yet. I sat down and educated him about my findings, discussing his collapsed bite, giving him the reasons why I felt he was continuously breaking his front teeth. And then I informed him about the suspected oral cancer on his palate and told him that he really needed to think about going to an oral surgeon for a biopsy. I gave him the name and number of one that I trusted, an MD, DDS, and told him that I would call the surgeon and introduce him personally before he went there. He refused again, paid his bill and left without another word.

I was frustrated, to say the least, because I knew that the lesion was not normal and that it might be a mucoepidermoid carcinoma, a very bad, fast moving and voracious cancer that can cause destruction of the palate, nasal sinuses, eyeballs and sockets as well. I was frightened for this man, whom I hardly knew.

I subsequently called the head of the pathology lab at the University of the Pacific Dental School, where I used to teach, and asked my colleague, whom I knew very well, to call this patient and ex-

BOX 6.1

The Chaos Theory

The **Chaos Theory** suggests that **management, the practitioner in this case, should place more emphasis on adaptability, initiative and entrepreneurial creativity to cope with a future that is inherently unknowable. ... The future is disorder.** To do an adequate treatment plan, it is relevant to draw upon the wisdom of this Chaos Theory and make order where there is none in all respects of the word... **order**. To do this with complicated dental issues, one must first assess one's ability to even move forward and plan to treat what the patient brings to you. Once a personal decision is made to proceed, then an outline of what treatment precedes the first item on the agenda: a full examination, including whatever radiographs must be taken or utilized in order to come to a personal consensus about caring for the patient.

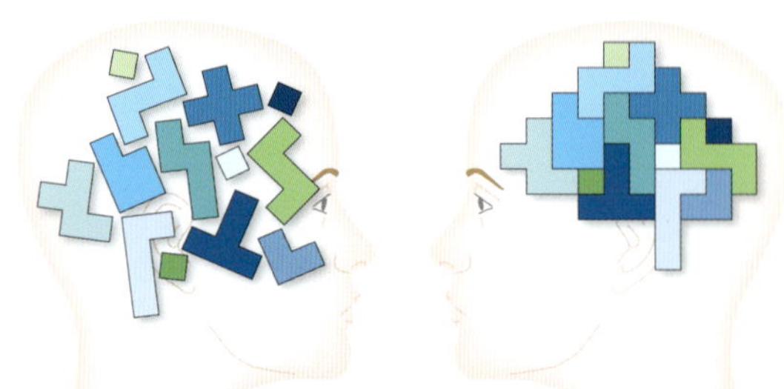

plain his concern as well as mine. He did this and encouraged the farmer to seek out a biopsy with my referral source. It took two more calls to other friends of mine who were well versed in pathology to get this man to my oral surgeon. Long-story short, he had his biopsy, and it was as I suspected, a mucoepidermoid carcinoma. He was encouraged by the surgeon and then me again, to go back for a wider excision, which is common for these things, but he refused. For this man doing anything other than what he wanted to do was a nuisance and a waste of his time. I could see that money was not the entire issue. I took it upon myself to call him daily until he gave in but decided to go to Kaiser Hospital, his HMO, and not my oral surgeon because of cost. He saw an ENT surgeon, who contacted me for information about the cancer. It seems my oral surgeon did such a good job that it was difficult to see where the tumor had been after the farmers palate healed. The ENT surgeon asked if I had anything I could send him that would help. I told him I did and sent him the measured photos, the radiographs, the examination sheet and the most important piece were the study models that had picked up the lesion itself in the impression. He had everything he needed. The surgeon later wrote me a note stating that I saved this man a lot of grief, because the cancer was caught early and with all the information I sent to him, the secondary surgery was minimized in terms of the **radicalness** of what it could have been. The patient kept his nose, eyes and sinuses intact and was free of cancer.

I knew the farmer would never come back to me because he did not like me "hounding" him about all of this, but I wanted to save his life, which I did. It was more important for me to do this one thing than be concerned about his tooth fracturing again, which I felt it might because I knew he would never spend the money to do a reconstruction to open his bite up and take the pressure off his front teeth. But I know that we should never second guess what a patient will or will not do. All we can do is increase their level of knowledge about what they bring to us and hope that something in their brain "clicks" and makes them think differently about how important their teeth really are in the scheme of things. I know what I did, and I am proud of myself for my actions. I did my due diligence.

In working with older, more physically compromised, more mentally confused and cognitively impaired patients, I have found that the **Chaos Theory of Management** (Box 6.1) is important to draw upon for the ability to make decisions out of disorder and confusion, on the part of the patient, and uncertainty, on the part of the practitioner.

6.1.1 The Outline of Treatment

The outline, firstly, is to assist the practitioner in his critical thinking regarding the needs to encompass both the discussion the practitioner has had with the patient and/or patient representatives about the findings and the necessary items that need to be treated. The practitioner must incorporate a "list" of treatment modalities that he or she is thinking about with respect to restoring the patient's issues. These can be discussed at a second consultation with the patient and their representative after the Outline is finished and the treatment plan(s) are written down for further discussion, consensus and approval. Included in this outline would be consideration for the following:

- Rehabilitation utilizing mixed modalities that are commonly used for restoring teeth, such as composite, amalgam, different types of crowns, partials, dentures or implants.
- "Rube Goldberg" types of tactics (meaning risky last chance treatment) in repairing basically irreparable teeth.
- Overdentures over remaining teeth: including necessary dentistry to get to that point, like endodontics, post support and cast copings with and without attachments.
- Bone grafting and extractions, gingival grafting to preserve or enhance attached gingiva, as well as periodontal therapy and education.
- Minimal treatment versus full mouth reconstruction/rehabilitation.

Case Study 1

56-Year-Old Patient

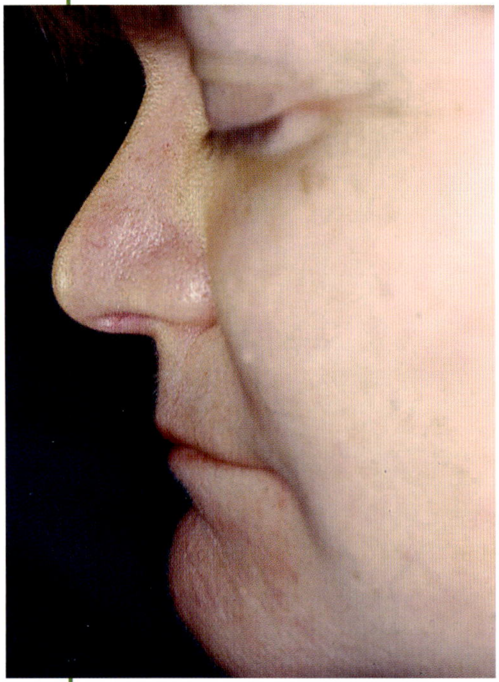

Fig. 6.1 Profile showing collapsed bite with thin disappearing lips.

This patient presented with numerous missing teeth, a collapsed vertical dimension, a 20-year-old "flipper" partial denture replacing her anterior maxillary teeth, decayed teeth, sub-standard porcelain to metal crowns, periodontal disease, poor homecare and minimal finances (Figs. 6.1-6.4). After the complete dental examination, study models and radiographs, a list was made of the dental findings and discussed with the patient. She was given several treatment plans regarding her issues, as well as options that she could "mix and match" for her treatment. She did not want a porcelain fixed bridge, nor a full denture. We discussed some options after narrowing down her wants and desires. I made an outline for myself of these issues and how I was going to go about prioritizing her treatment needs and a timeline for both of us to follow. I emphasized that this was not written in **stone** because the unknown can happen while being treated. This then goes back to the Chaos Theory of disorganization, not knowing how things will come out during the treatment and at the end. Meeting someone's expectations is a difficult task, and they must be clear. It is also important that the patient understand your expectations as well in order to minimize any conflict in your relationship. Write them down in your chart notes for each of you. A situation may occur for one or the other of you, which may necessitate reading them again, out loud, to clarify a possible misunderstanding or disagreement about something down the road of your treatment with each other. This will save you much heartache and potential legal issues in the end.

After this patient's examination, hygiene visits and consultations to discuss my Outline of Treatment and Timeline, she decided to opt for an overdenture on the maxillary arch (Figs. 6.5, 6.6). Her maxillary crowns were decayed underneath and needed to be replaced. I suggested both implants in the edentulous areas and new crowns, or fixed bridges as an alternative and as a secondary treatment plan due to her finances, an overdenture with copings and a bar for support, which she quickly accepted.

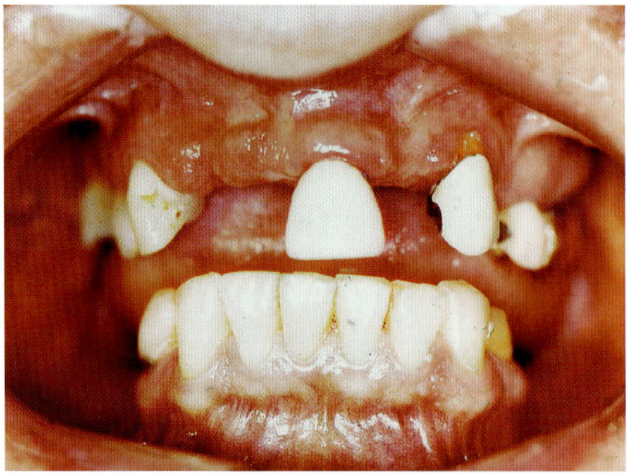

Fig. 6.2 Pre-treatment photo.

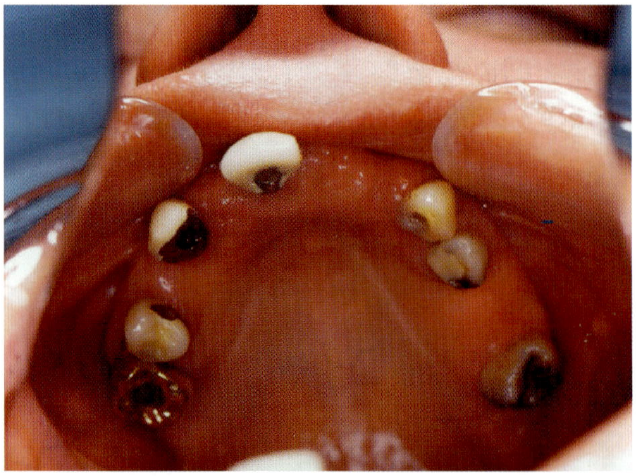

Fig. 6.3 Pre-treatment maxillary arch.

This patient was incredibly pleased with her result and stated that it exceeded her expectations (Figs. 6.7, 6.8). She felt the money she paid out was worth the time spent to seek out her new treatment and correct the disease processes going on in her mouth. Unfortunately, with her new and improved self-image, she proceeded to divorce her husband and find a younger partner who would lift her spirits and recognize her "new-found beauty".

We, practitioners, cannot undo what patients will not let us do and we cannot predict what the patient will or will not do post-treatment or even after a consultation prior to dental treatment.

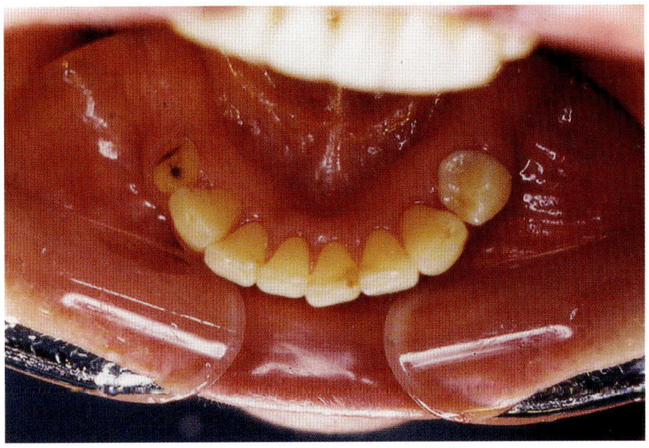

Fig. 6.4 Pre-treatment mandibular arch.

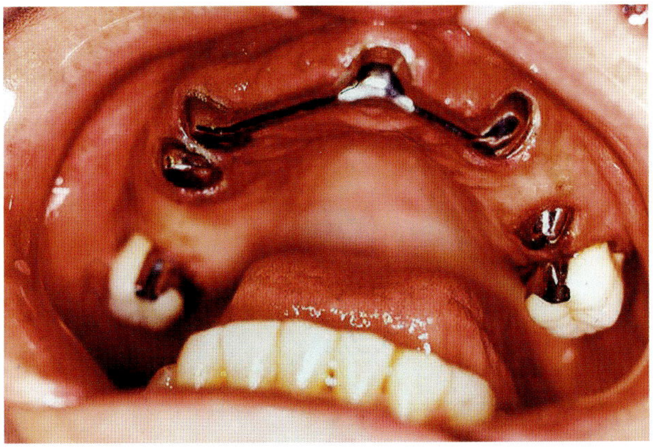

Fig. 6.5 Final restorative underlayment of the maxillary arch. Copings, bar connectors and precision attachments on new posterior crowns.

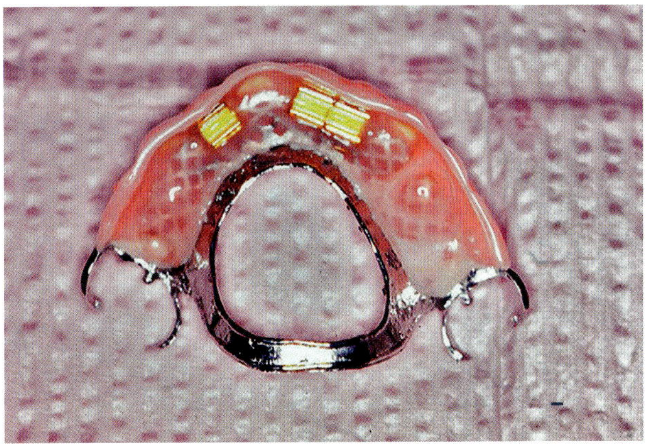

Fig. 6.6 Maxillary over-partial denture final restoration.

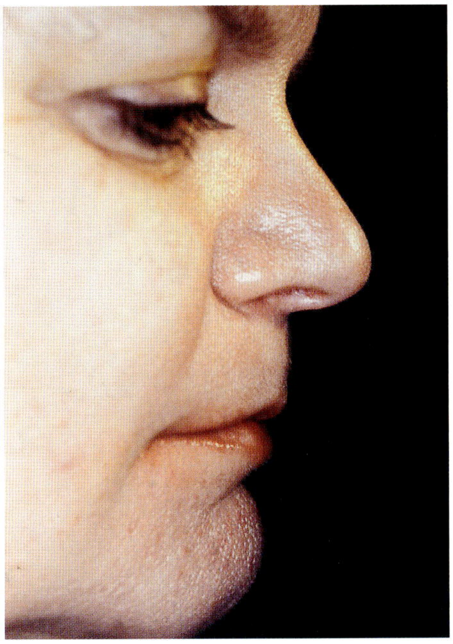

Fig. 6.7 Final profile photo.

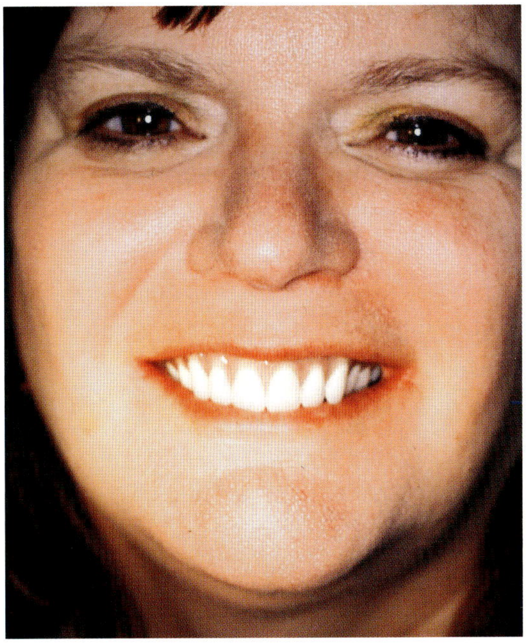

Fig. 6.8 Final smile without lower restorative.

Case Study 2

86-Year-Old Dementia Patient Who Only Speaks French (Now Deceased)

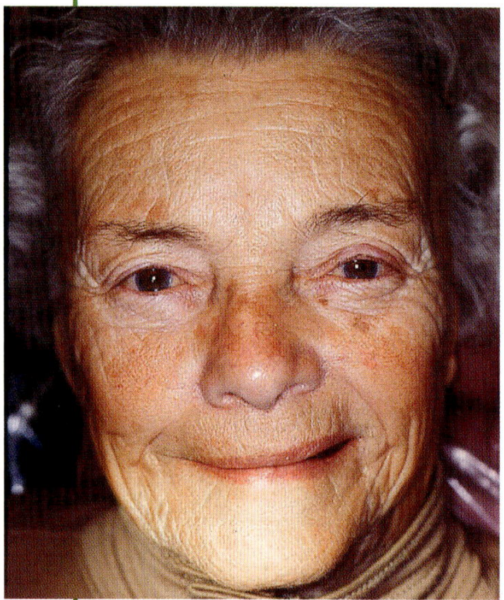

Fig. 6.9 Pre-treatment photo.

This 86-year-old woman (**Fig. 6.9**), now deceased, only spoke French. She came into my office with a young man who translated for her. However, he turned out to be a visiting medical student from France now going to Stanford Medical School as a transfer student, supposedly, and a friend of her family. He apparently was "engaged" to the patient after only being in the U.S. for 6 months, staying in her home, as well as being 32 years old. He was wearing a new Rolex watch and fine clothing on observation, which he bought with a gift from the patient. The patient was very well-off financially.

After my examination of this patient and my recommendations for a consultation, the young man spoke to the woman in French, which I speak little of, placing me at a disadvantage, and told me that he did not want the patient to spend the money for a full mouth reconstruction with implants and crowns. He wanted her to have an overdenture on both her upper and lower arches due to the lesser cost. In the meantime, I had some suspicions about this young man, in as much as he was controlling this patient's every move, as well as her money and dictating her treatment. The patient seemed to go along with her so-called fiancés suggestions for treatment. I later found out that the patient was paying for the young man's medical education as well. This told me that the young man had coerced or tricked the patient into giving him money on the pretense of loving her and wanting to marry her, thereby taking advantage of her with the knowledge of the fact that the patient was cognitively impaired.

I ended up doing the treatment he said she wanted. It was difficult, to say the least, and he paid cash for everything. There was both a marked improvement in her esthetics, bite and function. The patient seemed pleased with the treatment. I explained that she needed to return every four months to maintain her hygiene; however, I did not see her again for "four plus years", at which time she was brought in by a social worker.

After the initial treatment I did call the office of Adult Protective Services to report my suspicions as a mandated reporter of any kind of abuse. They were not allowed to tell me anything about what had happened after I reported the suspicions I had about the young fiancé.

When the social worker brought the patient in to see me some four years later, I found out that the young man had "hood-winked" the woman by lying about knowing her family, had not been going to medical school, which was a lie that he told her and everyone else he met with respect to being with her, and had no intention of marrying the patient. The police had apparently found out that he was a charlatan and had him deported and arrested upon his arrival in France. Meanwhile, the patient's dementia had progressed, and she did not realize that she even wore dentures, never taking them out to clean her mouth, nor did she see any dentist during her absence from my office. You can imagine what was underneath them at this juncture. Need I say more!

Note that the cast clasps on the exterior of the upper and lower dentures were placed there to help her remove the dentures due to the retention gained by the internal denture attachments. This treatment was less expensive than the other treatment I discussed and less invasive.

The woman had millions of dollars apparently, which the young man had designs on taking from her over time. Knowing that her dementia would limit her ability to make decisions for herself, as well as cause her demise soon enough, he would inherit her money at some point. I also found out that if I had not contacted Adult Protective Services when I did, they would have already taken a planned trip to the courthouse in Reno, Nevada, to get married.

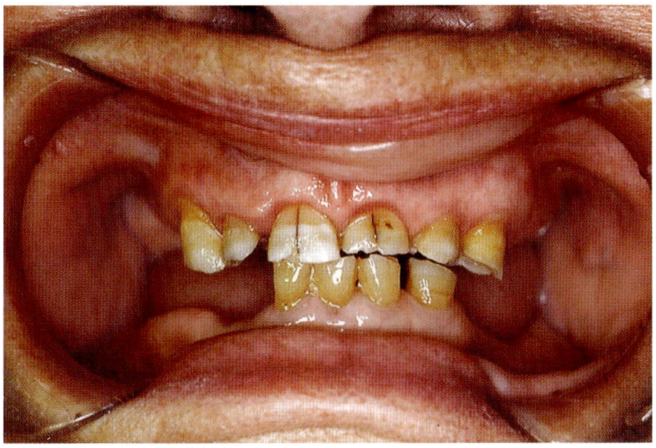

Fig. 6.10 Pre-treatment centric bite.

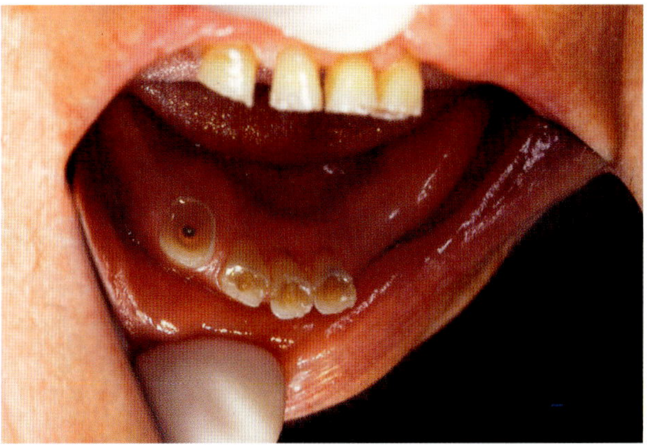

Fig. 6.11 Attrition due no posterior teeth.

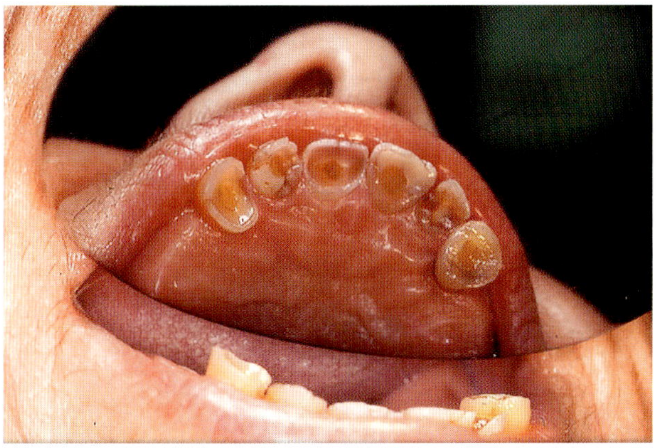

Fig. 6.12 Attrition on the lingual of the patient's upper teeth into calcified pulps.

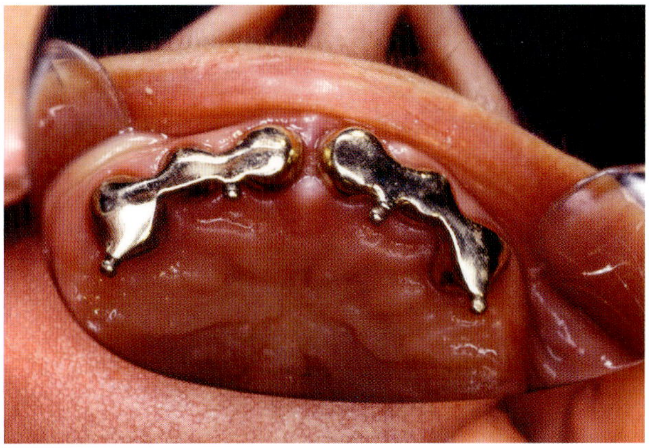

Fig. 6.13 Gold copings on her maxillary remaining teeth with attachments.

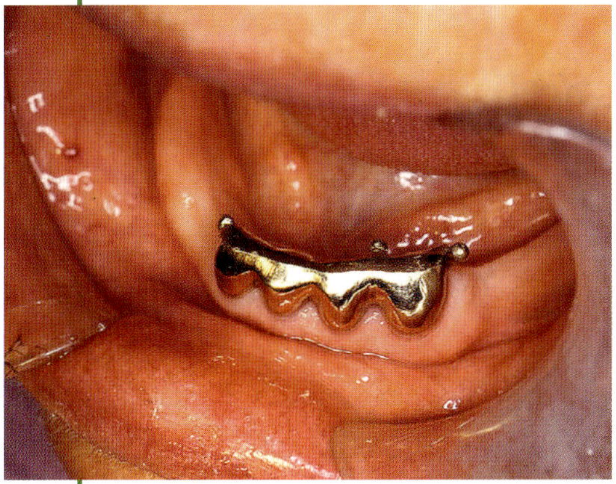

Fig. 6.14 Gold copings on patient's lower anterior teeth with attachments.

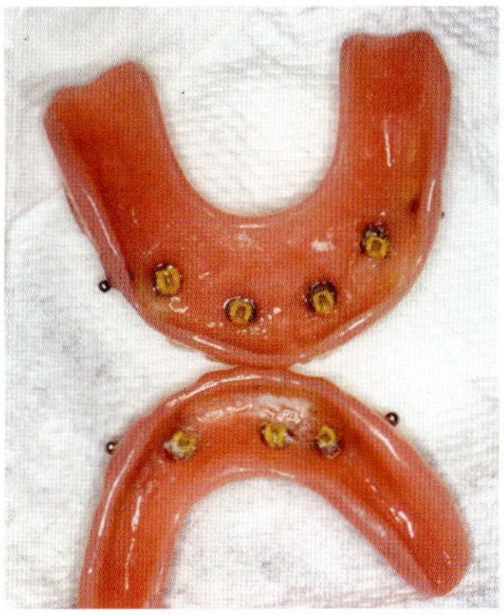

Fig. 6.15 Female attachments-upper and lower overdentures.

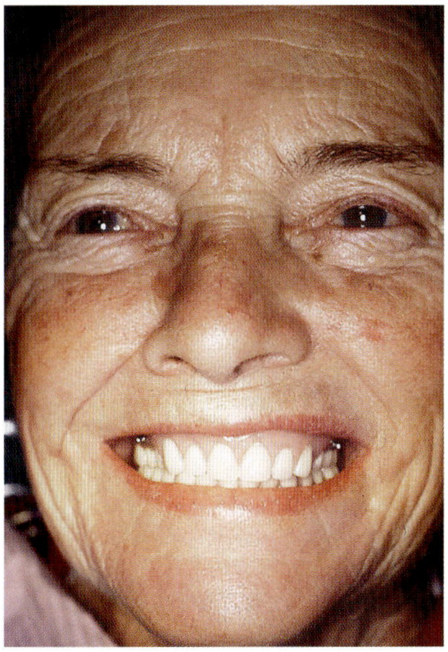

Fig. 6.16 Finished case of upper and lower overdentures.

She now had enough money to support her with caring people who gave her the necessary assistance to the end of her days (**Figs. 6.10-6.16**).

I had to sit down and think about this patient and what I had done to treat her, in lieu of the manipulation of the young man. I believe I did her a good service in treating her, as well as reporting what I suspected was a fraudulent person taking advantage of her. In hindsight, should I have not treated her and reported the fiancé first? I was young myself at that time and just learning, but I knew enough to realize that something was not right about the entire personal situation; however, I also knew that the dentistry was necessary and helpful in the long run. You can analyze your cases after-the-fact for years to come and never know if you did the correct treatment in the face of all the information you had in hand. But it is a good habit to get into doing. That is how we learn what to do and what not to do in the face of adversity. It is all about experience. I tell my students that there are no mistakes, only experience. Good judgment comes from experience, and experience comes from bad judgment.

This case shows the importance of including a **social history** with all the other histories that we take and utilize to analyze the pieces of the "puzzle" that each patient brings us. Being at a disadvantage by not speaking the language of the patient is difficult, besides dealing with a charlatan caregiver, who was supposedly someone the patient knew for a long time in this case and trusted (according to the young man). It Is important to assess all the information we receive and then analyze if you need more input in order to make a good **Outline for Treatment**. Each case is its own entity and brings with it a different essence and learning situation before, during and after treatment. Do not be afraid to ask yourself questions about your feelings in these matters and about whether you feel comfortable treating any patient. Your biggest challenge will be yourself in the end.

Case Study 3

65-Year-Old Woman with Esthetic Concerns

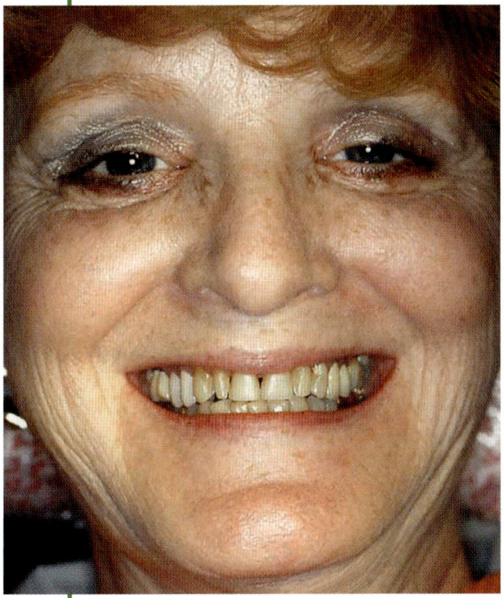

Fig. 6.17 Pre-treatment smile.

This patient (**Fig. 6.17**) was the office manager of a dental practice in my area. The dentist that she worked for called me and asked me to do a work-up on her for treatment. He stated he knew of my ability to do cosmetic dentistry and that I was an equitable and honest person. He then told me that he felt it was a conflict of interest for him to treat her because he was going to ask her to marry him. He did mention that he was in his late seventies and felt that he could not do the kind of work he knew that I did at this point in his life. The patient was in her mid-60's.

I agreed to see her and do a treatment work-up once I ascertained what his intended wife wanted to do to her mouth. She made an appointment for me to examine her, bringing recent full mouth radiographs and study models her dentist/future husband provided for her.

The patient was an attractive woman in good general health, yet desired to change her smile to be even more appealing and younger looking to her future new husband, a dental practitioner, whom she had worked with for almost 30 years as his office assistant and now manager. She had generalized recession with bone loss, poor homecare, especially in the lower anterior area, as evidenced by the presence of calculus and some failing restorations. After my examination, study models and photos, I did a wax-up on a duplicate study model of what I thought she would look like with porcelain laminate veneers. She immediately accepted treatment without any further discussion and told me that her "intended" would pay for all the work I was to do.

The day she presented for treatment, she had two black eyes, bruised cheeks, a swollen nose and steri-strips on her face in various places, as well as a bandage under her chin wrapped upward over the top of her head. She would not let me take photos of her at this juncture in her treatment. Apparently, there was some urgency in her desire to have a face lift, a rhinoplasty, a chin tuck, and a partial eye lift and whatever else she could do to cosmetically improve on her beauty in a timely manner, since the wedding was only weeks away! Did she have to do this before my treatment with her I asked?! She made an immediate statement upon getting into my dental chair and that was "Whatever you do, don't touch my face!" I retorted, "How am I supposed to restore your mouth and front 10 teeth in the upper and six teeth in your lower jaw without touching your face!?" I told her I could not do the work until she was completely healed. She told me that she had a timeline "crunch" necessitating having all this treatment at once. She apologized for surprising me with her plastic surgery adventures. After her persistent emotional cries and crying, I broke down, against my better judgment, and did the preparations and impressions of her teeth after I prepared them without touching her face, other than her lips. I found it exceedingly difficult not to be able to do my best work, I thought, not being allowed to rest on any part of her face, especially not being able to retract her lips at all. I got the job done, but it was most exhausting for me and my staff. At that point I was upset with myself for not charging more for the treatment after the fact.

Because I only restored the upper and lower anterior teeth, I was not able to fully equalize her occlusion, which would have required removing some of the gold onlays and crowns her dentist/employer/future husband had previously placed many years before. Since she had recession on her upper and lower anterior teeth, I had to extend the veneers onto the root surfaces of her teeth without disturbing the minimally attached gingiva that she had, making her teeth appear slightly longer than they were before, and hidden somewhat by her lips when she smiled (**Figs. 6.18-6.21**).

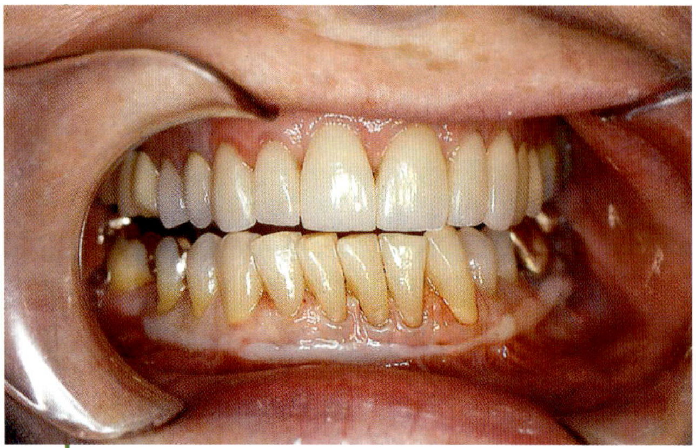

Fig. 6.18 Pre-treatment close-up on lower anterior/finished max veneers.

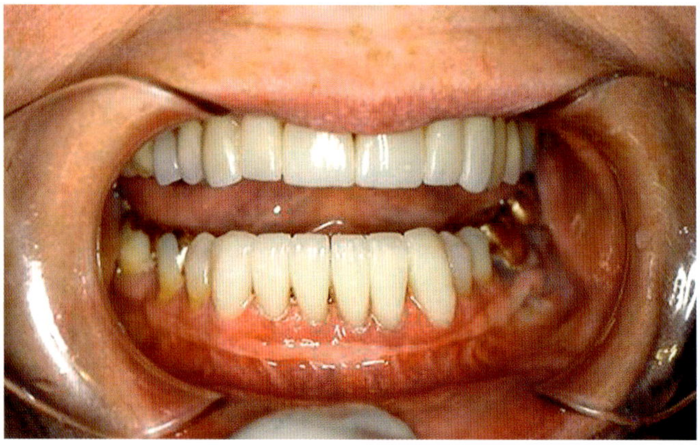

Fig. 6.19 Final placement of the porcelain laminate veneers.

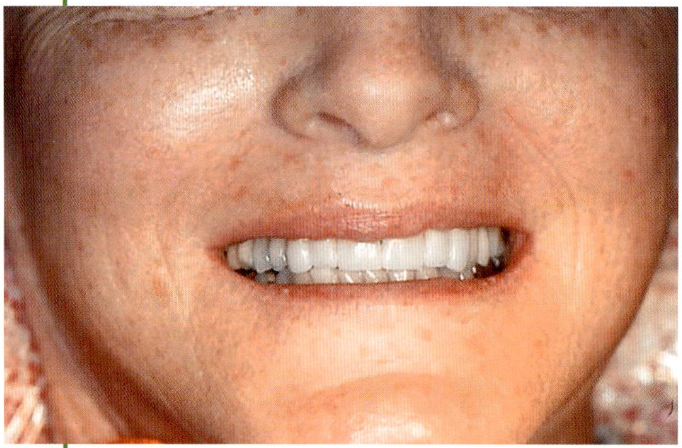

Fig. 6.20 Post-dental treatment and facial cosmetic surgery.

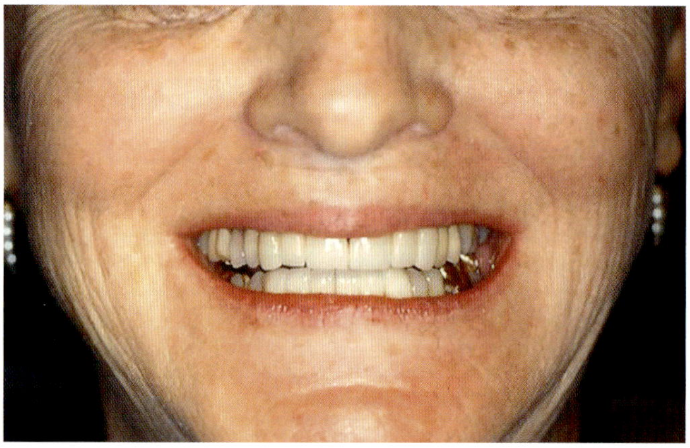

Fig. 6.21 Photo of the patient's smile after dental treatment and plastic facial eye surgery and other facial enhancements.

I learned from this case not to try to do any "favor" for another dentist in treating his future wife without really getting to know her first. Yes, I did a history on her, but did not discover her neurosis about her lack of beauty, her personal habits regarding this neurotic urge that apparently was a persistent one, and her feelings of personal inadequacy. I believe there may have been a demand by her future husband as well for her to be younger looking and even more attractive than she already was in a more natural way. These things can come back to haunt one in the future, both the patient and the dentist for agreeing to do the treatment in the first place. I only did two favors for other dentists with cosmetics in my entire career. The second time I did it on an already magnificent, beautiful women who had orthodontic treatment and wanted her mouth to be ideal looking. I did a full mouth rehabilitation on her, and it was most successful.

Still, I had reservations about seeing this second patient for cosmetics, basing my treatment with her on the previous neurotic patient, who made demands on me that were restrictive and could have impaired my treatment of her with a less favorable result if I were not so skilled as to avoid this happening. As I stated before, **always study the situation before you endeavor to treat** and **know before you go**, with respect to your patient.

Case Study 4

80-Year-Old Man with a Collapsed Bite and Worn Teeth

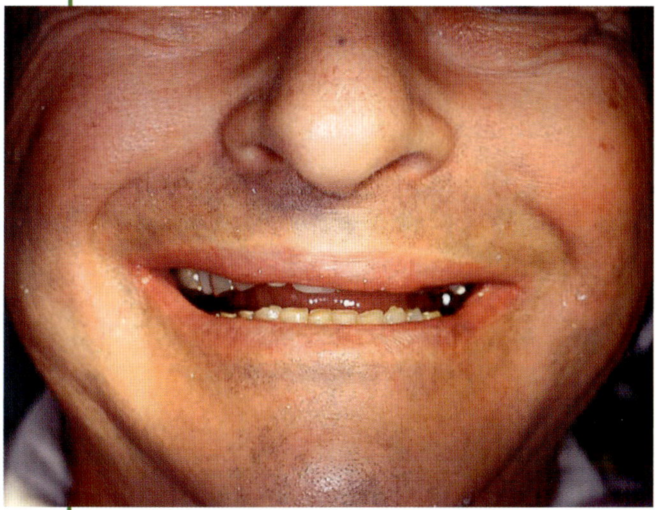

Fig. 6.22 Pre-treatment smile with worn teeth.

This 80-year-old gentleman (Fig. 6.22) was a physician and married to a slightly younger woman, aged 75, who had recently died. After his wife of many years passed away, he decided to sell his home, move into an independent living community and make himself more presentable so he could find another partner. He had some medical issues with hypertension and prostate hyperplasia, but nothing that would impede his having his teeth restored to a more esthetic situation (Fig. 6.23).

This patient was an ideal person to work with dentally. He had a high dental IQ, a relatively healthy mouth, knew what he wanted and had the means to do the treatment financially. He was "**goal oriented**". This is an important concept in restoring any person's teeth.

Firstly, one must have the **intrinsic knowledge** of what they desire. In the case of this physician, he desired to look more handsome and youthful. Secondly, one needs **persistence** in maintaining and following through with their goals. Obviously, he made an appointment after thinking about what he wanted to do with his critical thinking about himself. All too often "Life gets in the way of one's best intentions" and our goals somehow get pushed aside. The same thing happens with our "**inner-child**". Life and the restrictions put on us as children through adulthood, in terms of rules, laws, mores and other modalities that restrict our nascent playfulness and curiosity, happen. If we are lucky enough to remember what our unrealized goals are, we can go back and harness those goals and make plans to achieve them. The third item one must have then is **a plan**. In this case, since I restored this man's now deceased wife's mouth in good fashion, he felt he should follow suit and see me for his concerns, in essence this was one of his goals, he decided what part of his plan he wanted to complete, and he followed through with it (Figs. 6.24-6.28).

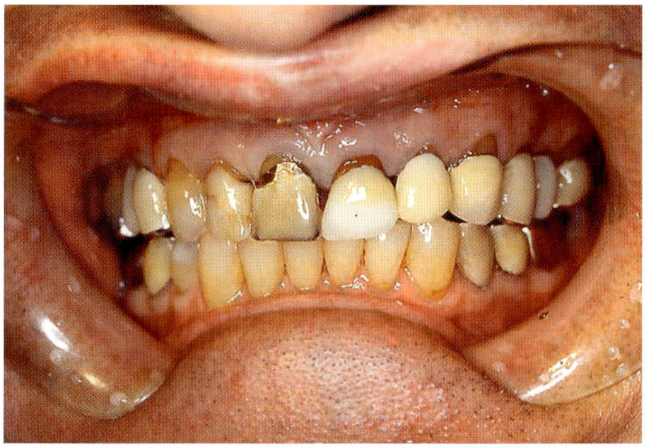

Fig. 6.23 Pre-treatment photo showing worn crowns, recession, decreased vertical dimension and poor esthetics.

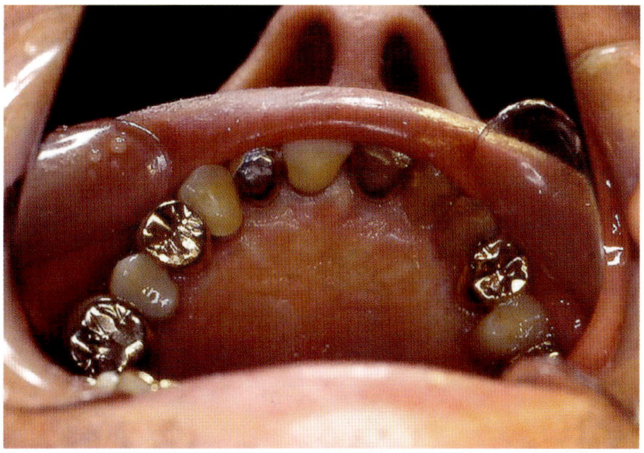

Fig. 6.24 Pre-treatment palatal view of the maxillary anterior teeth.

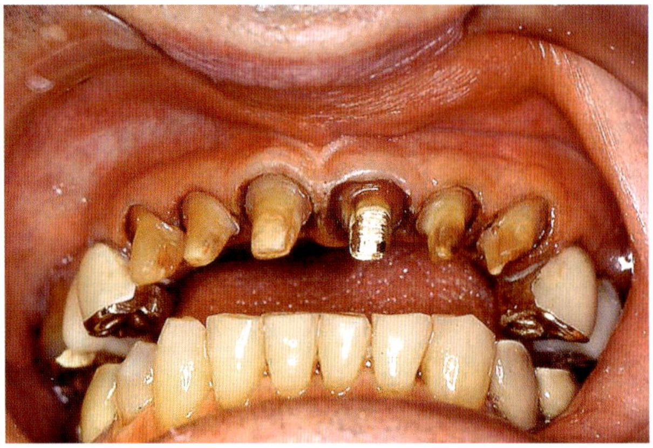

Fig. 6.25 Maxillary anterior preparations for new crowns.

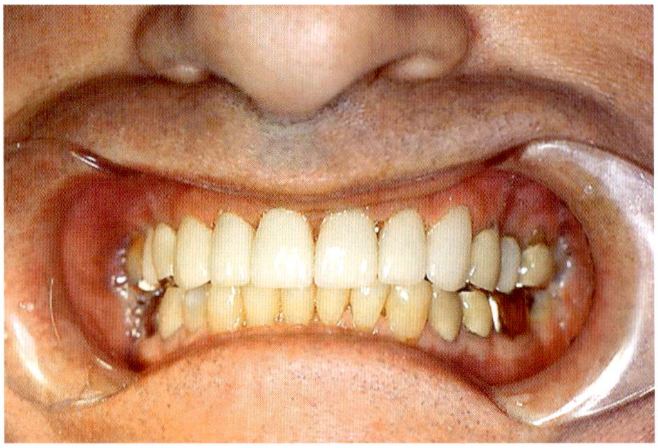

Fig. 6.26 Placement of new anterior crowns with much improved esthetics.

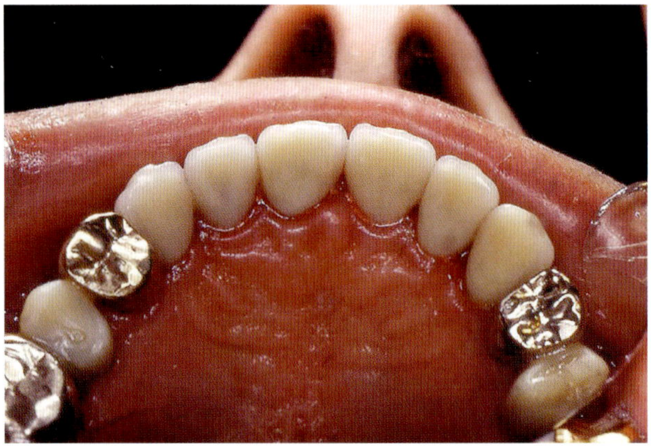

Fig. 6.27 Completed all porcelain crowns cuspid to cuspid-palatal view.

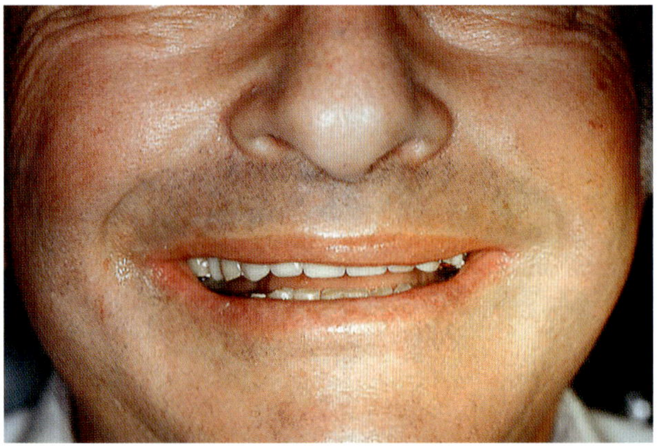

Fig. 6.28 New smile for the Doctor... a "Happy Camper".

All too often people do not make plans, especially if they have an emergency dental issue. It is more of an immediate need. We are looking at fine lines between, needs, wants and desires when making plans and we must **prioritize** all these things in the process of completing our goals. This is the number four in the scheme of following through with the decision-making process. Finally, **trust** is the ultimate decision-making factor with respect to completing one's goals. There must be **mutual respect** between the practitioner and the patient to have trust for one another. Once these things are clear in one's mind, the patient can move forward in completing their goals. In this case, the doctor was willing to become the patient and have his desires recognized and his appearance improved.

Case Study 5

84-Year-Old Woman Who Wanted to "Eat Apples Again" (Now Deceased)

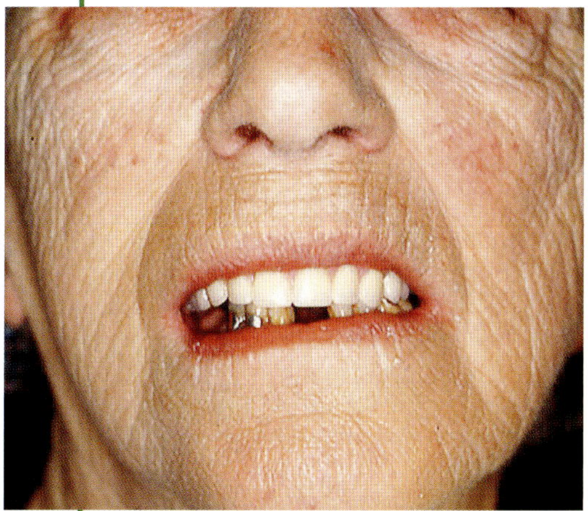

Fig. 6.29 Pre-treatment smile.

This lady wore a full upper denture (**Fig. 6.29**) and had many missing teeth on the mandibular arch. Her goal was to eat apples and taste them again by biting directly into them. For years she had to "mush" them up to eat them like apple sauce, telling me that she had dreamed of the day she could "bite" into an apple and hard food and not have her dentures dislodge. She had an unremarkable medical history, except for some previous eye surgery in her left eye and, upon dental examination, she had probably the best bone-retained edentulous ridges I have seen in a long time. She had mostly calcified roots on her lower teeth with no active caries and no upper teeth. The most important issue here was her inability to be social due to her oral concerns. As a "shut-in", she would run the risk of becoming cognitively impaired, depressed and subjecting herself to a depressed immune system as well as malnutrition. Her goal was mostly over her functional issues, as she was not aware of how her lack of edibility of certain foods affected her nutritional issues, mental health and overall general health in the end.

This lovely patient had issues with retention of her upper denture when biting into almost anything. The denture was large and since she had basically no posterior lower teeth, I discussed a lower overdenture with her because she wanted an implant supported overdenture on her maxillary arch. Balanced occlusion was the goal here. I had given her at least five treatment options and she mixed and matched what I had given her with respect to her financial ability to pay for treatment (**Figs. 6.30-6.32**).

Her lower teeth were beveled at the gingival crest (**Fig. 6.33**). She had calcified roots on teeth #20, 21, 22, 27 and 28. Teeth #23 and 26 were endodontically treated and had an amalgam core placed into them and then beveled. Both teeth #22 and 27 had Zest female attachments cemented into them. There was no evidence of decay on any of her remaining teeth. A lower overdenture was fabricated with Zest anchors that "snapped" into the cemented female attachments of the cuspids which were sunk into the calcified root canals. This was relatively inexpensive for her and functional. This was her primary goal in getting the treatment in the first place.

The maxillary arch was a complicated issue for her. She debated long and hard between getting dental implants and fixed prosthetic crowns or copings with implants and a full, screwed-in overdenture for maximum retention. This meant that she would have to come back every four to six months, have the upper denture unscrewed and her

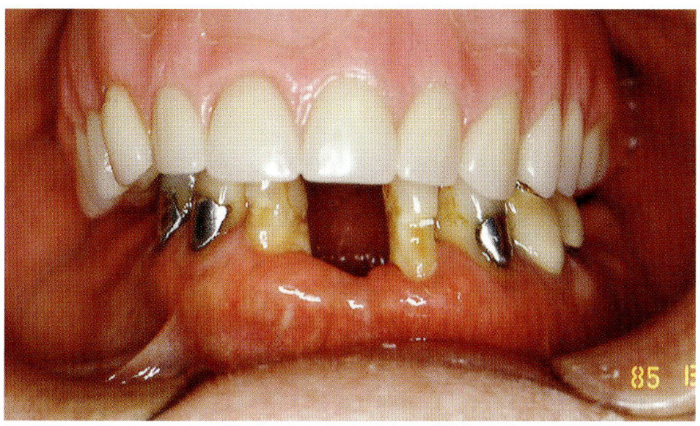

Fig. 6.30 Maxillary denture and missing lower anterior teeth.

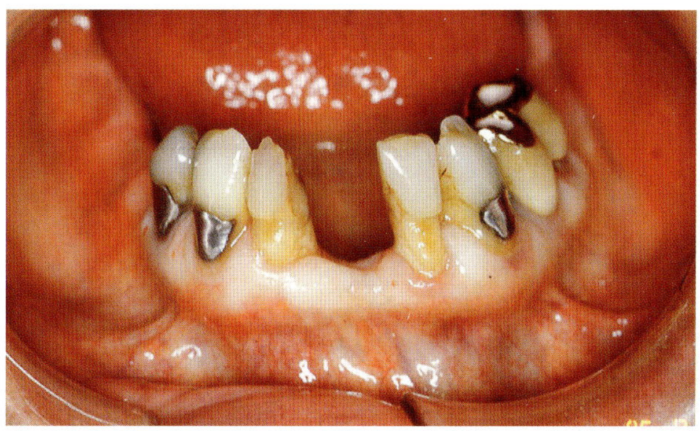

Fig. 6.31 Lower arch with missing teeth, bone loss, fractured teeth, failing restorations and recession.

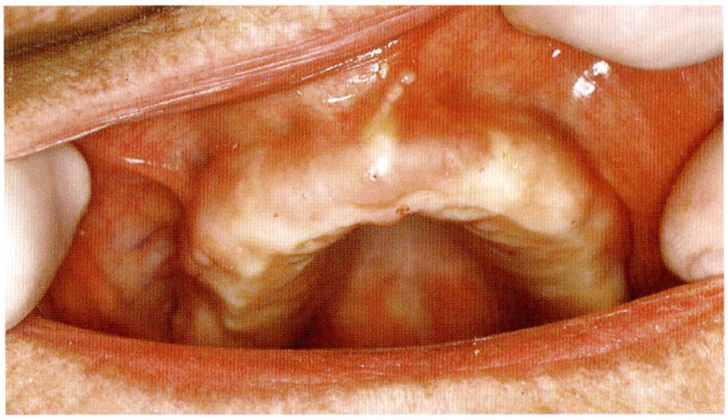

Fig. 6.32 Large bony maxillary edentulous ridge.

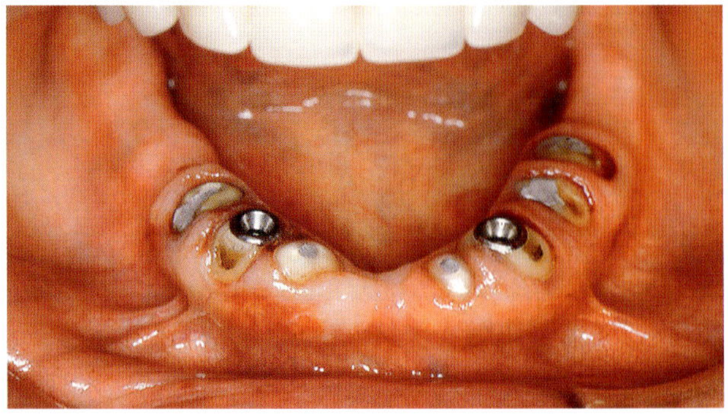

Fig. 6.33 Lower ridge restored conservatively.

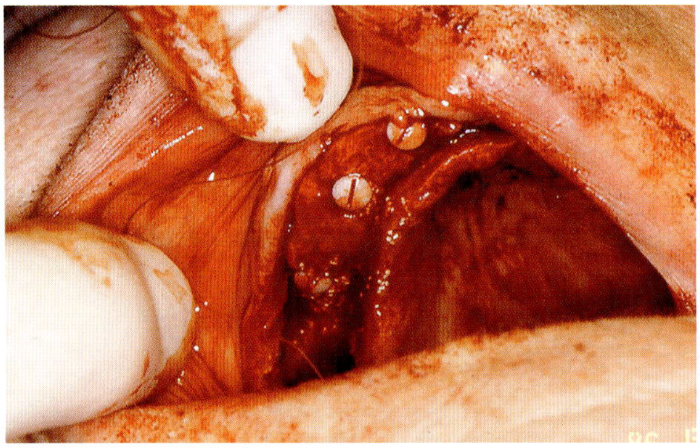

Fig. 6.34 Photo of placing the implants in the maxillary arch. (Calcitek® Implant with internal hex design.)

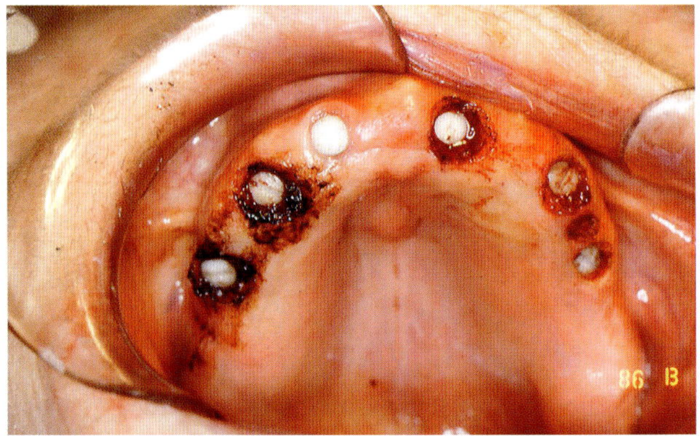

Fig. 6.35 Second stage surgery uncovering the implants with healing screws in place.

implants cleaned, and then have the denture screwed back in and acrylic placed over the screws. In the time frame that this case was done, we did not have CBCT (Cone Beam Computerized Tomography) to determine the exact position of placement of the implants based on four axis (horizontal, vertical and two oblique views from either side of the ridge) and a stent to work through made from the CBCT itself. The CBCT told us the width, length, depth and angle of the ridge, so there was no guessing as to where to place the implants. In this case, we had to use our two-dimensional radiographs and our Panorex, as well as making a full flap to expose the ridge, and our fingers and eyeballs for placing the implants (**Figs. 6.34-6.38**). In our more modern world, using an Itero® guide makes it easy, fast and efficient. There are no incisions, only a tissue punch through the guide with a healing attachment placed at the end of the procedure, making this a one-step surgery as compared to a two-step surgery in the past, whereby the implant needed to be uncovered and a healing attachment placed 4-6 months post-placement.

This patient went through a lot of effort to have this treatment and it was a success because it met her goals. She could finally eat solid foods, especially an apple, without any hesitation or expectation that her denture would fall out of her mouth (**Fig. 6.39**). She was able to eat in public again and be social, this being an especially important factor in maintaining continued good health and longevity for all of us, but especially for this patient. Her speech was good after adjusting her vertical dimension and finite occlusion and she had teeth that were "her" size that functioned well and were esthetically pleasing to her. She did come back every four months for me to remove the screws in her implant abutments, so I could clean them for her. This went on with this schedule for about one and a half to two years. Unbeknownst to me, and possibly to the patient, was that she had some form of underlying, undiagnosed cancer that caused her death about two years after she had her dental work completed. All in all, she was incredibly happy, content and could not thank me enough for what I did for her. Her goals were met, and I was happy for her.

On the other hand, this treatment was very intense due to the number of steps one had to take to get the result I did. It was a difficult learning situation for me in the end.

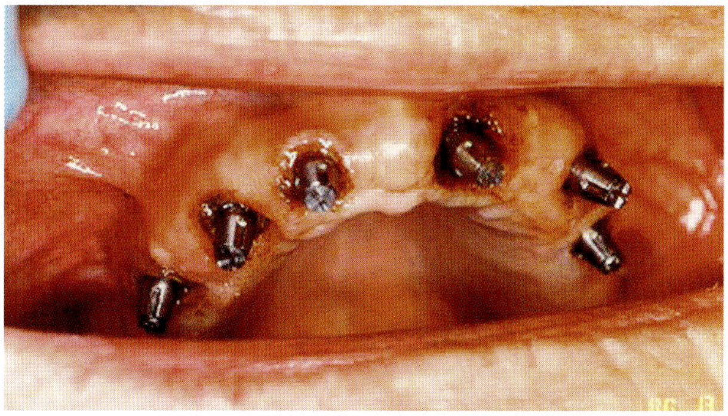

Fig. 6.36 Abutments placed in the maxillary implants.

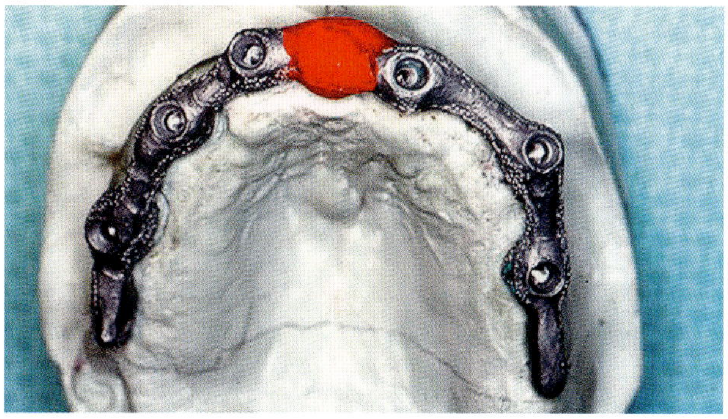

Fig. 6.37 Fabricated overdenture bar.

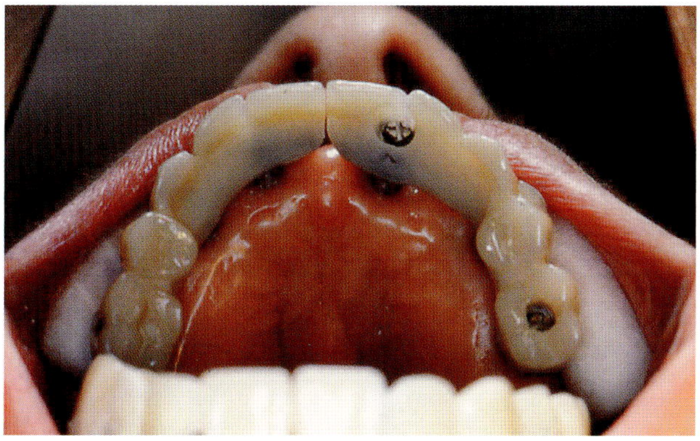

Fig. 6.38 Fabricated fixed implant supported overdenture off the palate with screws into implants.

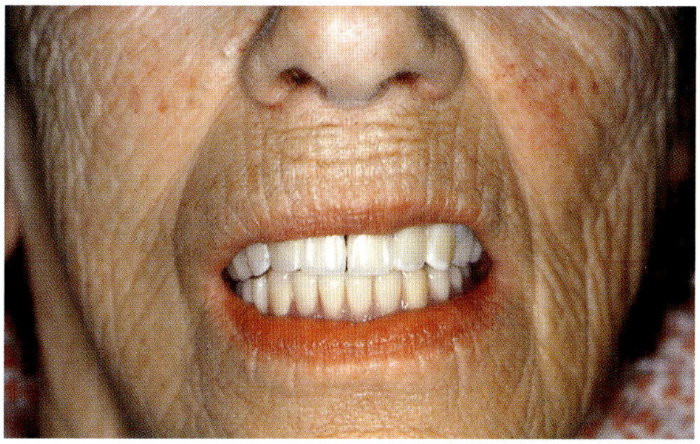

Fig. 6.39 Final photo of completed treatment.

Initial study models were taken and mounted, as well as studied. Radiographs were taken and studied. An Outline of Treatment recommendations was made for five separate treatment plans from fixed restorative over implants in the form of crowns and bridges, as well as fixed restorative on the lower arch, as well to another type of upper full denture and a partial denture on the lower arch. It was difficult for the patient to decide about what she wanted based on her budget, even though she had the resources to do the "top-of-the-line" treatment. She wanted to leave some of her savings to her children and this affected her decision making with respect to this treatment.

Her main goal was to bite into an apple again... She trusted my education on the subject at hand and each treatment plan I presented. She trusted my mixing and matching what treatment might be best for her budget as well. Ultimately, making an adequate decision for herself. However, she needed to be educated about the hygiene consequences for each treatment she selected or asked questions about. I told her no matter what, to protect her investment, her hygiene schedule would be every four months. I also told her and taught her about flossing with threaders under the maxillary overdenture using interproximal brushes and fluoride gel on her lower teeth. I taught her how to clean her female attachments on the lower arch, as well as the rest of her teeth and her lower overdenture. I gave her the knowledge she did not have to set her own goals by adopting my information and integrating it into her own personal hygiene processes.

Research has found that when the goal level is held constant, which is implicitly assumed under **Expectancy Theory**, higher expectancies lead to higher levels of performance. Across goal levels, lower expectancies, associated with higher goal levels, are associated with higher performance levels.[1]

The concept of self-efficacy is extremely important after a full mouth rehabilitation. When goals are self-set, people with high self-efficacy set higher goals than do people with lower self-efficacy. They also are more committed to assigned goals like a hygiene regimen and find and use better task strategies to attain the goals, as well as respond more positively to negative feedback than do people with low self-efficacy.[2] When patients are trained in the proper strategies, those given specific high-performance goals are more likely to utilize those strategies than people given other types of goals; hence, their performance improves.[3]

These concepts are good to remember in the face of teaching patients about themselves and how important it is for "them" to adhere to their own goal setting around prevention of oral disease.

Case Study 6

55-Year-Old Edentulous Woman with an Atrophic Mandibular Ridge

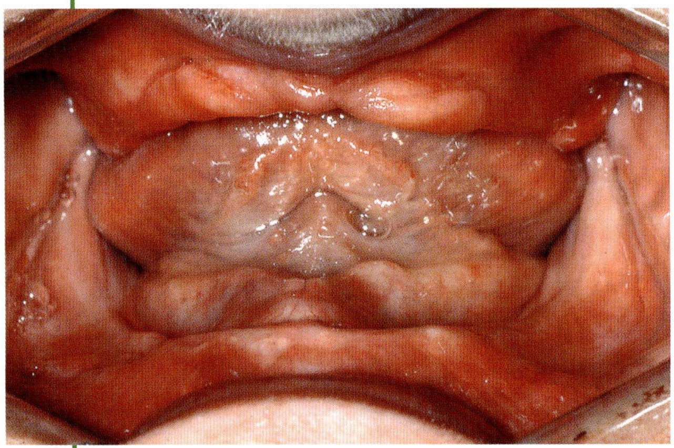

Fig. 6.40 Pre-treatment photo showing minimal bone support and no attached gingiva.

This patient (**Fig. 6.40**) presented with a "floating" lower denture for at least 25 years. In all that time, she never had a reline or a replacement. Most dentures should be relined periodically when physiologic changes happen, such as weight loss or gain due to any reasons and be considered for replacement anywhere from 5-7 years for them to fit properly, maintain continued oral health and function, as well as not be the foci of a plethora of bacteria and fungi that can live within the porous acrylic base, possibly causing a multitude of systemic diseases. Patients and clinicians need to be aware of the capacity of denture-borne microorganisms to cause oral/systemic diseases. Patients who wear removeable prosthetic dentures, overdentures or partial dentures need to be educated about sanitizing procedures to reduce the reservoir of microorganisms, not only in the mouth, but embedded in their prosthetic devices. Scrubbing an acrylic base of these prostheses produces a myriad of "micro scratches" that increase the surface area for microorganisms to colonize.[4] Soaking dentures in a "denture cleaner", like Polident® or Efferdent® for 20 minutes a day or more, is recommended for proper oral hygiene. Scrubbing dentures is NOT recommended because it makes micro-scratches in the denture acrylic, giving oral bacteria and fungi a greater surface area in which to propagate, thus, causing the possibility or increased oral and /or systemic disease to arise.

She was a nurse and had a high dental IQ. She had worn dentures since her twenties and, at this point in her life, she wanted something more stable in her mouth, as well as something more esthetically pleasing. After a consultation with an oral surgeon, he suggested that to accommodate this patient's lack of bone and attached gingiva, it was in her best interest to consider a mandibular staple implant, that is, a subperiosteal and intramandibular type implant (**Fig. 6.41**) requiring an incision under her chin (**Fig. 6.42**) and the placement of the "staple" through the inferior part of the jaw at the symphysis into the mouth. This is quite a different kind of implant and a more radical procedure, much more complicated than a single intrabony implant placement procedure. The patient agreed to his recommendation for treatment after numerous questions about discomfort, length of healing time, cost, stability and anything else one can think of to ask.

These titanium abutment posts are connected to the submandibular bar (**Fig. 6.43**) and are screwed into the substructure posts. A skin graft was placed around the abutments in order to increase the size of the attached gingiva and give stability to the surrounding tissue as much as possible. Impressions were taken and a gold Hader Bar with attachments was fabricated (**Fig. 6.44**) and cemented to the abutments to support an overdenture (**Fig. 6.45**).

Although this case was planned and instrumented at the behest of the patient and the mechanics that were done were successful, the case turned out to be a failure. These things do happen. It was not so much a failure by the oral surgeon, who did the surgery, or me in doing the prosthetics, as well as assisting with the surgery; the failure was in

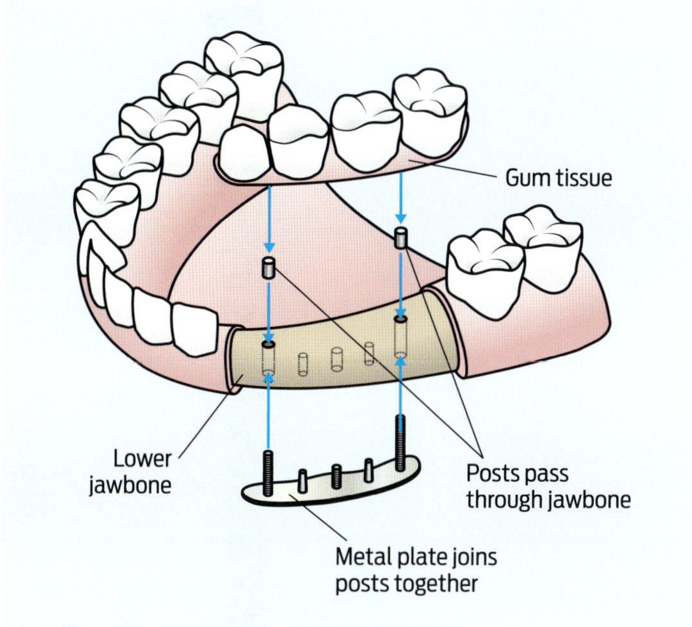

Fig. 6.41 Schematic illustration of the subperiosteal/mandibular staple implant placement.

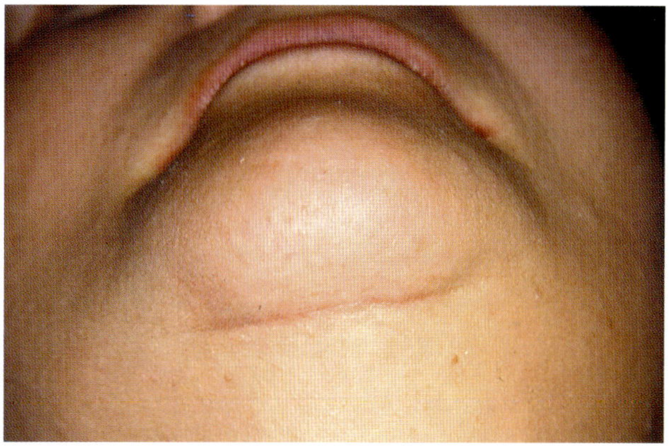

Fig. 6.42 Placement incision with a submental access.

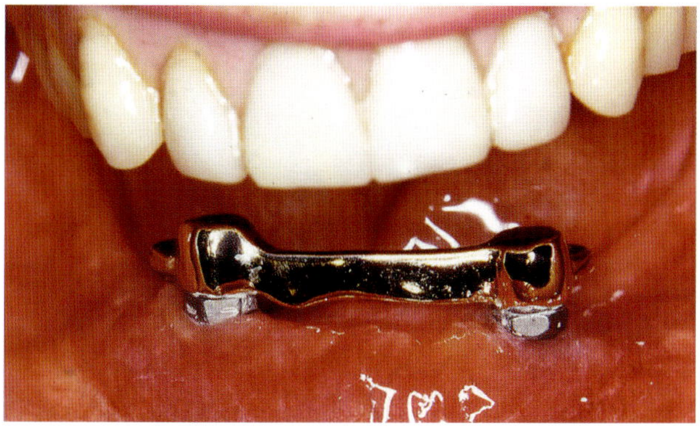

Fig. 6.43 Intraoral posts of mandibular staple implant with skin graft for tissue stability.

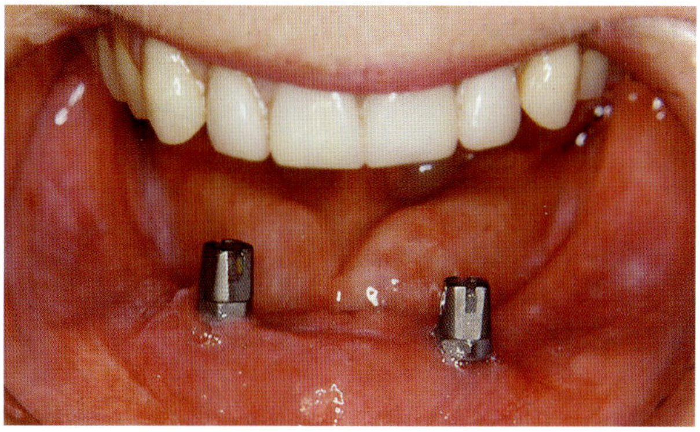

Fig. 6.44 Cast Gold Hader Bar with attachments with healing skin graft.

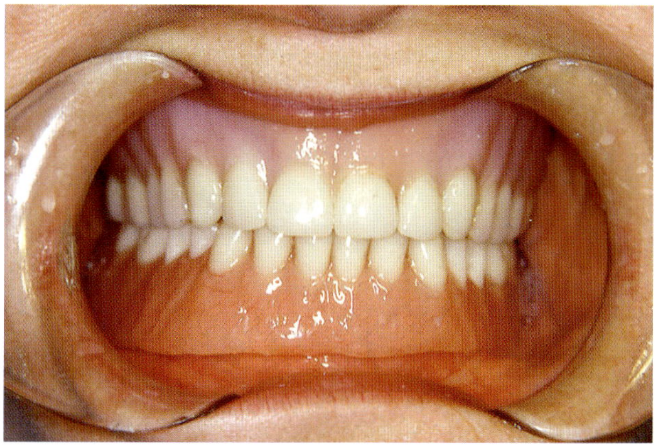

Fig. 6.45 New upper denture and lower overdenture with increased vertical dimension and enhanced esthetics.

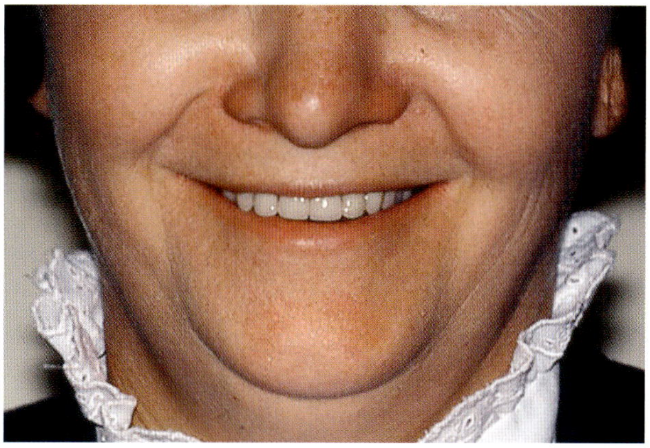

Fig. 6.46 Smiling patient with completed prosthetics.

the instrument itself, that is, the Transosteal Implant or Mandibular Staple itself. This patient was incredibly pleased with her results as were the operators who made it possible. She got herself transferred to a hospital in Oregon and left California to start a new life for herself with her new job and her new "looks" (**Fig. 6.46**). Almost a year to the day that her surgery was completed, the vertical strut on one side of the Mandibular Staple fractured and broke in half. She had called me to tell me her sad story. I do not know the how's and why's of the matter, whether she was hit in the jaw or was trying to bite something that was too hard for her; there was no way to discern what caused it because neither myself nor the oral surgeon were with her when the fracture occurred. Eventually, the patient saw another oral surgeon in Oregon and had the Mandibular Staple replaced. I never saw or heard from her again. Failure or not? There is no room for failure, but it happens. Failure to me is only experience, which assists me in my ability to make good judgment calls when treatment planning or discussing treatment with my patients. This is learning in its highest form. This was the one and only mandibular staple overdenture I did in my professional career.

To me, this case was a philosophical failure, in as much as this patient had a great result from my end of treatment, but the length of time that she could enjoy her goal of becoming more beautiful and functional was not the expectation that neither the patient, the oral surgeon nor myself had for her. Nothing lasts forever, but this was too short a time interval from the time that her treatment was finished to when it had to be redone. In my head and in my heart, I knew that I did a good job. There is no accounting for equipment failures or technical failures in dental materials, it is an unpredictable entity for the most part. I felt badly for the patient and told her my feelings about the situation. She was understanding and accepting, which allowed me to assuage my sadness and disappointment from this incident.

Case Study 7

68-Year-Old Male with Missing Teeth and Congenital Malocclusion

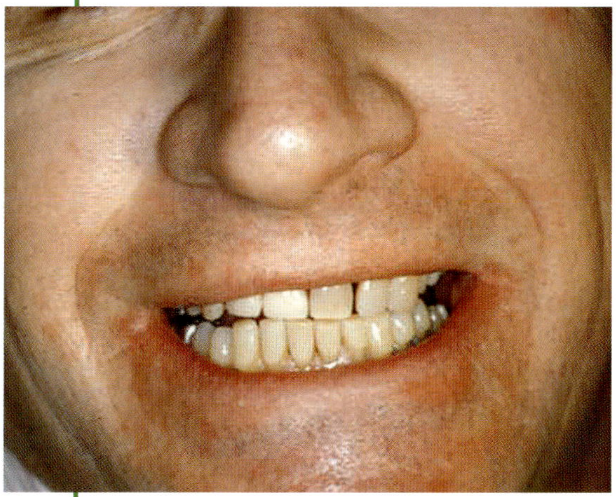

Fig. 6.47 Pre-treatment smile.

This patient (**Fig. 6.47**) was a very tall and large in stature, successful businessman. He had previous trauma to his mouth and unequal bony ridges on the maxillary arch as well as on the mandibular arch. He had trouble keeping his maxillary stay plate in place and was tired of the way he looked. After a full examination, radiographs, study models, "outlining" my findings and making numerous treatment plans, we both came to a consensus after listening to his wants, desires and goals for oral care options.

This was an extremely complicated case (**Fig. 6.48**). The patient wanted something more stable and esthetic. I discussed his seeing my oral surgeon to get an opinion on upper and lower osteotomies to even out his ridges and equalize how his jaws could align in a normal manner, which they were not even close to at this juncture. Finances were not an issue with him, but because these types of surgeries are so costly, he wanted to know if his dental insurance company would help foot-the-bill, which they ultimately did not. Under the circumstances, he wanted me to do a radical full mouth rehabilitation, which was and would be both challenging for me to do with a combination of dental implants, maintaining his remaining teeth for support, and making copings for some of them and crowns and esthetic porcelain restorations for others, as well as equalizing his occlusion in a mouth that did not fit together well from the beginning.

This seemed like a recipe for disaster. But I was young and adventurous and had the attitude that I could tackle any issues that came my way. Little did I know that this patient and myself would be linked together forever more after this treatment (**Figs. 6.49-6.53**).

The patient wanted to be conservative and, instead of fixed bridges, he changed his mind and opted for a precision lower partial denture (**Fig. 6.54**) at the last minute. Which I did for him (**Figs. 6.55, 6.56**). He had the money to do anything he wanted but told me in confidence that he was going to buy a house and get married again to a younger woman and that his teeth took a back seat to pleasing his newly married wife.

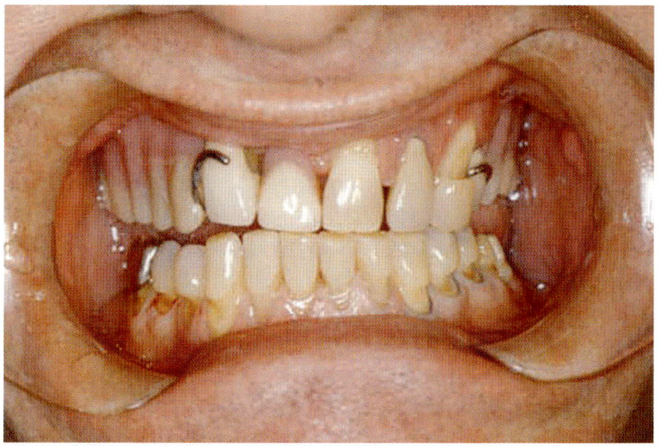

Fig. 6.48 This was his centric bite with his upper stayplate-partial denture and lower teeth exemplifying recession, attrition, malocclusion and failing restorations.

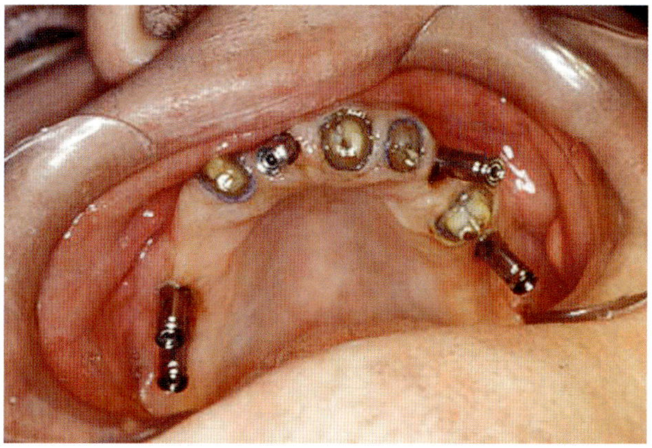

Fig. 6.49 The maxillary arch after placing a minimal number of implants (5) in the edentulous areas and preparing his remaining teeth for copings with attachments.

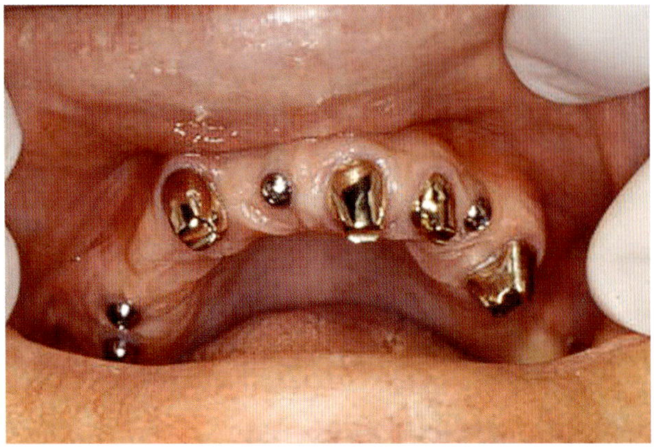

Fig. 6.50 Maxillary arch with mixed prosthetics: gold copings with rests and Healing screws on five implants to be utilized for retention of the final prosthesis.

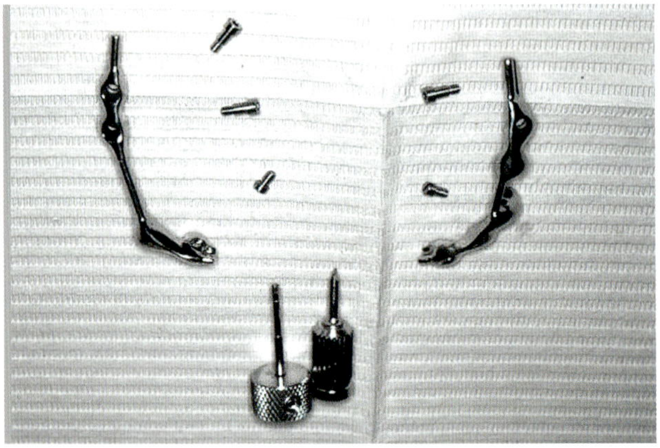

Fig. 6.51 Superstructure for maxillary stabilization, including custom screws for placement of the bars into the implants for stability.

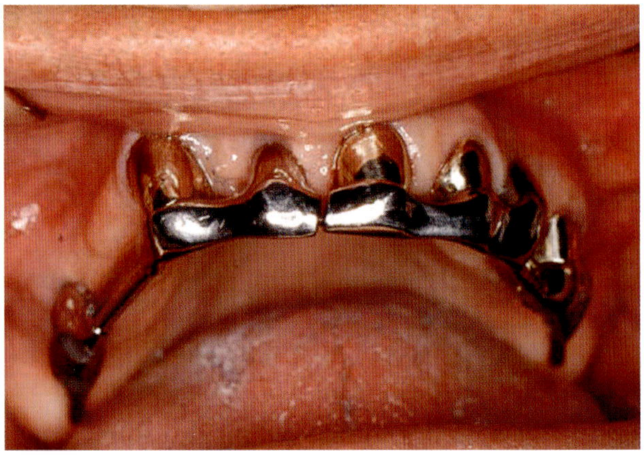

Fig. 6.52 The finished superstructure screwed into the underlying implants.

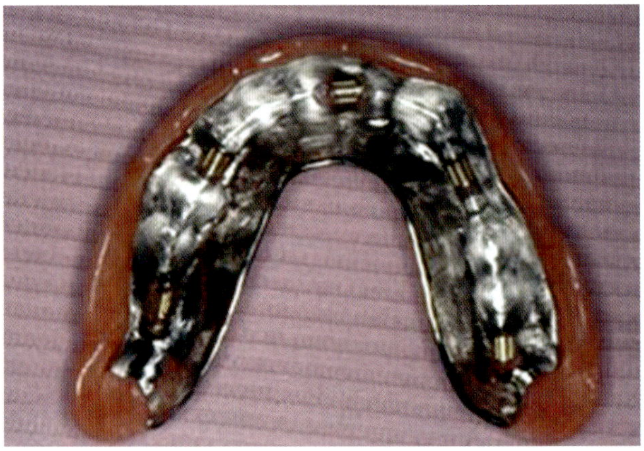

Fig. 6.53 Maxillary overdenture with retention clips for the superstructure supported by implants.

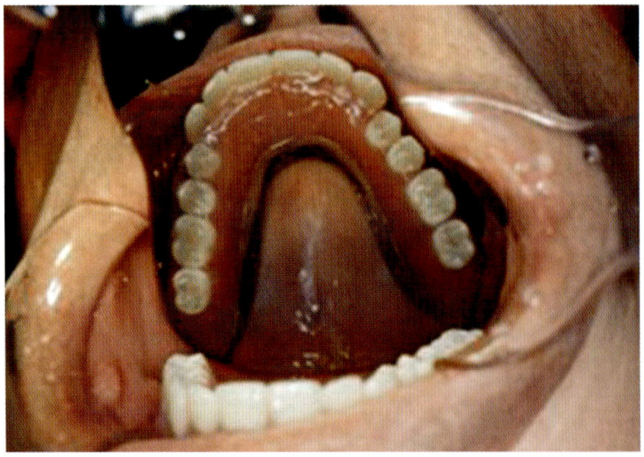

Fig. 6.54 Maxillary overdenture attached with open palate.

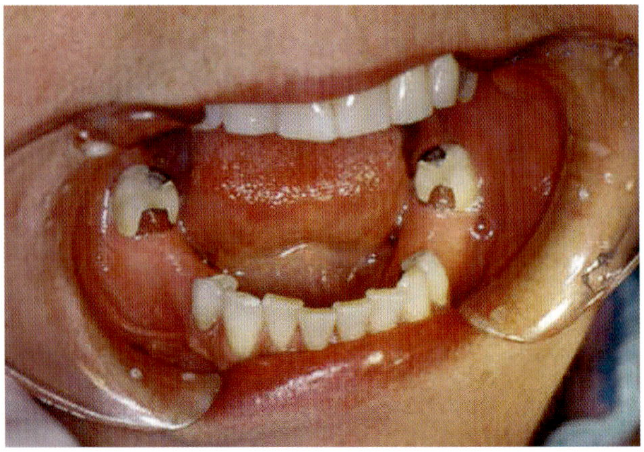

Fig. 6.55 Lower distal new porcelain fused to metal crowns with precision attachments.

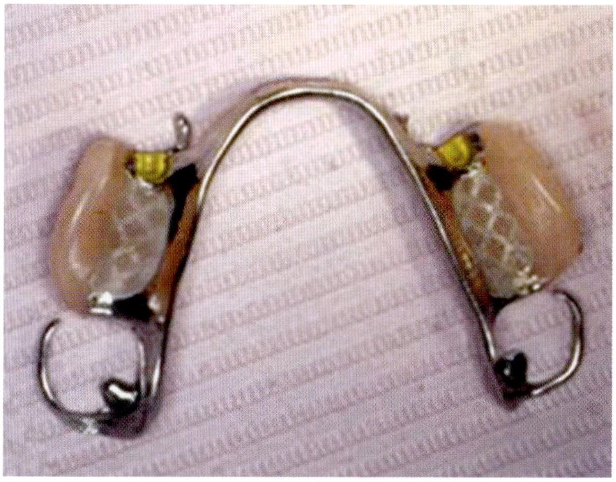

Fig. 6.56 The precision lower partial denture with attachments and clasps for retention.

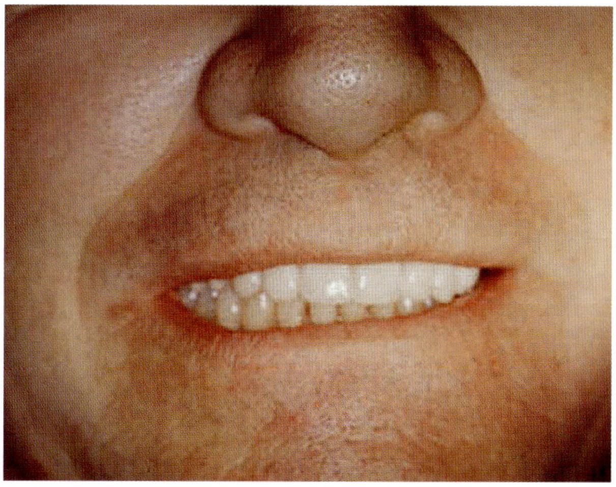

Fig. 6.57 Final placement of upper precision overdenture and lower precision partial on new crowns.

The patient was most pleased with the results of his treatment choices and my work (Fig. 6.57). One thing to remember is that when you do something to restore a mouth this complicated and involved on a person who shows uneven arch form due to genetics, acquired uneven bite and the patient asking for changes throughout treatment, it is extremely difficult to look forward to total and absolute satisfaction. You, me and our patients with this kind of complex treatment are basically "married" to each other for life. The fact that this patient had mild cognitive impairment may have been the chief reason he asked for so many changes in the first place. The other was a more material reason at the onset of his wanting to buy an expensive house and property to live on with his new wife. Lastly, he just wanted to look younger. Function was not even brought to the fore by this patient.

With respect to the dental materials I used to restore this gentleman's mouth: the attachments wear out and must be replaced periodically; bars break under repeated aberrant force should that force not be corrected; things fail due to lack of continuing professional hygiene recall and strict homecare coupled with dental recall examinations. This patient already told me that his teeth come second in the scheme of things, so I knew in advance toward the end of his treatment that it would be a difficult job to get him to be compliant. His noticeable mild cognitive impairment from the first time I met him to when I began treatment, should have been a clear sign to me that I needed to be on my "toes" in treating him and presenting a treatment plan that he could understand, managed, and not be changed in mid-stream.

He bought a house far away from my practice and did not come back for hygiene as instructed. He only came back to have things "fixed" that broke or needed replaced or adjusted periodically, as I have indicated. Eventually, he stopped coming back to my office for continuing care. I must say that I was saddened, but relieved from the burden of constantly having him expect me to fix things that he did not take responsibility for in the care of his mouth as he was instructed to do. The "divorce" between us, in essence, was destined to happen, and I was grateful for it when it did. My motto here is that "**we cannot undo what our patients won't let us do**".

Case Study 8

55-Year-Old Man with Multiple Medical and Dental Issues

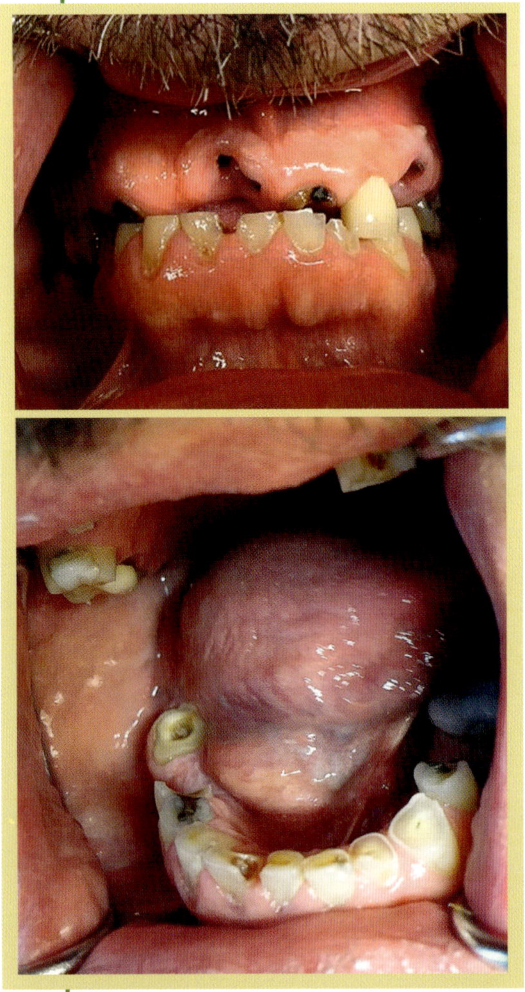

Fig. 6.58 Pre-treatment photos.

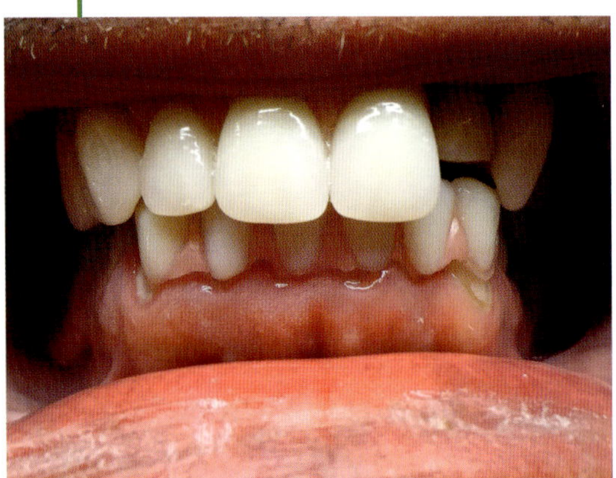

Fig. 6.59 First set of overdentures over existing teeth to open the bite and take Tomograms of his TMJ.

This patient (**Fig. 6.58**) presented to my dental office after having seen at least seven other practitioners who turned him down regarding treatment. I had several conversations with him before I examined his mouth. His social history included: a divorce; not dating; a daughter in her 20's; working as an IT specialist and part-time musician. He had no history of drug use, although he was a smoker and had an occasional alcoholic beverage on social outings. His parents were both alive and elderly and he had a good relationship with them. He admitted to being lonely and he stated that he did not feel well most of the time due to not being able to eat very well, occasional gastric reflux and pain in his mouth.

I discussed his goals, which included getting his mouth restored in good order, as he wanted to commit to doing this treatment. He stated that his parents would help him with the cost of treatment. I did his dental examination and found that he snored and had trouble sleeping. He woke up periodically gasping for air, which he stated he saw and heard in a dream, no less! I told him that if he dreamt of this, he was doing this action. I was sure that he had OSA (Obstructive Sleep Apnea). The wear patterns on his lower anterior teeth were into the pulps of his teeth and these were both calcified and decayed. The wear pattern also indicated that he had some chronic issues with gastroesphageal reflux disease. I referred him to a Gastroenterologist and to an Ear, Nose and Throat specialist for opinions on these two issues.

His dental examination also showed the following: bruxism; generalized caries; missing teeth; broken and fractured teeth; loss of vertical dimension; generalized, chronic geriatric periodontal disease with acute inflammation; localized recession; pulp exposures and periapical lesions; poor homecare including heavy stain, calculus and plaque, which were generalized throughout his mouth. After outlining his treatment in my mind and then putting it down in writing, I could visualize how I would approach his treatment in an orderly fashion. The first thing was to eliminate disease, getting his OSA and gastroesphageal reflux disease under control. Then working on his periodontal disease and increasing the level of self-efficacy he had so that he would get into the "habit" of regular recall and increased homecare. This would be an effort to create a good and permanent habit of keeping his teeth and gums healthy and protecting the prosthetic treatment investment he was about to embark upon.

I then wanted to remove all "hopeless" teeth and enhance his ridges with bone grafting, if necessary, to keep the ridges intact for possible implant placement as needed. After this was all finished, I would send him for Tomograms of his TMJ to determine where the condyles were in the fossae when he was in centric occlusion (Fig. 6.59). I then had to arbitrarily determine how much I was going to open his vertical, which called for me to make an acrylic over denture in the upper and lower arches, retaking a tomogram to see if the condyles were now centered in the fossae. If so, I would take my measurements, adjusting the vertical dimension, the overbite and the overjet, the speech patterns and his ability to determine if he looked something like this set-up when he had a full compliment of teeth. This procedure was incredibly involved and difficult because I was doing this in my head, transposing to paper, correcting myself and treatment projections as I went along, and then would discuss this with the patient before I attempted to start treatment. I wanted him to know all the nuances of every step in the outline I had created for him.

The patient and I sat down to discuss all the details of his medical history, dental history, his habits, the findings of his referrals and subsequent treatment, the outline I had prepared for his treatment plan and all the details that went into it for his care. I think he was stunned and did not know what to say. It took several hours of consulting to discuss these things and for me to listen to his concerns; finally, getting to "Yes" after a most detailed discussion. I had a dental assistant in the room taking copious notes for the chart and I had prepared a contract with estimates for treatment and cost. He went over everything and agreed to treatment. Before he did this, I emphasized that should he start this treatment and stop somewhere, anywhere along the way before finishing the treatment, he would not end up with a good result. He needed to be aware of what would happen in the face of adversity due to all the pre-existing issues that were not addressed, and that these issues would continue to exist if they were not treated, and his mouth brought into an ideal occlusion in the end. He understood and agreed to my care. I proceeded to take several sets of impressions again for study models to manufacture his overdentures that would open his bite up and help find his centric occlusion in as near a position to where he once was prior to all the tooth destruction he had acquired.

Once finding the center of the fossae for the condyles, I adjusted his bite into a better occlusal situation and made another ideal maxillary temporary appliance for him. I removed the porcelain crown on tooth #10 to improve his smile (Figs. 6.60-6.62). The left upper lateral incisor was covered by the denture and had a previous endodontic treatment on it. The patient was much happier with his looks after I did this one simple thing. I had asked him about his expectations before starting. He told me that he wanted to look better, eat better and be healthier. With these things in mind, I continued with my treatment outline.

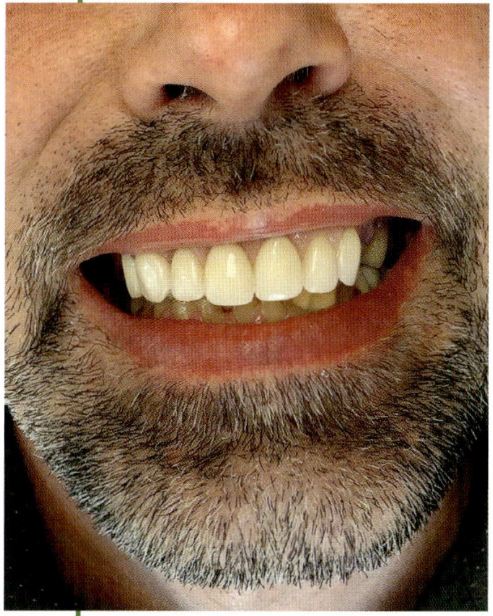

Fig. 6.60 Overdenture covering remaining upper teeth, replacing the crown on #10 for better esthetics.

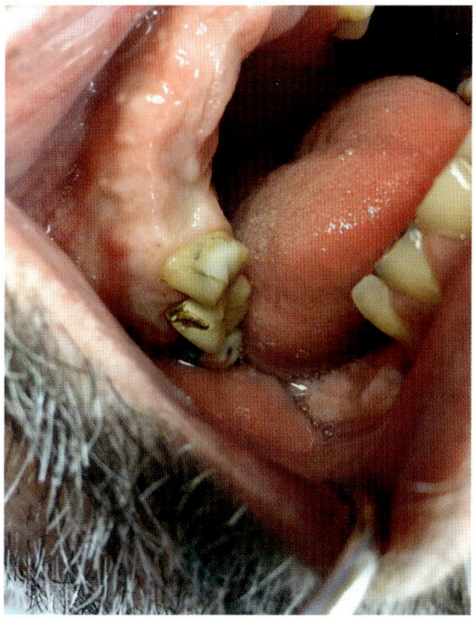

Fig. 6.61 This photo shows the healing extraction sites on the right side of the patient's mouth.

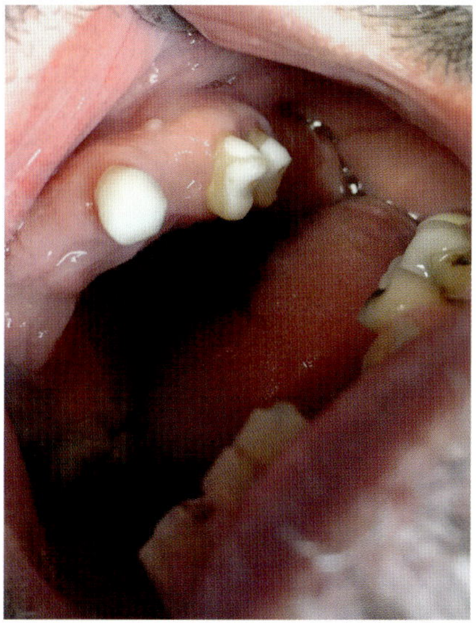

Fig. 6.62 Another view from the left side of his mouth showing the results of his periodontal treatment, extractions and tooth #10 treatment.

It is important to note that simply opening the patient's bite to an ideal vertical dimension for him, allowed him to look better, feel better and speak better. He had to relearn how to eat his food and I asked him to cut it up in small pieces until he got into chewing properly again. There was much more to be done at this point and the periodontal work and extractions were next in line for his treatment.

All this time he had been undergoing treatment for OSA and received a CPAP machine for his sleep apnea. He had quit smoking by then and was sleeping better and physically feeling better too. The GI medical doctor had given him some dietary instructions as well as some medication for his gastric reflux issues. He was on his way to a successful overall health rehabilitation.

The patient refused implants on the upper arch due to financial strain placed on him and his parents at this juncture, thus changing the treatment plan. I was forced into making a large "roundhouse" type Zirconia bridge in the upper anterior area. He had plenty of ideal bone for implant placement; however, as I have said in the past "you can lead a horse to water, but you cannot make him fish!" I needed to "back-up 10 and punt" now and rethink the treatment plan that I had to go over with the patient in lieu of his changing the plan. This took a lot of time and energy on my part and rethinking with respect to what the patient might do next to change the plan I had initially presented to him. Fortunately, he did not change it after this episode, and I discussed with him what the change would mean for him and the risk he was taking by placing mores stress on this long span bridge which would be fabricated for the front part of his maxillary arch. He understood and reapproved the plan in writing.

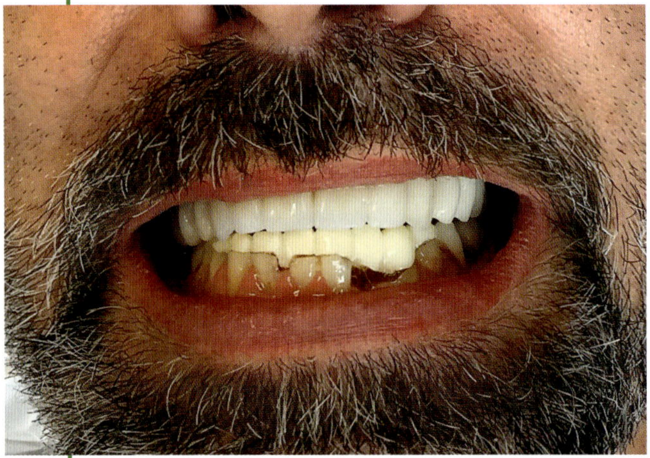

Fig. 6.63 A new temporary processed acrylic set of teeth on the upper arch and a new lower acrylic appliance as well to maintain esthetics after a failed attempt at an endodontic procedure in the lower left anterior and to maintain his vertical dimension and hold his centric steady.

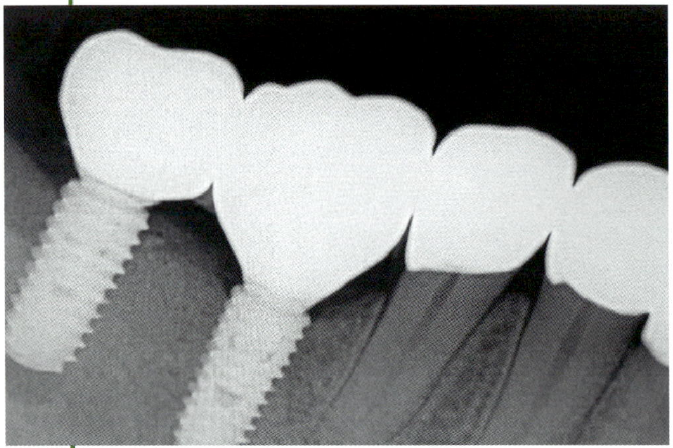

Fig. 6.64 A radiograph of the lower right posterior area showing his loaded implants and the height of bone maintained by them in his previous extraction sites. The Zirconium crowns can be seen as well, showing them with smooth and perfect margins as restored.

Teeth had been prepared on the upper and the Zirconia crowns were going to be made against the lower acrylic temporary overdenture in ideal occlusion (Fig. 6.63). Once they were cemented in place on the upper arch, the anterior six teeth on the lower arch would be restored to hold an anterior guidance position for the jaw.

Looking at the jaws of a person, once you visualize the condyles centered in their sockets, you can draw a line across connecting them in your mind's eye and then draw two straight lines forward to the centric bite of the front incisors that produces a drawing of a "Golden Triangle" if you will. These three points are what need to be centered and respected when restoring and opening a bite. The two centered condyles and the anterior guidance are the basis of a solid and healthy occlusion. Without this combination, the bite will be off, the occlusion will be less than perfect, the joints will become painful over time and the patient will not tolerate it. The bottom line is "study the situation before you treat" and make sure you have all your positions in correct alignment while restoring a full mouth to its optimum balance and function.

The patient was tolerating everything perfectly and doing what he should be doing until his changing his mind about

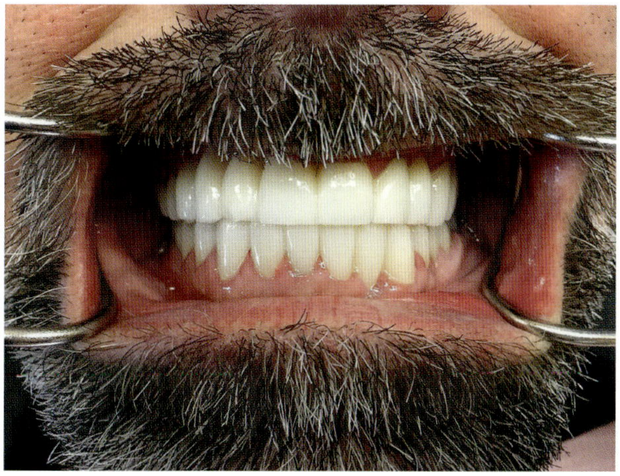

Fig. 6.65 Finished restorative after two years.

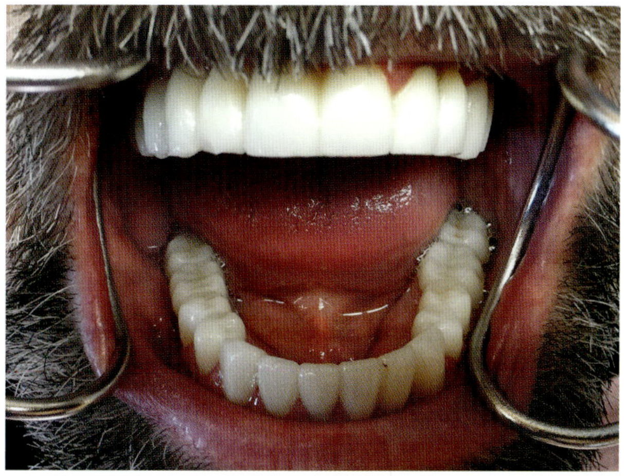

Fig. 6.66 The finished all porcelain case in both arches, except for teeth #30 and #31. These implants have screwed in PFM crowns. (In case they are damaged in some way in the future and have fractured porcelain, they can be removed for a simple porcelain repair rather than having the patient pay for a new crown.)

the upper implants. This forced me to change the treatment plan. I sat down with him at this juncture and determined that his father had been diagnosed with cancer and his mother told him that they could no longer afford to assist him financially... in the middle of treatment!!

The patient became distraught, hurt, sad and angry. An entire gamut of feelings I had to illicit from him and discuss until he felt better. I reassured him that we would work this out together so he could finish his treatment. This is **mutual problem solving**. It reassures that patient that he or she is not alone in this process. In essence, he knew he could trust me and that I was honest and open with him respecting his issues and feelings, as well as being his "partner" in this rehabilitation. It took longer than expected though, but we eventually finished him at about the two-year mark. I had previously placed two implants in the lower right posterior area for future restorative treatment and they sat there for a long time, which was alright, considering I was getting good osseointegration from them (Fig. 6.64). In the meantime, the patient was making payments that we set up for him in an affordable and regular manner as we waited until there was enough money paid down for the lab fees to continue his care in a logical series of baby steps.

We prepared the lower six anterior teeth for crowns and a small bridge to replace #23 that had been extracted, while keeping his posterior temporary parts of his overdenture, thus maintaining his vertical dimension to the ideal occlusal height. Once his lower crowns were placed, we completed one lower side and then, after cementation, we finished the opposite side, all to maintain his centric occlusion and his vertical dimension.

It is important for me to take pre-cementation films and post-cementation films on all my crowns. I want to make sure that the margins are down and smooth before the cement goes in and that the margins are smooth and down with no excess cement under the gingiva after I cement the crowns (Figs. 6.65, 6.66). This reassures me that the patient will have no ill effects from the cementation process and can maintain his gingival health.

This patient returned for hygiene recall and examinations regularly for about one year and then dropped out of sight. I believe that he was depressed and despondent about his father's situation with cancer and impending death. He was taking care of his daughter and had other responsibilities as well that kept him busy. All in all, I think that his recidivism in self-efficacy was a result of resorting to alcohol again for his drug of choice to relieve his emotional pain.

As practitioners, it is incumbent upon us to "care" for our patients; however, we can only go so far. I learned a long time ago that "we can't undo what our patients won't let us do". This was one of those times. There is not a day that goes by that I do not think about the positive change I created for this patient, which met his personal goals. But in the back of my mind, I still think there was something more that I missed that ignited his unwillingness to continue with his dental care and visits. I guess I will never know the answer to this statement, but I will know in my heart that I did my best to bring about a positive change to his life.

"Failure is not falling down but refusing to get up!"

Chinese Proverb

Case Study 9

75-Year-Old Male with Moderate Bone Loss and Mobility #22-27

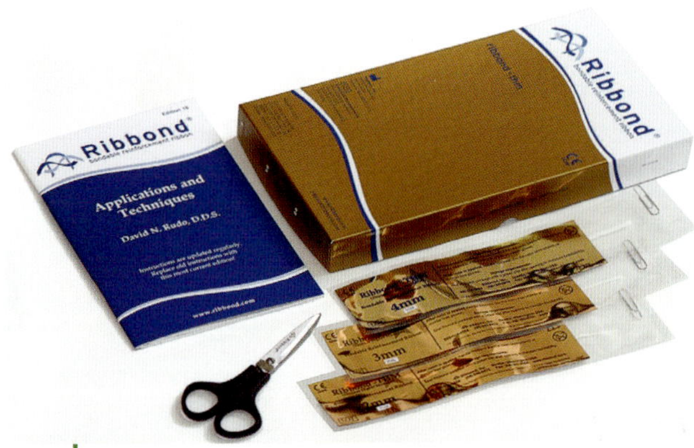

Fig. 6.67 Ribbond® is a periodontal/orthodontic splint material that comes in varying widths.

My patient presented with a chief complaint of mobility on his lower six anterior teeth. He stated that the mobility has been increasing slowly and now he came in as he was afraid of losing his lower six anterior teeth. Radiographs showed 30-50% bone loss with clinically Class II mobility. His homecare was excellent, and his gingiva was within normal limits, his "saving grace". I discussed using Ribbond® splinting material and he agreed to treatment (**Fig. 6.67**).

The teeth were cleaned and then a 1 mm groove was placed on the lingual surface at the level of the contact points from #22-27 (**Fig. 6.68**).

Foil was then cut into a ribbon about 5 mm wide and placed and burnished against the existing teeth to determine the length of the fiber we needed (**Fig. 6.69**).

A 1 mm wide piece of fiber was placed on top of the foil and cut to length. The groove was acid etched with 30% phosphoric acid etch for 20 seconds (**Fig. 6.70**), rinsed off and dried. A bonding material was placed over the etched surface and then the Ribbond splint material, made of Kevlar® material, was placed in the groove (**Fig. 6.71**), covered with flowable composite and cured for 30 seconds. The anterior six teeth were now one piece and "solid as a rock" (**Fig. 6.72**). They were stabilized against any forces placed upon them.

This technique is very handy, relatively inexpensive and a conservative treatment to save mobile teeth; save teeth that might have otherwise been extracted; save teeth that might have been avulsed due to force of some kind, like eating or biting into something hard, or a fall injury; keeping teeth from moving out of position, causing occlusal and bite force trauma and saving teeth that might be inadvertently lost from eating hard foods. I have also used this material to make bonded post and cores in endodontically treated teeth, as it is durable and inexpensive to use on a patient with limited means. It can also be used on patients to hold in a pontic or temporary crown and used to reinforce a fractured tooth, as necessary. I am mentioning it here because I have used the material for many years on older patients, who have limited finances, and it does maintain their teeth longer than if they had not had this used on them at all.

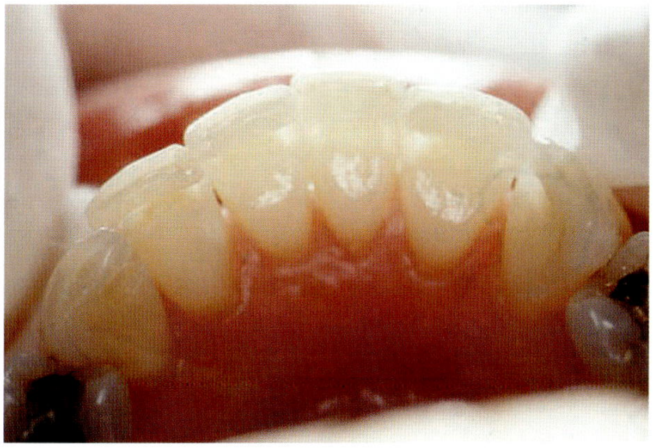

Fig. 6.68 The prepared lingual groove at the contact areas.

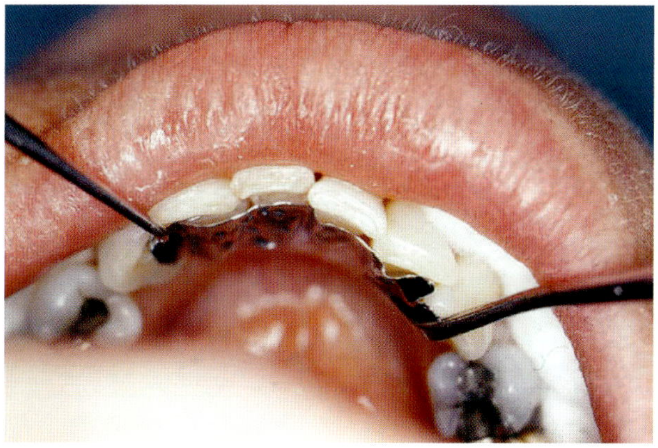

Fig. 6.69 Foil placed to get the exact length of Ribbond needed.

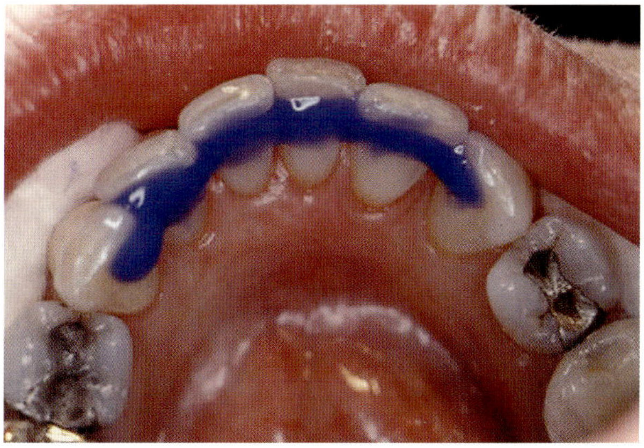

Fig. 6.70 The etch process.

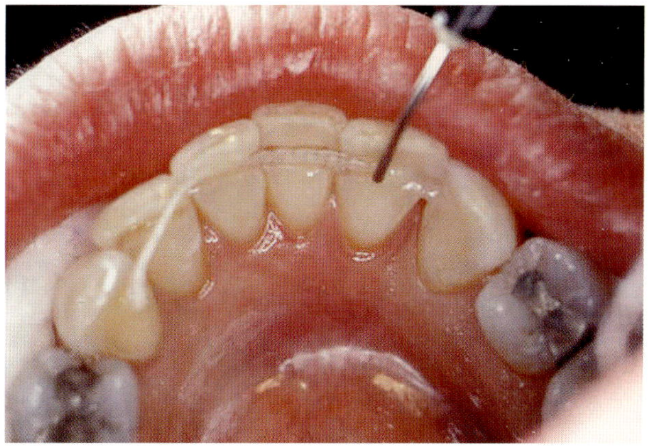

Fig. 6.71 Placement of the Ribbond strip.

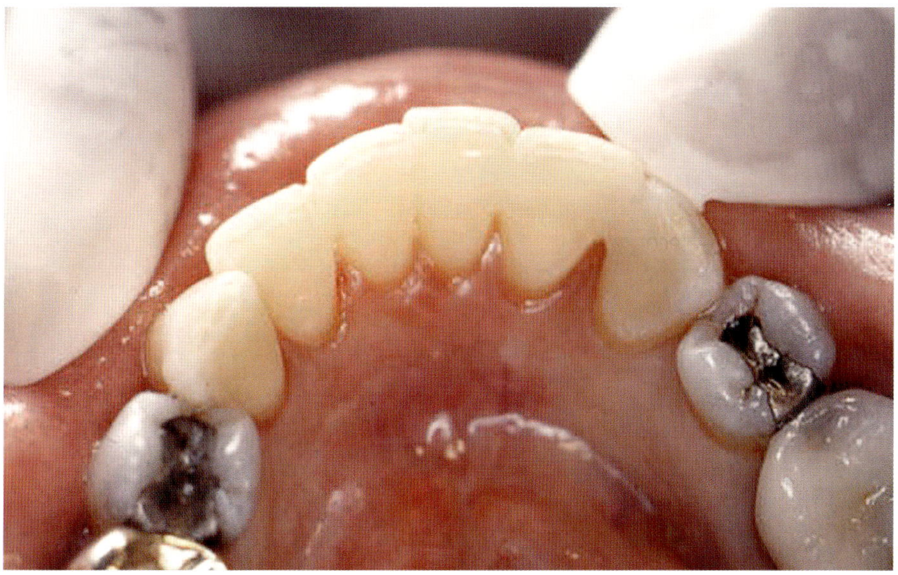

Fig. 6.72 Final bonded, esthetic Ribbon splint on the lingual of teeth #22-27.

Case Study 10

80-Year-Old Male with Missing Lower Anterior Teeth and Mild Cognitive Impairment

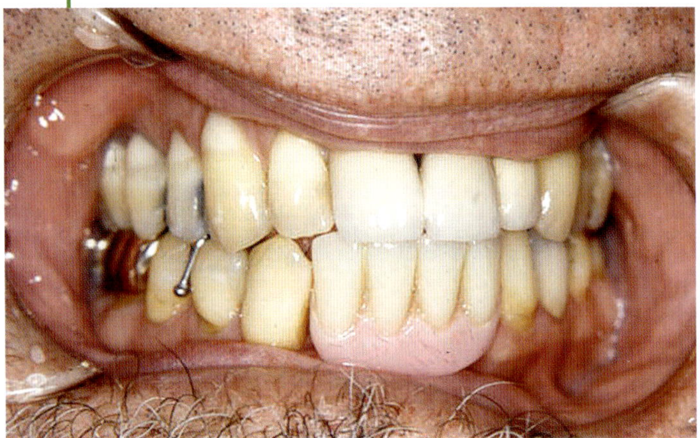

Fig. 6.73 Pre-treatment photo.

This octogenarian lost his lower teeth over time to breakage and extraction by another dentist. He had some mild cognitive impairment at the time I first saw him as a patient, but not enough to impede his decision-making process. He had a lower anterior stayplate fabricated by his previous dentist (Fig. 6.73) and was tired of it due to his inability to adjust to eating with it and keeping it clean. He also told me that he did not like the looks of the stayplate and was afraid of "swallowing" it! He also commented that he did not like his previous dentist because he felt that he did not listen to him.

The Maryland Bridge that was fabricated had "holes" placed in the wings. The patient had the means to place a six-unit bridge in place of the stayplate, but he did not want to minimize the integrity of his cuspids, nor did he want to incur the extra fees as he was on a fixed budget. I suggested a Maryland bridge to him, explaining the technique and what I had to do to prepare his two lower cuspids to receive the bridge. He agreed to this treatment. The goals of his treatment were to not have to be concerned about swallowing his teeth, saving money, being more functional and improving his esthetics.

I conservatively prepared two "wings" in the mesial lingual surfaces of his lower cupids (Fig. 6.74) and took an impression and a shade for his Maryland bridge (Fig. 6.75), as well as an opposing impression and bite registration. I temporized the wing preparations with a glass ionomer until delivery.

I had them done and made the wings thin enough to be buried in the wing prep and covered with composite for stability (Intradental bonded wings) (Fig. 6.76).

The patient was instructed on hygiene care and was most pleased with the function, the looks and the feel of his new bridge (Fig. 6.77). The fact that he spent less money than he could have, thus getting a "good deal" was something

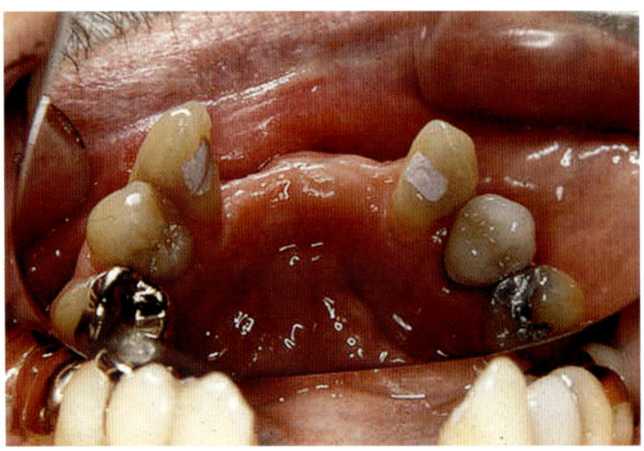

Fig. 6.74 Lingual retention wings temped with ZnOE.

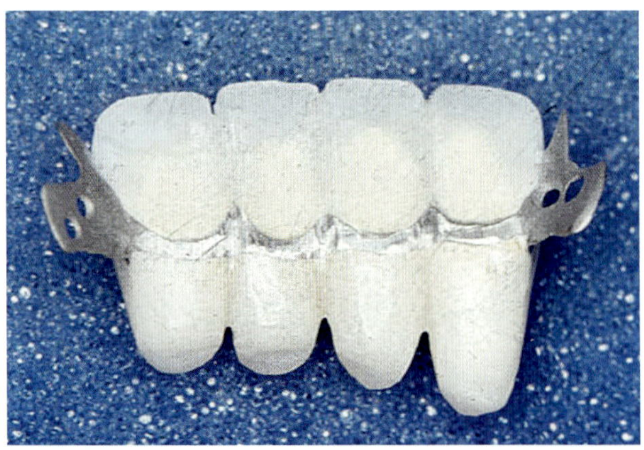

Fig. 6.75 The Maryland Bridge that was fabricated had "holes" placed in the wings.

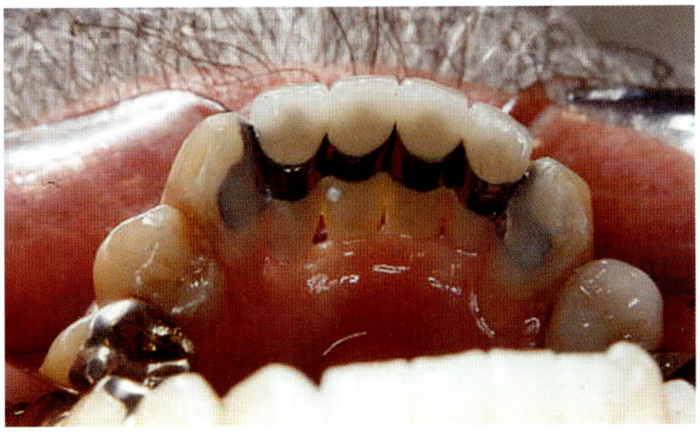

Fig. 6.76 The bonded Maryland Bridge in place.

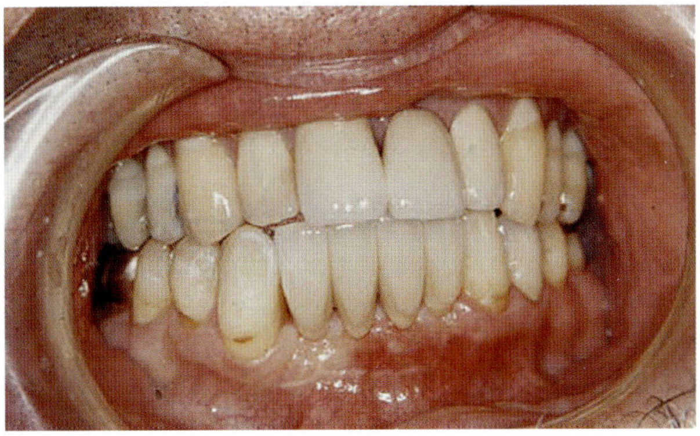

Fig. 6.77 The patient's smile photo of the bonded Maryland Bridge #22-27.

he smiled about when he stated this to me and walked out the door. He was excited about the esthetics. Since he was a widower, he could now date again with confidence, so he proclaimed!

This bridge stayed bonded in place for over five years before he knocked it out chewing on a spare rib. The bridge was cleaned, re-etched and re-bonded. It lasted him a lifetime, until his death at age 98.

As a conservative method of treatment on a "fixed" budget, for patients with and without supplemental insurance, this option always seemed to be useful as an alternative treatment plan with minimally invasive dental treatment modalities. Normally, I would offer the patient the options of

1. Implants and crowns or an implant supported bridge;
2. A full bridge from #22-27;
3. A removeable partial denture with supporting clasps (Figs. 6.78, 6.79), much better than the stayplate he came into the office wearing when we first met him, and then,
4. the acrylic partial denture (Valplast®).

This partial denture can meet most people's esthetic needs. It is also flexible to a point and seemingly more comfortable for that reason than the more ridged metal and acrylic partial denture. The cost for this partial is a little more than the standard partial. The clasps are colored acrylic to match a patient's gingiva as well. It is durable and esthetically pleasing.

It makes for a good option, along with the standard metal to acrylic partial when money is a major object in planning treatment. Most dental laboratories make this oral appliance.

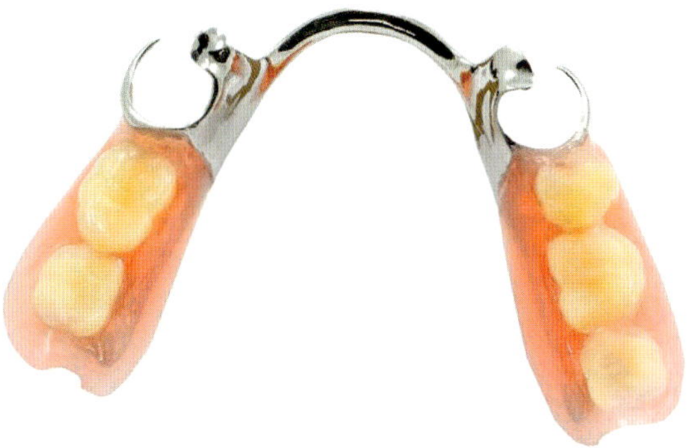

Fig. 6.78 The typical removeable partial is being used much more today than in the past as a viable option for missing teeth and tight budgets. Many people do not like the metal showing in their mouths and have opted for an all-flexible acrylic alternative, the Valplast® Removeable Partial seen in Figure 6.79.

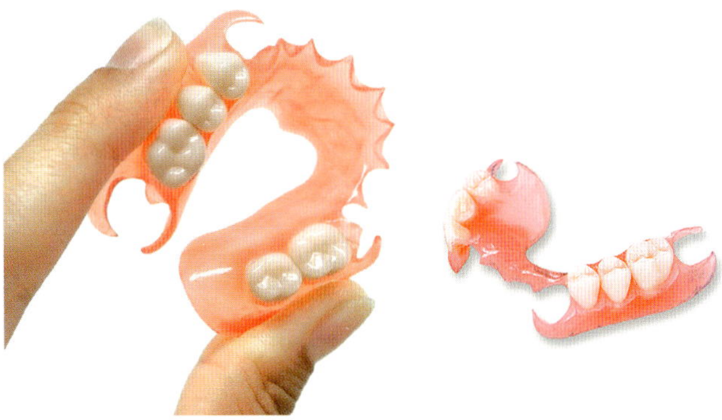

Fig. 6.79 The Valplast® Removeable Partial.

Case Study 11

A 75-Year-Old Man with Chronic Periodontal Disease and COPD

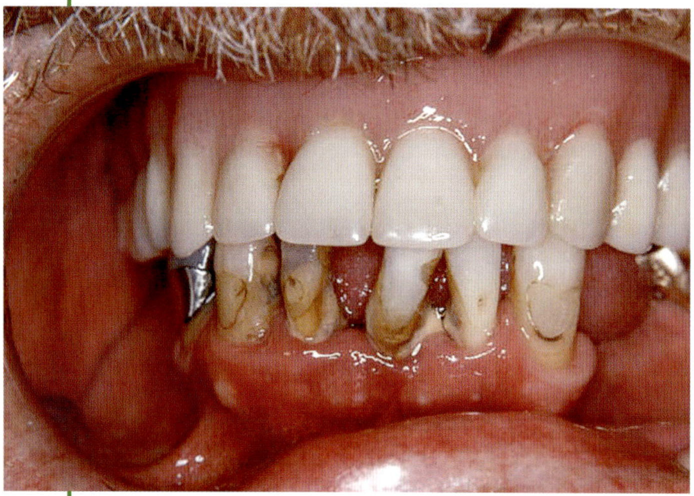

Fig. 6.80 Deceased patient.

The patient in **Figure 6.80** had a history of heavy, chronic smoking. He developed COPD (Chronic Obstructive Pulmonary Disease) and continued to smoke as evidenced by the stain on his upper denture and lower teeth and heavy calculus build-up (**Figs. 6.81, 6.82**). He drank alcohol as well and manifested a low dental IQ with a resultant poor self-efficacy when it came to dental homecare and recall hygiene. I discussed extracting his lower teeth or saving what I could and doing an overdenture utilizing the lower left posterior molar for a retention clasp. Or giving him a full denture should he understand his logistics for tooth survival under the circumstances, or make a positive change in his behavior to keep the teeth that we could. He opted to just keep his lower cuspids and use them as stops and retention teeth, along with keeping his posterior gold crown.

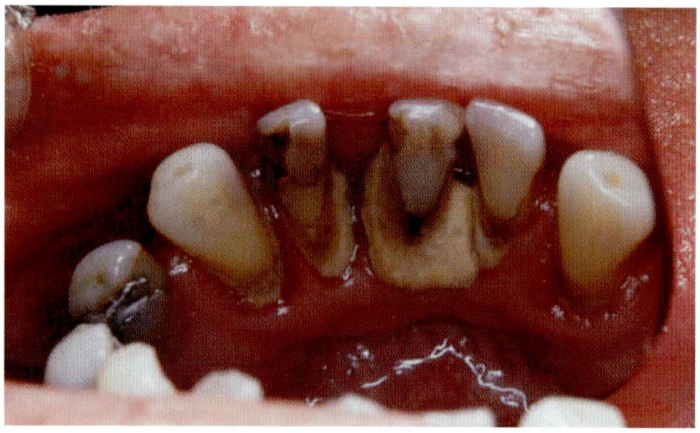

Fig. 6.81 Chronic Geriatric Periodontal disease. Lower lingual teeth view.

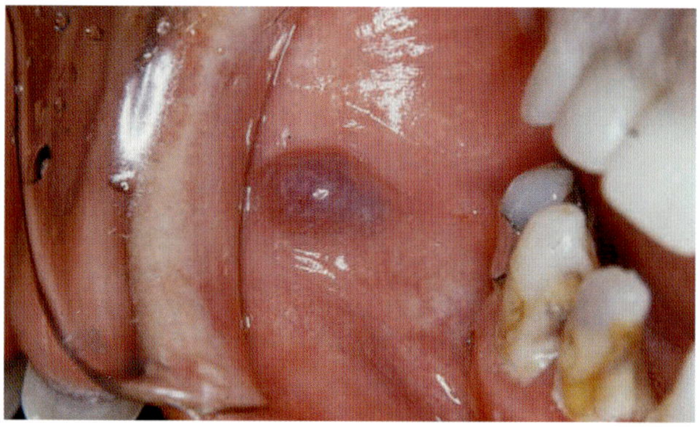

Fig. 6.82 View of his right cheek where he had a varix (cluster of vessels) and heavy calculus build-up on his remaining posterior teeth.

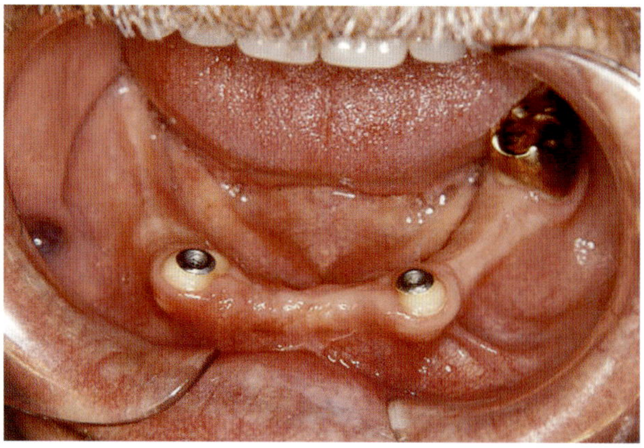

Fig. 6.83 Saved teeth #18 (Gold Crown) and #22 and 27 with Zest® intra-tooth cemented female attachments.

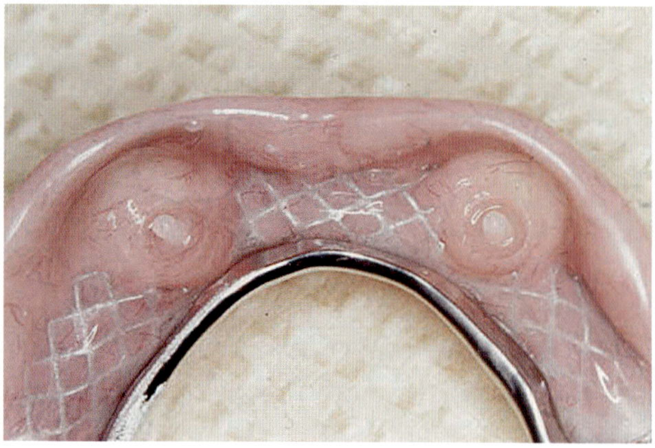

Fig. 6.84 Underside of the lower overdenture with male Zest® attachments.

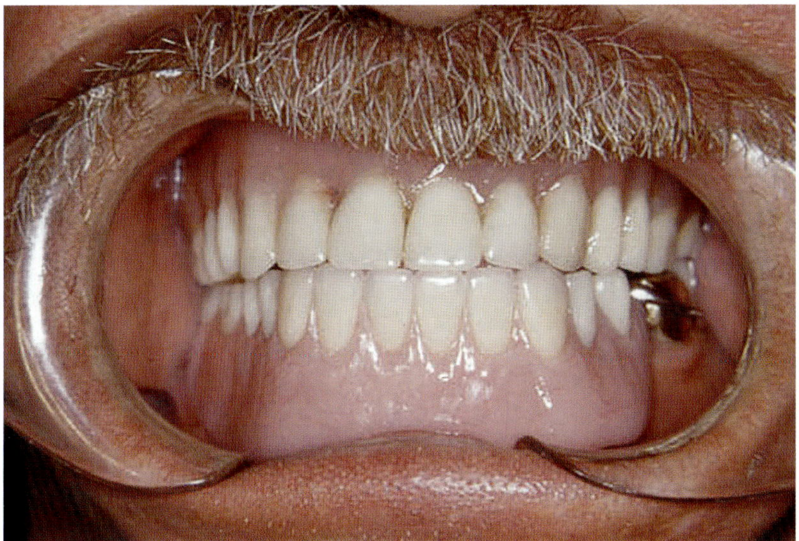

Fig. 6.85 New lower overdenture with Zest® attachments and a clasp on tooth #18.

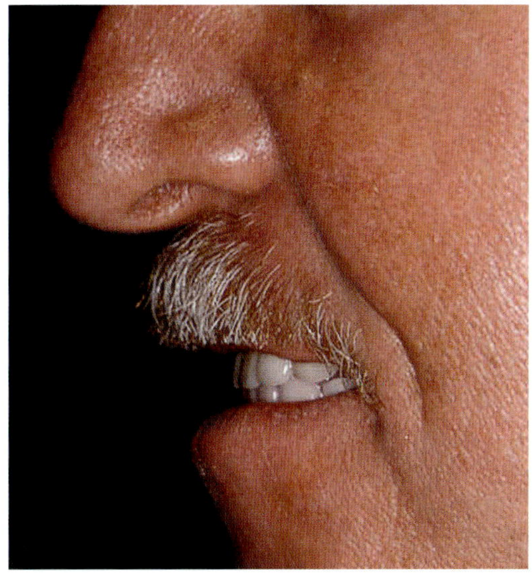

Fig. 6.86 Finished lower overdenture in centric occlusion.

The success of this patient's treatment depended upon his ability to consider quitting smoking, which he did not do, and increasing his self-efficacy, which he did not do either. He eventually broke both male attachments and had gold copings placed over #22 and #27, as well as Ceka® attachments placed on the occlusal surfaces of those teeth (**Figs. 6.83-6.85**). These were used because they were thin and flat, not taking up too much vertical space.

The patient died a few years later from both COPD and lung cancer, which he did not know he had until it was too late to be treated. He chose this treatment for esthetic purposes and functional reasons, wanting a stronger and more durable dental option (**Fig. 6.86**). Money was not an issue for him. He moved away after I finished the gold copings and readapted his lower overdenture to them. I never saw him again for any follow-ups. He was a nice man and will always be remembered for his kindness.

In retrospect to reading the case studies, I find that it is not enough to do the work, but to understand why you did it and what you did to change a person's life in a positive manner. When we say something to another, it cannot be taken back. And so, it is with doing something for someone, like remaking a new crown towards rehabilitation of their entire mouth. Once it is accomplished, it is most difficult to take it back or in many cases, to redo it. I have tried several times in my professional life to undo a treatment with an alternative treatment when the first treatment failed. But I needed to go back to study the steps taken in what I did and try to understand why the treatment failed in the first place. Maybe it was because I really did not "hear" what the patient's goals were, other than expressing what mine were for them. This is a big mistake and a negative experience based on my sometimes-impatient desire to make things right, but who is to say what is right or wrong. It is all a learning experience and the "Practice of Dentistry", so to speak.

As I have stated in the beginning of this textbook, "**There are no mistakes, only experience. Good judgment is based on experience and experience is based on bad judgment**". So, go back when you are in doubt prior to treatment and rediscover for yourself what the patient desires and be a part of the solution of discovering how you can assist them in attaining ***their*** goals. After all, the most difficult part of doing dentistry is getting the patient to want what we think they need.

Now that you have gone over the cases I presented, you can judge for yourself whether you can change your tactics to elicit what a patient really wants when they come to your office and how you can get them to "Yes", after you study the situation and outline your treatment, then presenting it all in a form the patient can understand. It is only through proper and continued communication that we can find mutual understanding and common meaning between us and our patients. Studying your actions between yourself and your patient's treatment selections, understanding your motives for doing something, understanding the way you think, coping with adversity, and your ability to listen and respond to your patients will assist you in your quest to be a successful practitioner.

References

1. Locke EA, Latham GP. *Building a practically useful theory of goal setting and task motivation. A 35-year odyssey.* Am Psychol. 2002 Sep;57(9):705-17.
2. Seijts GH, Latham GP. (2001). *The effect of distal learning, outcome, and proximal goals on a moderately complex task*. Journal of Organizational Behavior,22(3), 291–307.
3. Earley PC, Perry BC. (1987). Work plan availability and performance: An assessment of task strategy priming on subsequent task completion. Organizational Behavior and Human Decision Processes, 39(3): 279-302.
4. Glass RT, Conrad RS, Bullard JW, Goodson LB, Mehta N, Lech SJ, Loewy ZG. *Evaluation of microbial flora found in previously worn prostheses from the Northeast and Southwest regions of the United States.* J Prosthet Dent. 2010 Jun;103(6):384-9.

Chapter 7

Communication: Can you Hear me? Are you listening? Can you Understand What it is I am Saying? "Please take your fingers out of your ears!"

"The biggest problem in communication is the illusion that it has taken place."
George Bernard Shaw

7.1 Definitions

Communication, from the Greek, means a "talking together". To me, communication is "the highway of life"! It is a pathway by which we use multiple and various vehicles to travel in different directions in order to reach a specific destination of sorts. **We communicate with all our senses.**

> **DEFINITION:** ***Communication*** *is a two-way, simultaneous transmission of thoughts, information and feelings, usually between like forms, which, when successful, leads to common meaning and understanding.*

In Dentistry, I think we sometimes tend to minimize our communication with our patient's when we feel it is only necessary to relay just the treatment we want to recommend and perform, as well as convey the cost of that treatment to get the job done. For the most part, most people, and I say this loosely, deal only on a "thing" level, essentially an "informational level" and not a "feeling" level. However, it is a known fact that most people make decisions with their emotions, that "gut feeling" they have that is most spontaneous and usually final. Recent research has shown that people who were instructed to make an intuitive, gut-based decision were more likely to report that that decision reflected their true values.[1] Researchers also found that participants of their study who made intuitive, gut-based decisions were more certain of their decisions and more likely to advocate for them. One researcher stated, "Our research suggests that individuals focusing on their feelings in decision-making do indeed come to see their chosen options as more consistent with what is essential, true and unwavering about themselves".[2]

7.2 Face to Face Learning

My point here is to show that when we just deal with information, we may miss out on total treatment options for one. We also need to understand our patient's and in order to do this, since we need to understand their feelings, their concerns, their hopes and desires, their fears and their wants. As I mentioned previously, as dentists, "the most difficult part of our job is to get people to want what we think they need". In order to do this effectively, we need to communicate on a higher level and a different level than one might have come to know. This is especially important when dealing with older individuals who are set in their ways, may

BOX 7.1

Different Ways to Take Information

1. **Visual Learners:** those who need to see pictures and graphs to visualize.
   How does one speak to an older person who is a visual learner? For the most part, try not to speak at the speed of light and expect them to follow your train of thought. Instead, use visual aids: models, photos, patient before and after pictures, illustrations, and your skill at drawing diagrams, as well as sketches of what you want them to learn and know.

2. **Auditory Learners:** those who need to hear the information.
   They can best be communicated with thorough discussion in a slow manner, reading aloud from paperwork you would like them to sign and then having them both read it back to you, as well as having them explain to you in their own words what they interpret from what they read. Showing these types of individuals, a photo of anything a visual learner might understand, would not be remembered after a short amount of time. Auditory learners will ask a lot of questions and will express their interest and enthusiasm for the process of reading all materials given to them.

3. **Kinesthetic Learners:** those who need to engage in an activity in order to grasp a concept.[5]
   They are most complex and make up a small percentage of the population. They tend to be most "antsy" and anxious about sitting still and looking at material as well as reading material. They have high energy and are quick to react. Kinesthetic learners, no matter what age, like challenges. Give them something to do regarding their treatment plan or care and they will be a good teammate. They really are "task-oriented" people. My older kinesthetic patients are given projects to do like monitoring their homecare with a diary or coming in on a specific time schedule to report how they are and what they have been doing. Keeping records of their dietary habits is another important project they can accomplish. They seem to like the challenge of these things and are not so disruptive by getting bored or tired of the "dental lecturing" we might give them due to their lack of not doing something they should be doing, such as their dental homecare. By being "***participatory***" in their care, they will be able to have a good sense of recall after 3-4 hours of up to 90% and at least 70% after 3 days of having learned and accomplished their given tasks.[6]

Both Auditory and Visual Learners have less ability to recall things that were shown or discussed after 3 hours with a 25% and 80% retention, respectively, and 10-20% and 65% after 3-4 days, respectively.[7] If one takes on a combination of these learning style factors, the retention rates of what has been learned goes up exponentially.

be cognitively impaired in some way and who may have much anxiety about being at a dental office for one reason or another. This means we need to learn or relearn how to communicate better and more efficiently and effectively with meaning, compassion and on a feeling level, all the while incorporating relevant information, teaching aids of one sort or another and visual and tactile stimuli in the process.

We are in a visually oriented society. Approximately 65% of the population are visual learners.[3] Ninety percent of information that comes to the brain is visual.[4] It is therefore incumbent upon us to "show and tell" what it is we are trying to accomplish with specific patient care. We can do this by incorporating the "puzzles" of our patients' histories, their concerns, encourage emotions of all kinds, use visual as well as text to explain things to them and consider their ability to afford what it is they want in the long run. A Professor at Stanford University, Robert E. Horn, has explained the reason for visuals having been found to improve learning by up to 400%, stating that "when the relationship between words and visual elements are closely entwined, we create something new and we augment our communal intelligence... visual language has the potential for increasing – 'human bandwidth' – the capacity to take in, comprehend and more efficiently synthesize large amounts of new information."

People take in information in different ways. The older one gets, the slower their reflexes of the body are that assimilate information on all levels; therefore, we need to understand the dynamics of each individual patient we confront for treatment with mutual respect, understanding and their ability to absorb information we will present to them. Each person takes in information differently. Box 7.1 provides a detailed description.

7.3 Listening and Active Listening

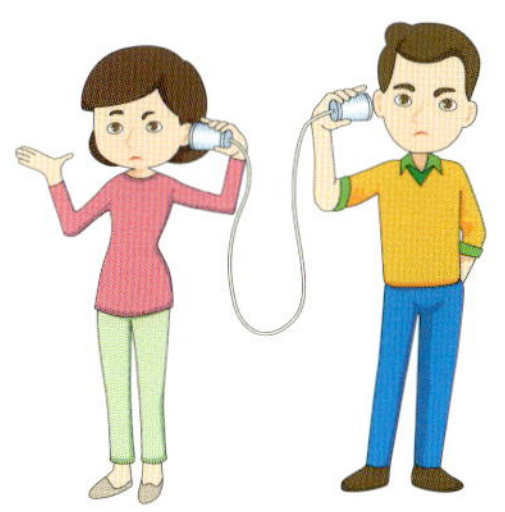

Older persons appear to not be listening at times if they appear disinterested in what we are saying to them. However, it may take them a longer time to process what is being said to them as they digest the information. We want to make sure that we first find out if they are hearing impaired. There is nothing like being embarrassed by the fact that we did not assess the patients' hearing at the onset of our relationship with them or during an examination of the head and neck areas. In our modern world, **hearing devices** have gotten smaller and **are easily undetectable**. So, it behooves us to both ask and look to see if our patient may have one of these issues. It will save you a lot of grief in the end. We also need to find out if our patients are sight impaired in some way, as this can also impede their ability to understand what it is we are trying to impart to them about their care. Both entities affect one's ability to listen attentively. We essentially listen with all our senses when it comes to learning.

7.3.1 What Is Active Listening and How Can It Be Used Effectively with Our Older Patients?

It is the ability to listen and then use an "I" message to respond to the emotion behind the words. For example, the older patient may say: "I have had a toothache for a long time and every time I eat, my tooth hurts me". The response might be: "I hear your concern. It sounds like you are both uncomfortable and frustrated about this tooth. Is this how you feel?" Rather than, "Have you tried taking aspirin or Tylenol® for your pain?" This is more of a sympathetic response and does not address the patients' feelings, rather only the information. Having a non-judgmental paraphrasing of what the patient is telling you is a form of empathy. Sympathy, in turn, is only an acknowledgement that the patient has a problem. It does not let him or her know that you care. This is a major difference in response and listening ability. **It is this empathic response that will "cement" your positive relationship with the patient**.

When I start a restorative procedure with an older, more compromised patient, I always ask first if they are comfortable. I start out showing concern for them as a person. I ask if they need a neck or head support or a blanket if they might be cold. If they do not respond in kind, I supply them with those things that I feel will make them comfortable in the first place. I give them permission to raise their hand or a finger, preferably not the middle one (Digitus Impudicus, from the Roman) to let me know if I need to stop my treatment, assuming they are not able to speak at that moment due to having a mouth full of dental paraphernalia. I listen with my eyes, ears, fingers, nose and intuition. All these things need to be honed over time, called the "experience of practice", in order to make quick decisions based upon responses that come forth from your patients over years of seeing them. An example of mutual respect in working with many older males and/or female patients alike who may find the urgency of having the need to use the restroom several times during treatment, due to prostate issues for men and urinary incontinence and prolapsed bladders in older women. This is an indication found on the medical history to keep your appointments short and give the patient plenty of breaks. It requires making longer appointments in the first place in order to accommodate these types of older individuals. **Physically challenged patients, cognitively challenged patients and medically challenged patients all need longer appointment times and special consideration when working with them.** This means that sometimes, for the most part, your fees will not cover the time you spend with these "special patients with unmet needs", especially when dealing directly with an insurance company or Medicare, both of whom have set fees for specific procedures.

7.4 Emotions

"The best and most beautiful things in the world cannot be seen or even touched. They must be felt with the heart."

Helen Keller

Remember to use the **EBW (Emotions Before Words)** mnemonic and you cannot go wrong. Emotion is "a natural instinctive state of mind derived from one's circumstances, mood, or relationships with others".[8] There are seven basic Human emotions:

1. Happiness
2. Sadness
3. Surprise
4. Fear
5. Anger
6. Disgust
7. Contempt

Anger being the strongest emotion amongst these other feelings. Diffusing a patient's emotional issues, especially anger, is a difficult and challenging state of being. We can break tension with humor, but it is not a good idea to do this when someone is angry with you. I might recommend the use of the EBW mnemonic, placing a recognition of anger at the forefront. An example might be, "I hear your anger and I sense that you are upset and frustrated with your treatment, is this how you feel?" With this statement I have tried to defuse the emotion being verbally tossed at me and not own it. I use a soft, lowered voice in the process of responding. I want the patient to own their words and tell me about his/her feelings so I can understand where it is this anger is coming from and how it got generated. If one tends to deal with the information only, nothing will get accomplished.

It is only through "**mutual problem solving**" that something positive will come out of the discourse. It might be best to let the patient vent all their anger by saying nothing, just letting them speak. Once spent, we might ask, "How can we both mitigate your anger and solve this unmet need?" This way you both will accept some responsibility for the issue at hand and it should work itself out. Doing anything other than this is doomed for certain failure and the possible loss of a patient or an entire family of patients and then some. If you let the patient vent, they may realize that you truly care about them because you were listening to what they are saying. In turn, they will be your patient forever.

I try not to use "red flag" words; those words that might incite more anger and/or anxiety, such as:

- pain = discomfort or the state of being uncomfortable;
- shot or injection rather than = sleepy drops or salve;
- problem = unmet need;
- hurt = frustration or uncomfortableness;
- I understand how you feel = I think I know how you feel (only because we are not inside another person's brain and cannot fully understand how they feel unless they tell us exactly). These are just a few examples. There are many more examples and the more you listen, the more you will hear.

The language we use and speak is most difficult; coupled with our non-verbal cues, it is even more difficult. **Know thyself and know your patient** is a good motto to follow. Listen with all your senses and learn the visual cues of body language, including facial expressions that can tell you a lot about how your patient is feeling, even if your patient is not saying anything verbally; they are saying things visually the entire time they are in your dental chair.

7.5 Body Language

Body language tells us many things about all our patients, especially our older patients. I always go out to the reception room (not "waiting room, as we don't want people to have to wait) to greet my patients to see how they are dressed, how they move, sit, walk to the treatment room and if they look at me when I say hello. These things or "cues" can tell us a great deal more about the patient: their mood, their attitude, their health, their ability to listen, their willingness to be there with you and more (Fig. 7.1).

Fifty-five percent of all communication is body language, that being body movements, face, arms, legs and expressions. Thirty-eight percent is tone of voice and only 7% is words.[9] With these statistics in mind, it is important that we understand how this affects our verbal communication, especially when the body may be speaking entirely different messages to what is being heard from the mouth!

Part of non-verbal communication are eye signs. Socrates has stated that "the eyes are the windows to the soul". We can learn a lot about a person by looking at their eyes and how they react to direct oral communication as well as things that may be happening around them. If we ask a personal question to an older, cognitively impaired patient we may find their eyes searching to the upper right (Fig. 7.2) to remember what they should say. They may not be able to remember, and rather than cause an embarrassing situation, I wait for them to tell me so. If they cannot remember what to say, then I ask them to close their eyes and visualize the word or the scenario they were trying to find in their "minds-eye". Once they do this and tell me that they can see what they want to say, I ask them to slowly grasp it with their tongue, in their mind's eye and speak it out. Nine times out of 10, they can do it. If you ask a personal question about diseases that a patient may have had in the past, and their eyes look upper left (see Fig. 7.2), they may be trying to synthesize an answer that is not true. This may be due to embarrassment or the fact that they do not want to tell you or cannot remember at all. Having your eyes in central focus while asking questions and getting answers is the best scenario for honest and open communication, so look for this by setting the example of not looking down and reading your questions, if possible; but by stating the question(s) directly with central focusing (Box 7.2) of your eyes into that of your patients.

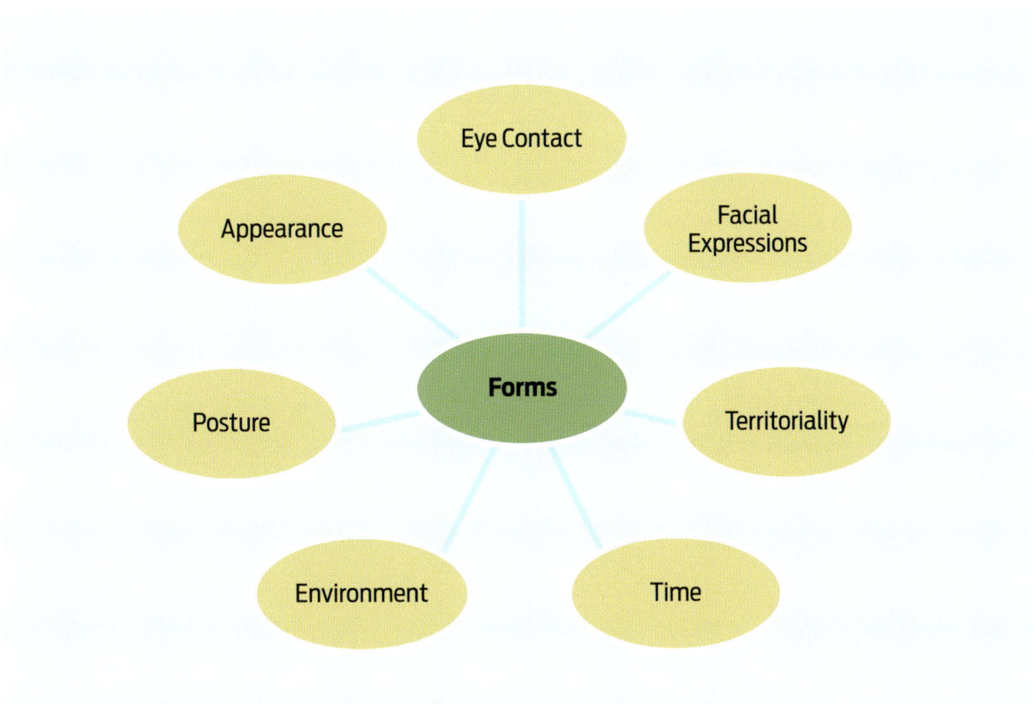

Fig. 7.1 Non-verbal cues.

Fig. 7.2 Eye signs.

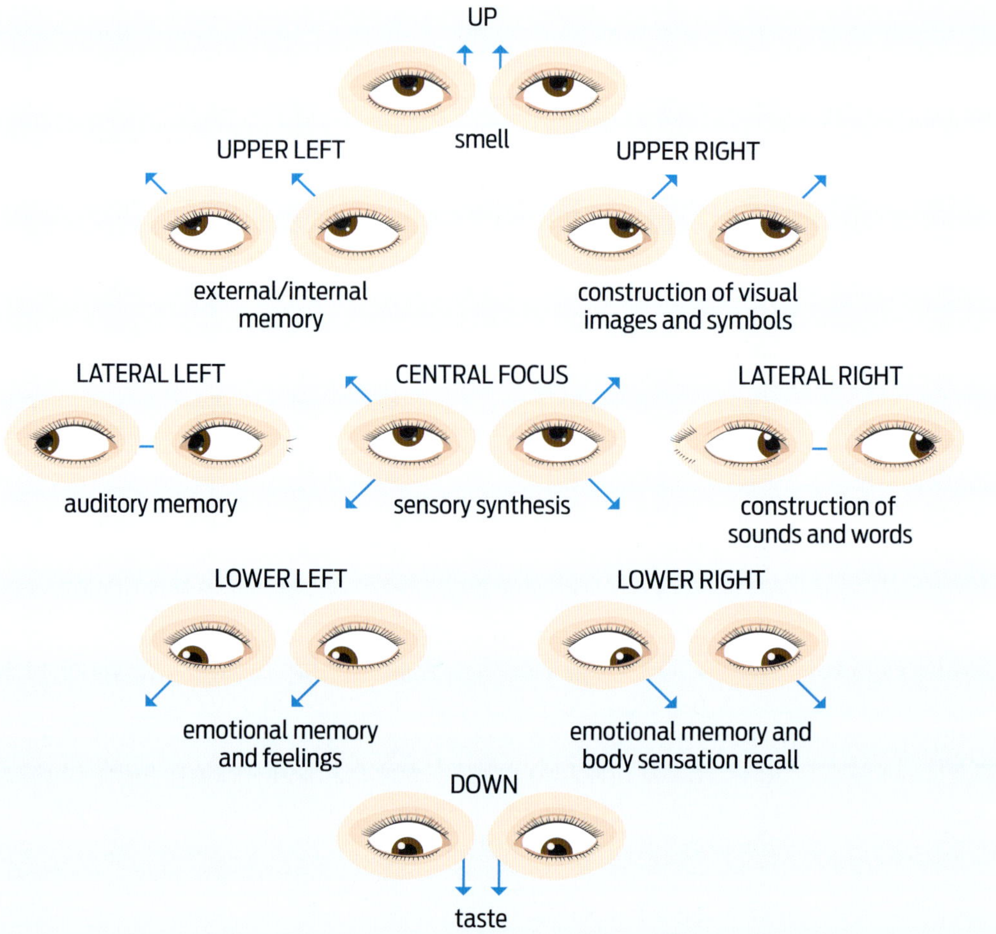

We can basically hear most things that are said to us, but we only listen to 7% of what we hear. Because of this fact, we need to use different techniques, such as repetitive information, asking for feedback, which is an active listening exercise and having the other person in the conversation define what it is they think they heard us say in the first place.

Once we understand the basic intent, tenets and content of communicating, we can practice our techniques in the safety of our homes, in our offices with staff or with a trusted friend and ask for feedback about how we performed. It is an eye-opening experience. We need to do these exercises in order to prepare for giving a treatment plan in good stead. Without the skill to listen attentively, use active listening for our responses, be empathic and interested in our patient as an individual person and respected patient that we hold on high, or not "lumping" them into a numbering system of impersonal automatons marching into our reception rooms, we will not be able to keep them as long-term patients. **Mutual respect** is what we want to achieve by doing all the right positive things. It promotes "trust". Mutual respect is allowing the patient to have thoughts, information and feelings different than our own.

BOX 7.2

What You See?

What is wrong within the following photo and what is right? Is it a good scenario or not?

The patient is 101 years of age (Fig. 7.3), a retired teacher with almost totally normal cognition at the time of this photo. She read at least five books a week. She had a hearing disability and wore hearing devices. She was frail and needs assistance walking. Basically healthy and spry for the most part. She wore a full upper denture and a lower precision partial denture. She had no anxiety about coming to the dentist. In fact, she couldn't come enough because it was a social outing for her to see her "friends".

Notice:

- The dental assistant took off her mask so that the patient could hear her better and/or read her lips at the same time as well as see her facial expressions.
- The dental assistant has several issues to deal with here. She did the correct thing by taking her mask down, but she needed to lower her chair to be at eye level with this patient or raise the dental chair to be at her eye level and turn the patient towards her. The patient is straining to see her face and has limited neck movements due to arthritis.
- The assistant also needed to remove her gloves, wash her hands and then hold the patients hand. **Our most intimate form of communication is touch**. The brain will absorb this feeling and allow an emotional response, such as the pressure of the patients hand(s) or the overlapping of the opposite hand over the top of the assistants hand in a caring manner. Under the circumstances, it is better for her to feel the other person's warmth and feel of the skin. I do this also in order to assess the patients' pulse, unbeknownst to them, especially if they are older and medically compromised. The assistant also has her right hand on the patients shoulder, which you can hardly see in the photo. It is a reassuring hand. However, whenever we touch a patient, no matter how old, we need to ask for permission to touch them and be sure to note this in the patients' chart that you got permission to touch their hand or arm, etc. Now it is in the legal record.

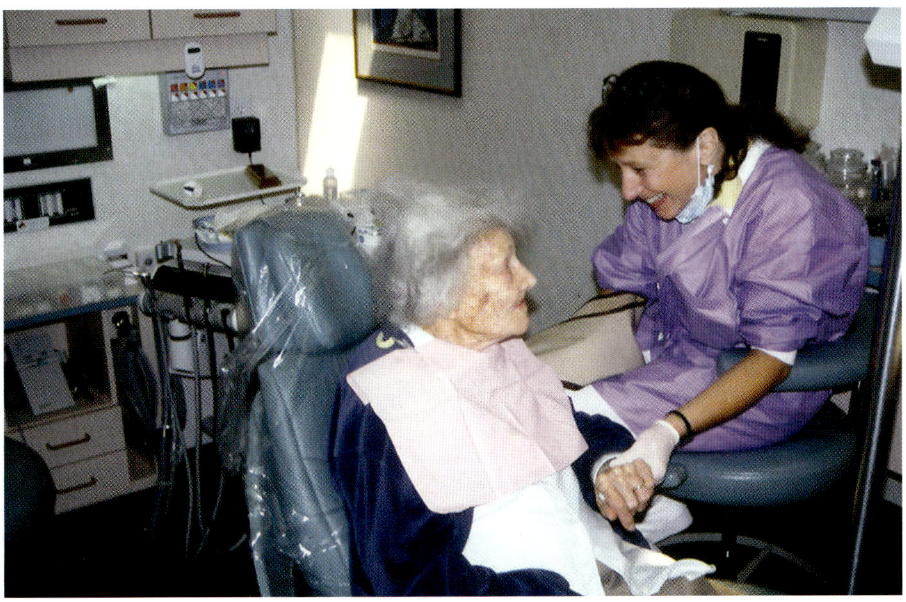

Fig. 7.3 Deceased 101-years-young patient.

7.6 Integrating a Dental Treatment Plan for Patients with Cognitive Impairment

7.6.1 Treatment Plan for Success

I usually make a **Treatment Outline** prior to doing a treatment plan so that I have a "road-map" of sorts to guide me in making the Treatment Plan itself.

> **DEFINITION:** ***Treatment plan*** *that can be written electronically or on a paper document that describes the patient's individualized diagnosis, strengths, disabilities, problems, behaviors, needs, long-range goals, short-term goals,* **treatment** *interventions, and* **treatment** *providers.*[9]

These documents are legal papers in the dental record of our patients. After presenting this paper to our patient or their guardian/caregiver, it needs to be signed and dated.

I always have the patient tell me in their own words what they read and heard after I read the Outline and Plan to them and go over these thoroughly, so that I might try to understand what part of the plan they did not understand, if any. I do the same with a caregiver or family guardian as well.

With cognitive decline it is most difficult to have total understanding of a treatment plan, especially if it is complicated. I need to find out what kind of a learner the patient is at the onset of the meeting. This way I can use the correct modalities to instruct them as they learn what it is that I feel they need based upon all the information I receive from them.

I usually read in short sentences and ask the patient to repeat to me what they heard and if they understood what it meant or what I was going to do for them with respect to current and future dental treatment. If they can read, I highlight each paragraph describing treatment as I go and have them read it. I alternate colors using a highlighter so that I know where I am at and do not repeat myself in order to not confuse myself or the patient. I do the same for the caregiver or family member guardian. It is a difficult and time-consuming effort as it takes a lot of time to process these things, especially if the treatment plan is complicated. If they are a visual learner, I use models, pictures, photos and even draw what I want them to understand. Sometimes I get a non-verbal agreement or acknowledgment with a head bob and a smile. Then, I know that this compromised patient understands. It is okay to record their answers and your discussion if you get permission from the patient or guardian. I had a dentist colleague who video taped all his consults with every patient and got a signed permission slip to do this for his records. After a while, he had these tapes transcribed and printed so the patients could read and sign them. This took less room than a storeroom full of video tape.

A simplified Dental Treatment Plan that can be used to fill in the blanks is presented in Figure 7.4. One might consider using this for a Treatment Outline before they work-up a more involved treatment plan; however, if the treatment is simple, one can use this type of form. Treatment plans are useful, and copies can and should be given to our older patients for their review and for "jarring" their memories about the proposed treatment if they are somewhat cognitively impaired. This helps them remember what treatment is recommended, necessary and dated for completion of the treatment as well.

How to Get to "Yes" with Your Treatment Plan

Some questions to ask yourself to begin this process:

1. Who are you working with?
2. Do you know their histories? Social, dental, medical, drug, family, economic?
3. Do you know their wants and desires?
4. Do you know their habits?
5. Do you know how they think?
6. Do you know how they feel about dentistry in general?
7. Do you have any rapport with them?
8. Does the patient know who you are?
9. Do you want to work with them?
10. Do you have the skills to treat their specific needs?

These are most germane and important questions in the scheme of things and should be addressed by you personally at the onset of meeting the patient and afterward as a reflection of where you intend to go with this patient after your examination and history taking. It is also important to

DENTAL TREATMENT PLAN
For use of this form, see TB MED 250; proponent agency is Office of TSG

1. **CONSULTATION DESIRED** ☐ **YES** ☐ **NO**
(If yes, complete Section III, on reverse side)

SECTION I - PLANNED TREATMENT AND SEQUENCE OF ACCOMPLISHMENT

Check items in column c to indicate treatment planned. If sequence of treatment is other than that printed in column b, use numbers (1 thru 10) in column c to show desired order

LINE	CODE a	TYPE TREATMENT b	PLANNED SEQUENCE c	ACCOMPLISHED d
2	**A**	URGENT		☐
3	**B**	PERIODONTAL		☐
4	**C**	PROPHYLAXIS SnF2 PASTE		☐
5	**D**	TOPICAL SnF2 REPEAT AFTER ______ MONTHS		☐
6	**E**	COUNSELING IN SELF CARE		☐
7	**F**	OCCLUSION		☐
8	**G**	SURGERY		☐
9	**H**	RESTORATIONS		☐
10	**I**	PROSTHESIS		☐
11	**J**	OTHER (specify)		☐

CHART
Chart ONLY missing teeth and TREATMENT TO BE ACCOMPLISHED
Do NOT chart existing Pathology or Restorations
e

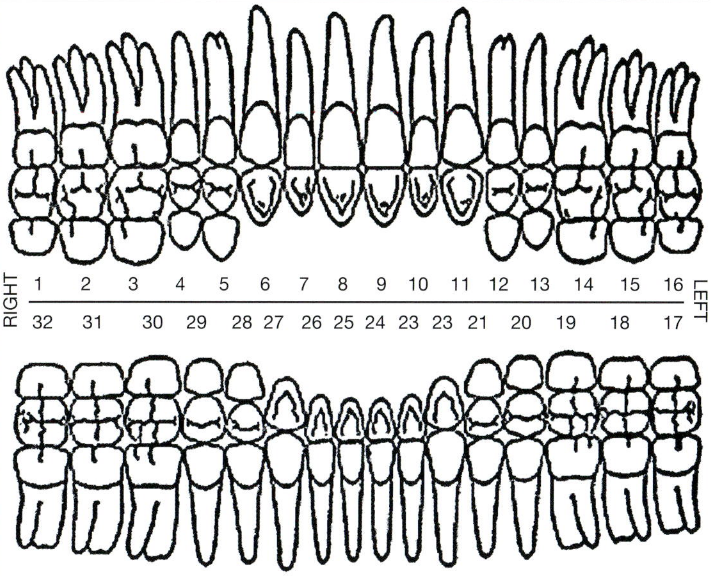

12. **REMARKS OR INSTRUCTIONS**
Use this space for additional clarification of recommended treatment or for describing treatment which does not lead itself to charting. Indicate nature of treatment and teeth or other tissues involved. Identify entry by code letter (Column a, above).

13. **DATE**	14. **TREATMENT FACILITY**	15. **SIGNATURE OF DENTIST RECORDING TREATMENT PLAN**

SECTION II - PATIENT IDENTIFICATION

16. **SEX**	17. **RACE**	18. **GRADE**	19. **ORGANIZATION**

20. **PATIENT'S LAST NAME - FIRST NAME - MIDDLE INITIAL**	21. **DATE OF BIRTH**	22. **IDENTIFICATION NUMBER**

DA FORM 3984, DEC 1972 REPLACES DA FORM 8-276, 1 AUG 62 WHICH WILL BE USED.

Fig. 7.4 Sample Dental Treatment form.

have your dental assistant and hygienist with you when you make the decision to work with an older, compromised individual because it gives them a chance to assist you in making your decision to treat or not to treat, and it allows them also to tell you their feelings about whether they feel adroit enough to work with you or alone with this category of patient.

Without your support system in play, it will be most difficult for you as the dental practitioner to do what needs to be done to satisfy your older patient. So, think about it...

What is your goal here?

- To sell dentistry.
- To provide ongoing care for your patient.
- To make a lot of money.
- To put another notch on your dental belt.
- Make yourself look good in the eyes of your peers and patients.
- Get on the "good" list with your suppliers as a faithful customer.
- To be esteemed in the eyes of your staff.
- To work up an older, compromised patient and then refer to a colleague.
- To get to "Yes" for your treatment plan acceptance.

What is the meaning of "Yes" here?

- Is it an adverb that expresses agreement...?
- Is it a noun meaning an affirmative reply...?
- It can be a noun that expresses one's willingness to BS their way out of a situation by giving an affirmative answer, but avoiding the commitment...
- It is possibly a stall tactic with the subliminal meaning that "I want to think about it...".

What does "I want to think about it" mean?

It means that the patient is rationalizing what he/she thinks they heard regarding your comments, but are conjuring up answers to appease themselves in their decision-making process in order to get to an answer that is acceptable to them.

The following is a rationalizing scenario:

1. I am scared due to "fear" of the unknown and cannot decide.
2. The risk involved frightens me. I should stop now before I am in over my head.
3. There is NO motive to buy. I do not see a benefit through the proposed cost presented to me.
4. Due to what I am hearing, I feel a lack of trust.
5. I feel a lack of understanding, due to what I hear. There is no consideration given to me (no discounts or breaks spoken about).
6. The price is too high for my means. There were no alternatives given.
7. I am sure I can get it done for a "cheaper" price elsewhere.
8. "I can't afford it anyway!" (the ultimate rationalization).

How do we make an impression on our patients to get them to "want" what we think they "need"? Tell them a story... (Box 7.3).

Johari Window

There is also a useful tool that I have used in getting to learn about myself and my patients; especially those patients whose treatment plans will be complicated and long-term. It is called the **Johari Window** (Fig. 7.5).

The Johari Windows are the "light" that will shine upon you and your patients. If you are brave enough to speak to your patients, staff, families, caregivers and the like about yourself and how they perceive you as well as your turn in doing the same with your patients and staff, the rewards will be having patients and associates for life. One may think they know themselves; however, when it comes to a perfect stranger asking about yourself after only a short period of time in knowing each other, it is a wonderful door that opens to give you a glimpse of how someone else sees you in a different light. The same for you and your patients.

Getting to "Yes" is a journey, but not without some pitfalls, a lot of hard work and effort. It takes a great deal of communication and interpretation, patience and understanding, but in the long run, it is worth every moment that you may spend on this exercise.

An effective way to communicate is to understand the process of how we understand messages and then again, how we process them. In the 1980's, a psychologist by the name of Avram King developed a method of understanding how one comes to make a decision through a **"Step-Wise" System**

BOX 7.3

Quality Outcome Assessment

"Imagine it and then create it..."

- Is the treatment **Conceivable**?
- Is the treatment **Doable**?
- Will the treatment be **Maintainable**?
- Will the treatment be **Sustainable**?
- Will the treatment be **Achievable** from what I know?
- Will the treatment be **Acceptable** as proposed?
- Will there be a **Positive outcome** for all concerned?
- Can I **Work backwards** from here...?

Factors of Success: **Change management...**

SWOT(T) Analysis

KNOWLEDGE = INFORMATION = POWER

(S) Strengths = Assets **(W) Weaknesses = Assets** **(O) Opportunities = Assets**
(T) Threats = Assets **(T) Trends = Assets**

1. **Change management** involves one's ability to effect change through efficiently using the tools they have and have learned in business, as well as with accessible communication techniques, **in** the application of a structured process and set of tools for **leading the people-side of change to achieve a desired outcome.**
   This is a particularly important part of getting to "Yes" in the process of defining your dental treatment plan and subsequent treatment.

2. **The SWOTT analysis** gives one a useful tool to determine the **Strengths** of your components and what you present to the patient and/or family members responsible for the financial side and decision-making aspects of treatment for their elders. One's **Weaknesses** are a listed asset because we can learn from our previous experiences on what not to do and how not to act or react to negativity, rationalizations and disinterest in our treatment plans that are presented. Change is constant and we must "bend with the winds of change" if we are to accomplish our goals. I always like to "strike" when the iron is cold! This means taking **Opportunities** to discuss things, ask questions, challenge thoughts and answers as well as present my opinions, based on provable facts, when they are least expected. This is a real asset and works to break down my resistant patients' attitudes and promotes their abilities to listen attentively and respond positively. These kinds of **Threats**, which can be detrimental to case presentation and acceptance, can be handled effectively by discussing the unexpected.

I have had many patients who have been resistant to change. I have challenged them and said caregivers in their thinking and asked them to explain themselves in being reticent about accepting or even considering my treatment plans. When I can show them that their threats are defeating their goal for recapturing their ultimate health, they usually respond positively after getting over the shock of having their thinking challenged. This is done in both a gentle, kind and communicative way with an acknowledgment of feelings attended to first, followed by useful and important information. Monitoring positive acceptance will set the **Trend** for effective use of the SWOTT analysis in future patients.

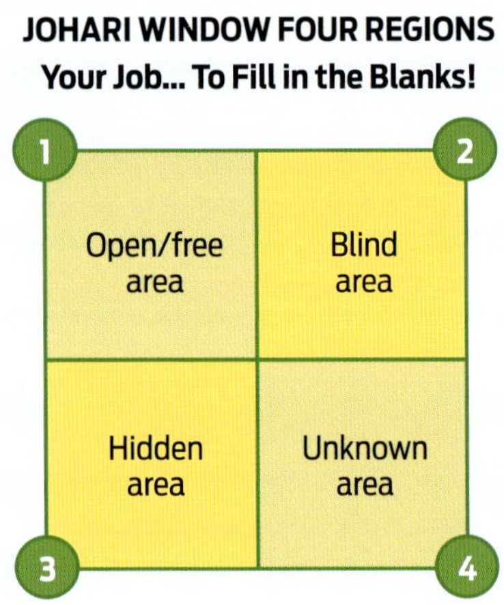

1. What is known by the person about him/herself and is also known by others – **open area, open self, free area, free self or "the Arena".**
2. What is unknown by the person about him/herself, but which others know – **blind area, blind self or "blind spot".**
3. What the person knows about him/herself that others do not know – **hidden area, hidden self, avoided area, avoided self or "façade".**
4. What is unknown by the person about him/herself and is also unknown by others – **unknown area or unknown self.**

Fig. 7.5 Johari Window.

to Learning (Fig. 7.6) and its importance in understanding the messages that were conveyed.

Decision making is a big part of knowing our patients and how they base these decisions on whatever information is conveyed and their subsequent interpretation of it that leads them forward in the process of getting to "Yes" or "No".

"The most important thing in communication is hearing what isn't said!"

You, as the sender of messages to your patient about his/her treatment plan, give certain facts and information gleaned from your examination of the patient and the history taking. The message is conveyed verbally and with visual and tactile examples of what it is you are trying to explain. The message is basically information in several forms. It is given out in a manner that best fits the person's learning style as discussed previously in this chapter, that is, Visual, Auditory and Kinesthetic.

The **information** takes a path in the patient's brain to the **stage of interpretation**. It is at this point that **judgment** is passed about that information, based upon this person's experience, as well as the knowledge and teachings from the dental practitioner and any other source of information stored in their brain. Once the information has been

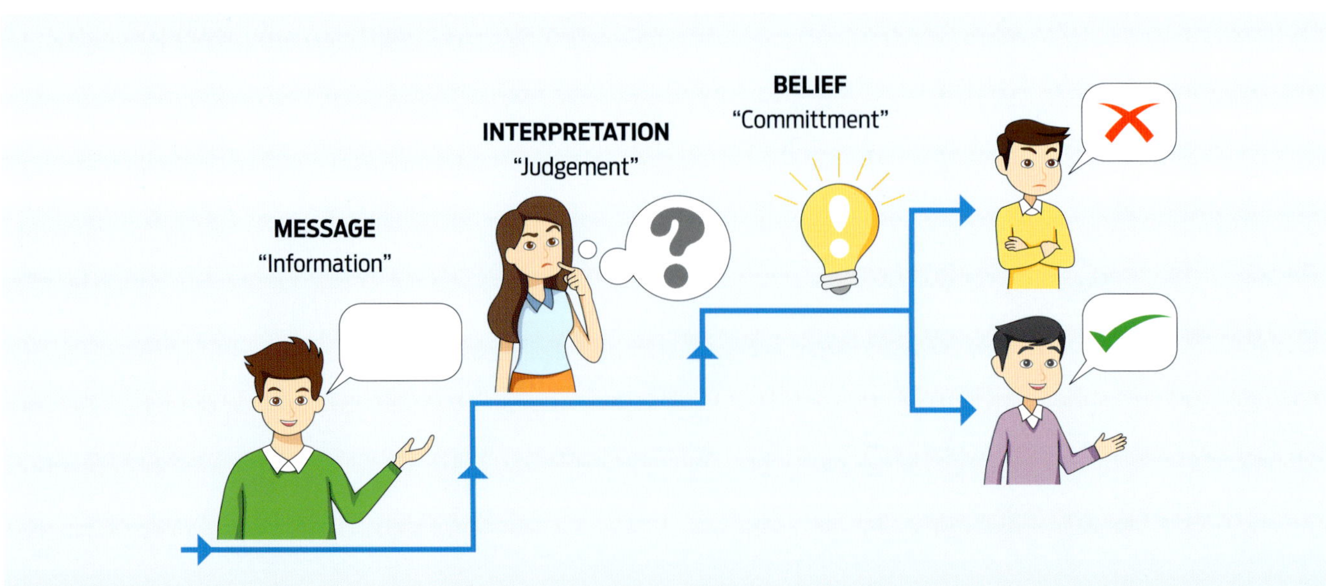

Fig. 7.6 A Stepwise System of Learning.

processed to a point of understanding, whether inferred or verbally communicated, this patient can form a belief about what it is they are thinking, in turn, making a **commitment** to either do the proposed treatment, alter the plan or not do it at all (Fig. 7.7). This mechanism of communicating will work-out well if the practitioner has followed all the steps I have mentioned previously in this chapter.

Informed Consent: Why, How and When?

Informed consent is a process of communication between the patient or patient's representative, and their health care provider that leads to agreement or permission for care, treatment, or services. Every patient has the right to get information and ask questions before procedures and treatments. The motto "**inform before you perform**" is what one needs to remember prior to doing any treatment whatsoever.

We live in a highly litigious society and one can never know who might turn around and file a lawsuit against a practitioner considering their "perception" that the practitioner or a staff member did something wrong to harm them in some way.

There should be an informed consent for every procedure we perform in our offices, including dental hygiene. I have not been in one office in over 50 years where there is an informed consent for dental hygiene given out prior to treatment, but that does not mean we should not have one. There are some clinics, schools and offices that have modernized their thinking and are now using an informed consent for hygiene procedures. Recently, I noticed in a clinic where I was teaching that an elderly woman had fallen asleep during scaling and root planning. While the hygienist was working away, this patient suddenly awoke seemingly startled as to where she was and whipped her head left and right in a frenzied manner. The whipping action of her head caused the operator to slip with the curette and inadvertently cut a line down the patients' lip across the vermillion border to the upper part of her chin. Not a good scenario. I was called in to mediate in Spanish with the patient and explain what happened. I gave the patient a mirror to show her the wound, which was superficial, no less a wound, and gave her a few packets of antibiotic cream to put on it at home, which I demonstrated for her. She was informed that if she wanted to go to an emergency room that we would cover the cost, but she declined. I had the hygienist write a narrative verbatim of the incident and conversation, and I did the same. These things can happen, through no fault of our own, but they must be recorded and there must be an informed consent that can list the possible side-effects of any treatment rendered, besides what the expected results from treatment should be. "**Protect thy staff and thyself and patient at all times**". If there are accidents that occur in the office or clinic, the patient should always be called to be questioned about how they are doing, after the fact, and if they need anything. The time date and conversation should be recorded in the patient record as well.

There are four components of **informed consent** including decision capacity, documentation of consent, disclosure and competency. It is imperative that each one of our consent forms have these entities in the context of information regarding a specific procedure. It might also be beneficial, even though time consuming, to have these stated in terms that a cognitively impaired patient might understand as well as their caregiver or family representative.

There are four principles of informed consent:

1. The patient must have the capacity (or ability) to make the **decision**.

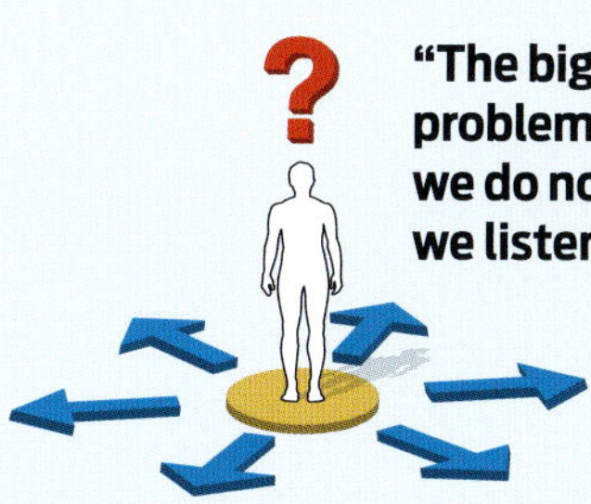

"The biggest communication problem most of us have is that we do not listen to understand, we listen to reply".

Note: if the patient is too feeble and mentally challenged to understand the process and if the practitioner was not able to thoroughly discuss the information at hand in a manner conducive to mutual understanding and subsequent decision making, then the practitioner must do this exercise with either the family or caregiver, or both, to come to an agreement about what treatment is necessary, relevant, and able to be achieved in a successful manner.

Fig. 7.7 Choices and decisions?

2. The dental provider must **disclose information** on the treatment, test, or procedure in question, including the expected benefits and risks, and the likelihood (or probability) that the benefits and risks will occur. All of this is **documented** and signed.
3. The patient must comprehend the relevant information.
4. The practitioner must voluntarily grant **consent**, without coercion or duress.

I like to add a 5th provision in lieu of the 3rd principle, and that being that **the language must be understandable, and the procedures must be defined in simple lay terms, coupled with pictures, if needed, especially for older adults that are not familiar with the dental language being used**. Without understanding, there is no way that the older, more compromised patient can make an educated decision about their care.

And for this last reason, getting a patient to sign an informed consent **without understanding**, is akin to fraud and can get the practitioner in a great deal of "hot water".

7.6.2 Decision-Making

The components of decision-making capacity are as follows:

- The ability to understand the **options** as presented.
- The ability to understand the **consequences** of choosing each of the options that were discussed.
- The ability to evaluate the personal **cost** and benefit of each of the consequences and relate them to your own set of **values and priorities**, assuming one can elicit such information and thoughts.
- The ability to understand the ramifications of not making a valid decision.

If the patient is not able to do all the components, family members, court-appointed guardians, or others (as determined by state law) may act as "surrogate decision-makers" and make decisions for the older patient who may be mentally compromised.

To have decision-making capacity does not mean that the patient will always make "good" decisions, or decisions that the dental practitioner agrees with. Likewise, making a "bad" decision does not mean that the patient is "incompetent" or does not have decision-making capacity. It also means that the practitioner can have his/her opinions and choices as well. If the patient or their representative(s) make a "bad" decision based on the practitioner's perception, and he or she is not happy with this decision, then the practitioner can choose not to treat this patient, but must refer to someone who might meet their needs or risk "abandonment," which is an offense that he/she can be sued for as well.

> **DEFINITION:** ***Decision-making capacity***, *or competency, simply means that one can understand and explain the options, their implications, and give a rational reason why one would decide on a particular option instead of the others (see Box 7.4).*

Here are three types of Dental Consent Forms. One is a simple "fill-in" the blanks and sign, and the others are more sophisticated in that they are more specific and cover the things I have mentioned previously in this chapter.

There are also even more specific forms for every procedure that we do as Dentists that can be used, which include everything necessary for a patient to read and understand what it is that they are signing and why.

Every form can be modified to fit your own style and needs. They should include Disclaimers as well, this being what the procedure is intended to do and the predicted results, but what the treatment will not do or what happens if it fails and why, as well as the responsibility of the practitioner in this case, versus the patient having done something to impede the success of the procedure as discussed. The individualized Consent Forms enclosed here all have Disclaimers in them for your edification.

7.6.3 Sample Consent Forms

A. Simple Consent Form

This consent form is quite simple and basic (see Appendix, Fig. 1). It is a short, fill-in the blanks or circle the procedure to be done but has no specific

BOX 7.4

Updated Tenets for Treating Geriatric and Special Needs Patients

With respect to the practitioner in the decision-making process, there heeds to be some consideration of certain principles for the ultimate protection of the practitioner in the process and his/her abilities to make the process for the patient an easier and more successful one. As far as the practitioner is concerned, one must follow the **Tenets for Treating Geriatric and Special Needs Patients**, which will allow for a trusting relationship and one that will be considerate of the thoughts and feelings of both the patient and their family, the practitioner, and the staff. They are:

1. Show mutual respect for the patient, always.
2. Use your power of observation to enhance understanding for both you, as the practitioner, and your patients.
3. Innate and learned knowledge is needed and necessary in the process of treating any patient. What you think you know, and which may not be the case therefore, causing one to learn or relearn the necessary "tools" to treat the patient at hand in good faith.
4. Know before you go...
5. Communicate effectively and appropriately and include both the patient, caregiver, family member, or Power of Attorney.
6. Educate your staff with respect to the issues that the patient brings with them and what the intentions of treatment are or may be. This will include your staff in the decision-making process, as well as help educate them about the treatment process.
7. Think "MID" (Minimally Invasive Dentistry).
8. When in doubt... STOP, LOOK and LISTEN to your inner self. Possibly rethink your treatment plan and situation and back-up to renew your efforts to regroup and refine what you intend to offer the patient. If this is not reasonable, then consider referral.
9. Do not be afraid to ask for assistance.
10. Be prepared for any medical, dental, or uncontrolled situation that might occur and practice scenarios with your staff. Remember, "Practice makes permanence".

disclaimers that could protect the practitioner should something go wrong. There is a small paragraph at the end with a short Disclaimer, but not effective enough, I feel, to protect oneself.

B. Involved Consent Form

This form is more complete with a lot of information that should be put in the form to protect both the patient and the practitioner (see Appendix, Fig. 2). It gives one the opportunity to define the specific work to be done and the possible consequences. It does give reference to alternative treatment, which is a wonderful thing from the treatment plan discussion to put into the consent form.

C. Advanced Consent Form

The more advanced form for this specific procedure covers all the bases of treatment, side-effects, if any, which are spelled out for the patients' understanding. It has a place for a "witness" to sign, which is important (see Appendix, Fig. 3).

Because the information is specific for each patient, treatment may vary, as well as the laws in each state may differ; hence, consulting with an attorney or other professional advisors may be in one's best interest and prudent for medical-legal information and interpretation.

Disclaimers are a valuable part of the consent form as well as the treatment plan. I suggest using these as much and wherever possible. Without a Disclaimer, there is no recourse to handling something that did not go as expected. Without a Disclaimer for the technique you are performing, one leaves themselves open for a lawsuit should things not go as expected. The patient can come back to you for damages. There is no guarantee that they will not do this anyway, but at least with specific Disclaimer information, you have some "legal" protection that was incorporated into the permission for treatment in the Consent Form.

In our litigious society, there is no guarantee that a patient, who may be friendly or a "friend," will not go after you in court for something they think should have gone better clinically. I had such a patient, who was a friend, in as much as she was the wife of a man whose Foundation sent me to China for Humanitarian dental, medical and nursing teaching and work for almost 13 years.

This woman, in her late 50's, was a very demanding individual and would call at all hours of the day or night should something break or chip or not feel right in her mouth, wanting to be seen sooner than later... meaning now, no matter what the time of day. I would try to fit her in or see her the next day if possible because I lived at least an hour or so from my practice office. (A friend of mine who is a Minister told me once that most people expect their clergy and their dentist to be there 24/7 for them and have no qualms about calling these professionals at the drop of a hat and at any hour!).

My patient had a maxillary central incisor with internal and external root resorption (Fig. 7.8). She had fallen on her face while hiking several times over at least the last 10 years, as well as got hit by something several times. The tooth was asymptomatic, but had deep pockets on the palatal of about 7-8 mm. The tooth root was disintegrating from "internal resorption", and the surrounding bone was being lost at the level of resorption as well due to the inflammatory process. I suggested the tooth be extracted and an immediate implant be placed (Fig. 7.9). I gave her a Consent Form with "all the bells and whistles" in it about failure, peri-implantitis and more to sign, which she did. The tooth with the impaired root was removed without anything fracturing or any bone being lost and no post-operative sequelae. I spent months making sure this implant would not fail. However, one day, my patient informed me that the gum was receding from the facial of the implant. There was plenty of attached gingiva around the implant, as it was never dis-

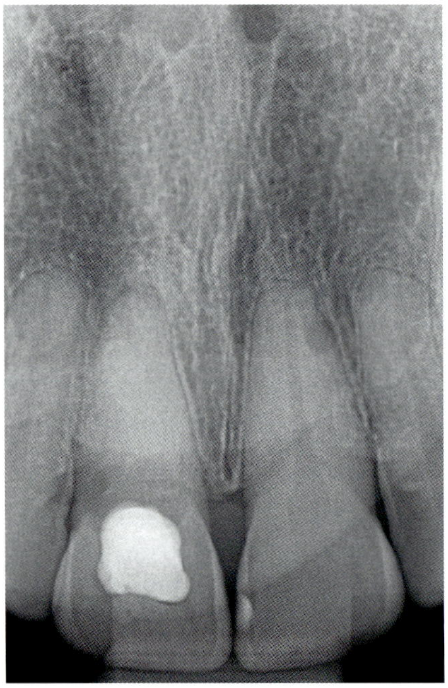

Fig. 7.8 Internal and external resorption of the right maxillary central incisor.

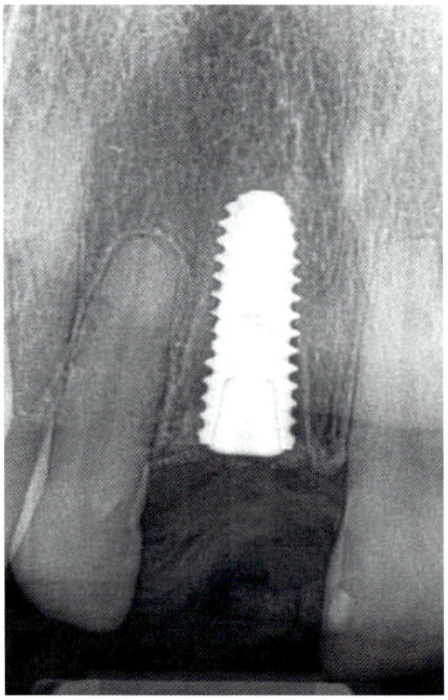

Fig. 7.9 Immediate implant placement radiograph.

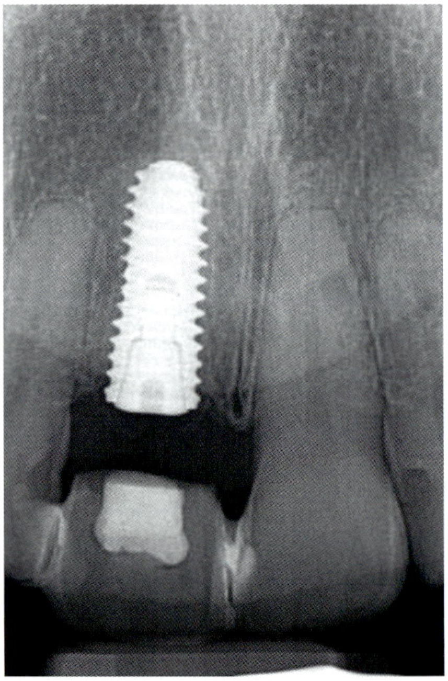

Fig. 7.10 Immediate implant placement and extracted tooth crown bonded as a temporary for esthetics.

turbed by me during the entire process. She had an extraction of the central incisor with no sequelae and the implant went right down the socket where the root had been. Bone was placed around the implant at the time of placement to seal any inequities between the socket and existing bone (Fig. 7.10). The area was covered by a collagen membrane and a primary closure was achieved with resorbable sutures. All was well until the recession.

Apparently her stayplate had broken several times and she was putting an excess amount of force on the tissue in front of the implant. Instead of coming to me, she went for a second opinion and was told the implant was not placed in the correct position. This started a real mess of verbal abuse on her part towards me and she threatened to sue me. This was a prime example of what I am talking about from personal experience, even with an Informed Consent and attached Disclaimer. This patient commuted from Paris, France, twice a year to see me dentally.

So, there is no real protection per se from this kind of action; however, in the end I was not sued, but forced to pay for this patient's next dentist to redo everything because of one millimeter of recession and her getting several other dentists, including a periodontist, who did know me, to tell her that what I did was not right. The issue was a psychological issue with this patient. She was neurotically demanding, set in her ways, expected her dentist to be on personal call to her 24/7 and her thinking was one-sided and unreasonable in my estimation. She was not rationale and I believe that she had unmet emotional needs, as well as personal issues that were the main source of her visible frustration, which she apparently took out on me.

7.6.4 Honesty

I was taught that there is one thing which should constantly be present in our lives and that is "honesty". Honesty is a major part of integrity, and with integrity everything good manifests on its own. Honesty also allows us to feel safe because it spawns fairness: where there is truth there is justice. But in some cases, such as the case I just described, that does not always happen, despite my overwhelming truthfulness, taking pride in my work and having integrity and the ability to admit a wrongdoing, if that is the case, which it was not in this previous scenario.

I once stated to my wife that if a patient sues me for something I did not do and we go to court, and the case is decided for the patient, they can take my money, but never my integrity. So, I fight for justice and what is right with respect to myself and for my patients as well. Honesty, the basis for truth, is or should be an integral part of everyone's make-up. It frees you like the cocoon letting loose the struggling butterfly, but not without a struggle to strengthen its wings. If there was no struggle inside the cocoon, the chrysalis would erupt as a beautiful butterfly, but because its muscles were not exercised prior to hatching out of the cocoon, possibly because someone opened it out of curiosity, the butterfly cannot fly and will eventually die from starvation.

Older people have years of experience and hopefully that is accompanied by wisdom. However, as we age, the hardships that befall us can be devastatingly harsh with respect to our physical and mental status, which, in turn, can affect our incomes, personal health, personal wealth, and the way we communicate. I have found some older patients to be somewhat manipulative and dishonest in how they present themselves to me as a practitioner. This could be due to mild cognitive impairment, embarrassment, or not understanding the situation they have embarked upon, or plain prevarication. It is important for all of us to be honest or seek an honest relationship when dealing with a person's overall health. Gandhi once stated, "To believe in something, and not to live it, is dishonest".

As dental practitioners, we cannot afford to be anything but honest in our communication with our patients, especially our elderly, more compromised patients. Allowing each person mutual respect, the ability to have thoughts, information and feelings different than our own, ultimately gives us trust. Without trust, there is no honest relationship, and our treatment is at risk and at a standstill, if we get that far. I can only repeat this short mantra: communicate, communicate, communicate on all levels, using all your senses to assist you in understanding your patient's and yourself with respect to each of them. Use good judgment and practice fairness to all who seek your wisdom and skill.

The Rotary Four-Way Test

Rotary International, the oldest service group worldwide has a motto called the Four-Way Test. It is used in things that we think, say and do. It was developed by a man, who eventually became the International President of Rotary, Arch Klumpf. He formulated the motto of the Four-Way Test after taking over a defunct "Pots and Pans" business that had essentially failed due to unethical business standards, poor management, dishonest relations, and unfairness with and toward the previous staff. The Four-Way test saved the business and helped it prosper. I use this test in all that I do and find it helpful in my Business/Practice and in my personal life, as I am sure you will too. I have been a member of this Club for over 45 years. It has changed my life as I have changed the lives of others in the process. Rotary is some 1,250,000 men and women worldwide.

1. Is it the TRUTH?
2. Is it FAIR to all concerned?
3. Will it BUILD GOODWILL and BETTER FRIENDSHIPS?
4. Will it be BENEFICIAL to all concerned?

Truth, Fairness and Goodwill all create better friendships and relationships. Overall, it stimulates **honesty** as a way of life. If you let it, it will be beneficial in more ways than one can imagine in your practice of Dentistry and in your life as well.

References

1. Maglio SJ, Reich T. *Feeling certain: Gut choice, the true self, and attitude certainty.* Emotion. 2019 Aug;19(5): 876-888.
2. American Psychological Association. In gut we trust when it comes to choices: Decisions recruiting gut feelings seen as reflection of true self, more assuredly held, study says; Science Daily, 10, Sept 2018. Accessed online 5-10-2021: www.sciencedaily.com/releases 2018/09/ 180910093528.htm.
3. Mind Tools, 1998.
4. Hyerle, D. (2000). A Field Guide to Using Visual Tools. US: Association for Supervision and Curriculum Development.
5. Louis, Molly St., How to Spot Visual, Auditory, and Kinesthetic-Learning Executives/ Inc.com; Accessed online, 5-10-2021 at https://www.inc.com/molly-reynolds/how-to-spot-visual-auditory-and-kinesthetic-learnini.html#:~:text=Approximately 65 percent of the, remember best through visual communication.
6. Joyce BR, Showers B. *Transfer of training: The Contributions of Coaching.* Journal of Education 1981; 163(2): 163-172.
7. Lecture of Professor Albert Mehrabian, University of California, Los Angeles.
8. The Oxford English Dictionary, Oxford University Press, Dec 1, 2010.
9. Treatment plan-DPHHS, Nov 15, 2015, DPHHS. Accessed online 5-102012 https: //dphhs.mt.gov-documents.

Chapter **8**

Sex and Oral Disease in the Compromised Older Patient: May be a "Touchy" Subject!?

"Consulting one day in the hospital with an older gentleman dementia patient, I heard a voice, turned around and found myself confronted by a woman who lifted her blouse and asked me to talk with her while she was completely exposed. With dementia, one's inhibitions are lost, and anything goes, including sex at any time or any place. I kept my "cool" and told her I would talk to her in a minute and would meet her in her room... she immediately left!"

8.1 Introduction

Mentally compromised older people are unpredictable, and one must be prepared to handle anything that comes your way with calm, rationality, a smile, all the while looking at the eyes of the person and speaking gently, and the entire time thinking about what to do next.

As we age, our sex lives change considerably (Box 8.1). In Western society, both older women and men in retirement communities, which comprises independent living situations, holiday clubs, and onboard senior cruise ship adventures, are part of a group who have more leisure time and financial assets than ever before and are probably enjoying sex more than ever before as well. In the process, we may see changes in the levels of fatigue, libido, time of having sex and arousal changes, erectile and lubrication issues, climax and discomfort issues, mobility problems and the subsequent side-effects of medication, including non-performance or performance for a shorter than expected time, heart attacks and difficulty breathing, causing fainting, stroke and even death if one overdoses on ED (Erectile Dysfunction) medication specifically. These things can continue to occur throughout ones aging process under several different scenarios, issues and partners.

Dementia will at some point, for some of us, impart added difficulty to every aspect of life, including sexual behaviors. The sexual, relational changes do not all happen at once, as one may think, or to all who suffer physically and emotionally from these changes. We cannot "lump" all aging people with cognitive impairment into the same slot of performance or love-making activity. There is no time slot, per se, when this cohort of people will start to fail, in as much as their sexual desires and performance are concerned.

The brain is the organ that is in control of every function known to the human species. It thinks about itself and how it functions. It has no feeling itself but creates feelings through both its nervous system and subsequent transference of chemicals, hormones and interactions as such, that tell the brain how to feel emotionally for our well-being and pleasure, as well as our sorrow and pain. When one develops a form of dementia, our sexual selves and behavior become part of a flowing inner-outer flood of feelings, thoughts, movements and actions that become less familiar to us over time. It is possible that we may retain our desires and subsequent actions but lose recognition of who was the object of affection that graced our presence previously, re-

BOX 8.1 Something about Sex

Sex is:

- A method of procreation.
- A primal urge.
- A pleasurable experience, or not.
- A method of spreading disease.
- A desire that may fade as we age.

What can sex do for us?

1. Sex releases endorphins, the "feel good" chemical which acts as a natural painkiller, lessens anxiety, and helps you sleep better (all of which makes you look younger, apparently!).
2. Exercise boosts circulation, which is good for the heart — and gives your complexion that after-sex glow, as well as a twinkle in your eyes, possibly.
3. Sex causes the human growth hormone to be released, making the skin look more elastic.
4. Regular sex can boost estrogen levels in women, which prevents skin dryness. It also keeps a man's prostate in check and allows for increased testosterone secretion.
5. Sex puts a smile on your face and a bounce in your step (especially when you know that everyone around you assumes you are "past it").
6. Psychologically, sex can keep you thinking "young".
7. Sex without protection is risky if you do not know your partner or care.
8. Sex can be a source of both oral and genital sexually transmitted infections (STIs) and diseases (STDs).
9. Should one suffer from erectile dysfunction (ED) at an older age, trying various things to arouse oneself could cause injury and serious consequences, especially those older individuals who are compromised physically or mentally.
10. Unprotected oral sex can be the source of oral and throat infections for both men and women.
11. Overall, sex is an expression of love and admiration for another person and oneself.
12. Sex for some is just a way of "burning calories", about 4-6 calories per session.

sponding possibly to just physical arousal and being less controlled or influenced by our former inhibitory reactions to our sexual behavior itself. Deeper memories from the past in the hippocampus region of the brain may exist, but may be fragmented, or intact or fully formed to the current place, time or partner. Sadly enough, our sexual desires may leave us in part or completely over time. As I have seen in the past, dementia coupled with memory loss can be unpredictable, volatile, and at times voracious. Our brains have the ultimate responsibility to help us understand what is happening in this process and supporting those persons with dementia. It is not just patients with dementia that need our observation and guidance, but those intact or with mild cognitive impairment, older individuals that are having or attempting to have sexual relations with one or multiple partners and not thinking that they need to protect themselves or even think about having each other tested for HIV and sexually transmitted diseases or infections prior to the intimacy and sex act itself.

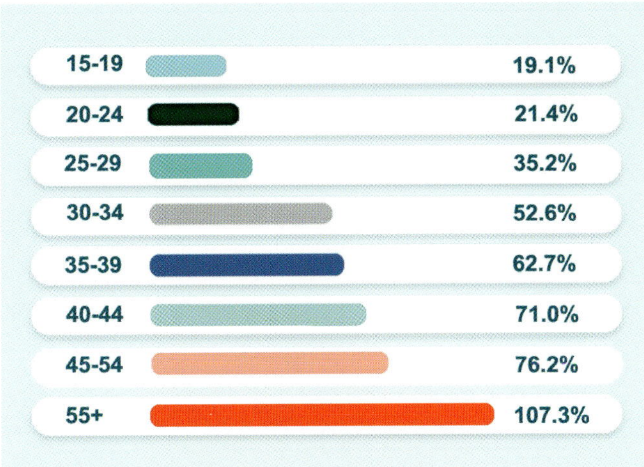

Fig. 8.1 Percentage increase in average rate of STDs by age group (2014-2018).[2]

There is not a lot of current research about sex and oral disease. However, there is a correlation between oral sex and oral health status knowing that oral sex can transmit oral, respiratory and genital pathogens.[1] One can see by the above chart (Fig. 8.1) that the rate of STDs in people over 55 years has been exponential and leads the other age groups and continues to be on the rise.

Table 8.1 shows the different infections and presenting features of sexually transmitted diseases. The infections and their method of transportation are shown and are all related to oral sex and disease.

Some head and neck cancers have been attributed to human papillomavirus (HPV), smoking, alcohol use, drug abuse, genetics, environmental issues like pollution, stress, carelessness, and erectile dysfunction prescriptions. HPV is primarily responsible for oral cancer due to oral sex practices. Unprotected oral sex is a major cause of disease transference from other parts of the body in all persons. It has been recommended to use covers for the genitalia involved, as well as dental dams or cutting a condom and opening it up to place over one's mouth for oral sex.[3]

The issue here is "will a mentally or physically compromised individual be able to protect themselves during a heated sex act of any kind, but especially oral sexual in nature?". This remains to be seen and depends upon multiple factors including rituals of meticulous oral health care habits, executive functioning skills, cognition, ability to learn about disease and how to protect oneself from acquiring it, as well as cooperation between partners.

8.2 Oral Health Issues in Older Adults

Many oral health issues affect us as we age:

- **Untreated tooth decay.** Approximately 96% of people aged 65 years or older have had dental caries, that being 1 in 5 (20%) have untreated tooth decay.
- **Periodontal disease**. A high percentage of older adults, about 2 in 3 or 68% of adults aged 65 years or older have this disease.
- **Tooth loss**. Nearly 1 in 5 (20%) of adults aged 65 years or older have lost all their teeth. Complete tooth loss is twice as prevalent among adults 75 years and older (26%) compared with adults aged 65-74 (13%). The loss of teeth and wearing dentures can affect one's ability to chew properly or eat efficiently and can adversely affect the nutritional aspects of total body health. This can also have social implications, loneliness and subsequent depression. More recently studies have shown tooth loss itself being a nidus associated with the onset of dementia.
- **Oral cancers**. Especially found in older people whose sexual practices involve experimenting without concerns for protection and caution. Cancers of the mouth (oral and pharyngeal) are primarily diagnosed in older adults; median age at diagnosis is 62 years.
- **Chronic disease**. Older individuals with chronic disease, such as arthritis, diabetes, heart diseases and chronic obstructive pulmonary disease (COPD), may be more likely to develop periodontal disease, but are less likely to get dental care than adults without these chronic conditions. Medications taken by older adults may also cause xerostomia, which, in turn, can cause dental decay and inflammation.[4]

In 2016, there were nearly 45,000 new cases of cancer of the oral cavity and pharynx diagnosed in the United States and more than 10,000 deaths. This figure has tripled in 2021. The 5-year survival rate for these cancers is about 61%. The mortality

Table 8.1 Sexually transmitted infections

Infection	Method	Presenting features
Human immuno-denciency virus	Cunnilingus, Fellatio, and Analingus	• Life-threatening sexual transmitting disease. Hamper immune system especially CD4 cells. Secondary and superinfection proceeds • No specific cure though HAART has some significant effects
Gonorrhea	Fellatio	• Sexual transmitted disease • Sore throat • Burning sensation and discharge from penis • In extreme cases cause infertility and tubal pungency in women • Increases HIV load • Treatment with antibiotics under proper medical visualization
Syphilis	Analingus, Cunnilingus, and Fellatio	• Sexual transmitted disease. Easily passed through contact with open sores (commonly called chancres) on the penis, anus or mouth (white spots in mouth) • Sores, warts and rashes of syphilis infection are painless. Left untreated syphilis can eventually cause brain damage, heart disease, blindness and death. Open syphilitic sores or chancres provide an easy entry and exit for HIV and can increase viral load • Antibiotic coverage and periodic medical check-ups will be the line of treatment
Chlamydia	Fellatio, Cunnilingus, and Analingus	• STD caused by the *Chlamydia trachomatis* bacteria and affects women more than men. Common features include pain while urinating, smelly vaginal or penile discharge, spotting after intercourse, can be found in the throat, but less commonly than gonorrhea • In extreme cases cause severe damage to women's reproductive system, including permanent infertility • Increases HIV viral load. Can be cured by proper medical treatment
Herpes	Fellatio, Cunnilingus, and Analingus	• An STD caused by herpes simplex virus is the most common cause of genital ulceration. There are two types of the virus: Type 1 affects mainly the lip causing cold sores and Type 2 causes blisters on the genitals • Sores and blisters (usually on the lips, genitals or anus) are very infectious and painful • Research suggests that having genital herpes can more than double your risk for HIV infection • Some individuals with herpes usually have periodic outbreaks throughout their lives • Treatment can reduce the frequency and severity of herpes outbreaks, but there is no cure
Human papillomavirus-genital warts	All modes of oral sex	• HPV infection and genital warts are the most common STDs. Warts usually appear on the penis or in the anus but may also occur in or around the mouth or lips. Genital warts may be more common and harder to treat • Spread through skin-to-skin contact. Contact with warts or HPV while most strains of HPV only cause warts. Some strains may cause oral or throat cancers • Different cures are available, but the virus stays in the body. Vaccine available
NSUM	Fellatio, Cunnilingus	• NSU can cause burning when urinating and/or discharge from the penis • Infections of the throat can cause a sore throat • NSU may amplify viral load in semen making it easier to spread HIV • Manageable with antibiotics and hospitalization
Hepatitis A and E	Analingus	• Both these diseases can be spread through oral sex. Hepatitis A and E both are contagious viral infections of the liver • Common symptoms of hepatitis are fever, diarrhea, loss of appetite, dark urine, vomiting, jaundice and pain in the abdomen • Vaccination is available for prevention

(continued)

(continued)

Infection	Method	Presenting features
Hepatitis B	Fellatio, Cunnilingus, and Analingus	• It is most commonly transmitted by inoculation of infected blood, virus particles are found in semen, stool, and saliva, as well as blood. There is clear evidence that it can be transmitted through vaginal and anal intercourse, but it is unproven whether it can be transmitted through oral sex. Hepatitis B can cause weakness, dark urine, jaundice (yellowing of skin and eyes), and enlarged liver • Vaccination is available for prevention
Bowel organisms and worms	Analingus	• The bowel organisms *Salmonella*, *Shigella* and *Campylobacter* can all be transmitted • Abdominal pain and diarrhea • Treated well after microbiological stool examination
Intestinal parasites	Analingus	• These include *Amoeba*, *Giardia* and *Cryptosporidia*. Symptoms include unknown diarrhea, stomach cramps, bloating, increased gas, and nausea • Treated well after microbiological stool examination

HIV=Human immunodeficiency virus; STDs=Sexually transmitted diseases; HPV=Human papillomavirus; NSU=Nonspecific urethritis; HAART=Highly active antretrovral therapy. (Adapted from Reference 1).

rate from oral cancer is nearly three times as high in males as it is in females (4 versus 1.4 for every 100,000 people) and nearly twice as high in white and black populations as it is in the Hispanic population (2.6 versus 1.5 for every 100,000 people). Preventing high risk behaviors, that include cigarette, cigar or pipe smoking, use of smokeless tobacco, vaping and excessive use of alcohol, are critical in preventing oral cancers. Early detection is key to increasing the survival rate for these cancers. Oral HPV, the most common sexually transmitted disease, can cause cancers in the back of the throat, called "oropharyngeal" cancers, or if other factors (such as smoking or chewing tobacco) interact with HPV to cause these cancers.[4]

We must understand that the statistical nature of the statistical facts presented is over a wide variety of older people and under a gamut of quality-of-life issues such as people with decreased income, poor general oral health, varied living situations or living on the street, as well as those in long-term care facilities or homebound individuals, as well as those whose mental acuity is diminished.

Oral health is vital to the general health of all people everywhere. The mouth reflects a person's health and well-being throughout life. Oral disease can affect anyone, but because of the disparities in the lives of our older population, they may be more susceptible to oral disease than the norm.

National data for older adults show racial/ethnic and income differences in untreated dental disease and oral health-related quality of life issues.[5]

According to the Center for Disease Control Annual Sexually Transmitted Disease Surveillance Report, in 2020, cases of several common STIs have reached historic highs in the elderly populations in the U.S., including chlamydia, gonorrhea and syphilis (**Figs. 8.2-8.8**).

More than 115, 000 syphilis cases have been documented, an increase of 14% to more than 35,000 cases, which is the highest number since 1991. Gonorrhea increased 5% to more than 580,000 cases, the highest since 1991. Chlamydia increased 3% to more than 1.7 million cases, the highest ever reported to the CDC.[6]

There has been a drastic increase in the above three STDs in the elderly population, causing alarm for the older population who is at increased risk for other serious illnesses. The numbers cause concern as they imply that, with the increase of STDs among older populations, even more malicious disease such as AIDS become an increased risk as well.

Since the older population has essentially passed the stage of life for having to cope with menopause and andropause, the use of preventative measures, such as wearing condoms has decreased or altogether ceased, which essentially heightens the risk for increased infection, such as an STI.

(continued on page 148)

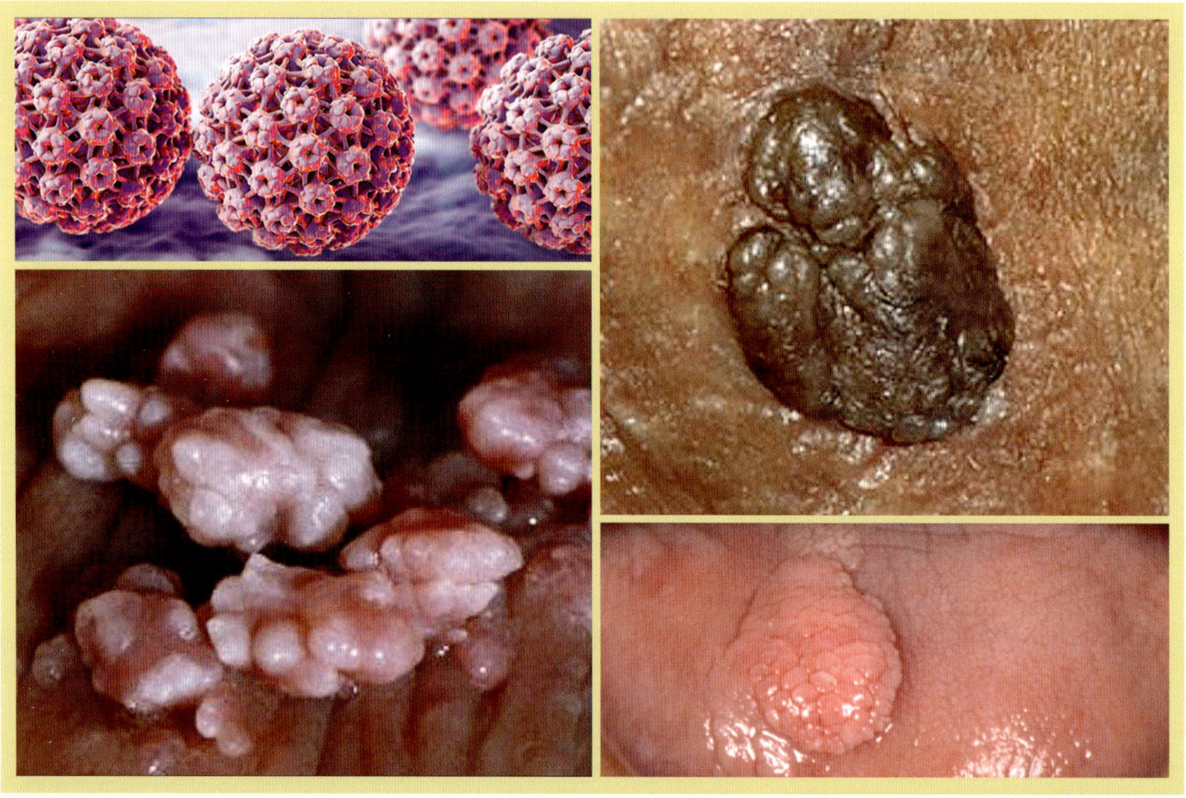

Fig. 8.2 Genital warts and human papillomavirus (HPV) on the tongue, the lip and face. (*Photo credited to WebMD.*)

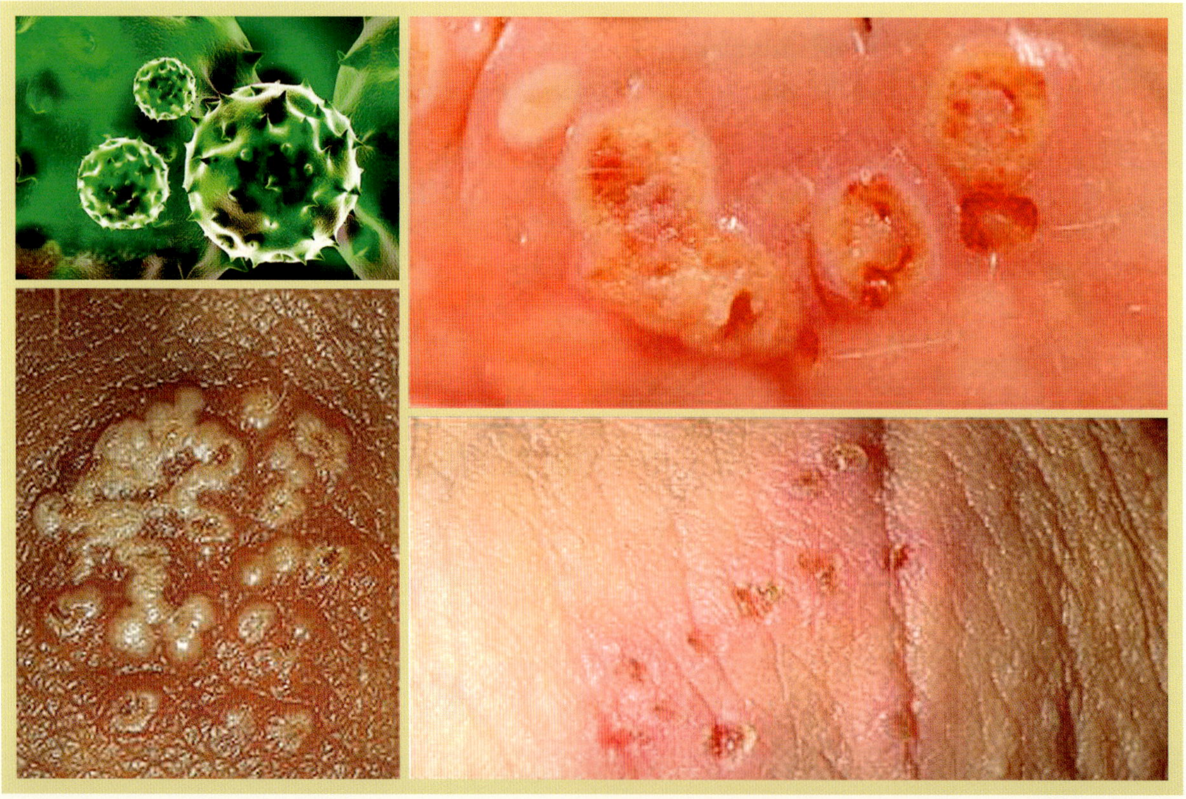

Fig. 8.3 Herpes simplex type 2 virus (HSV-2) on the skin and mucosa of the genital area. (*Photo credited to WebMD.*)

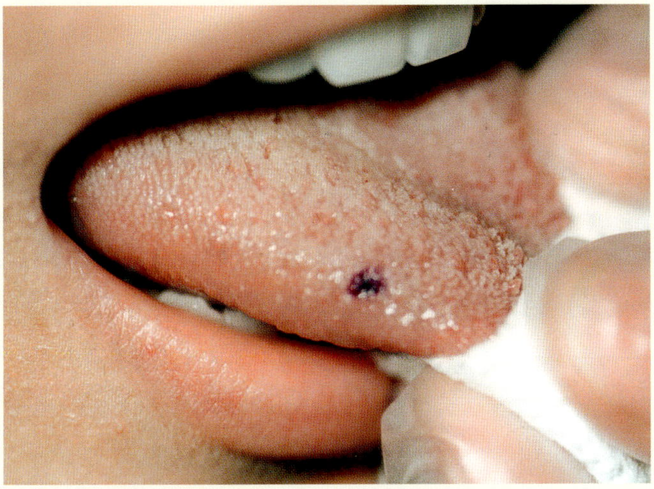

Fig. 8.4 Squamous cell carcinoma on the tongue using *ViziLite*®.

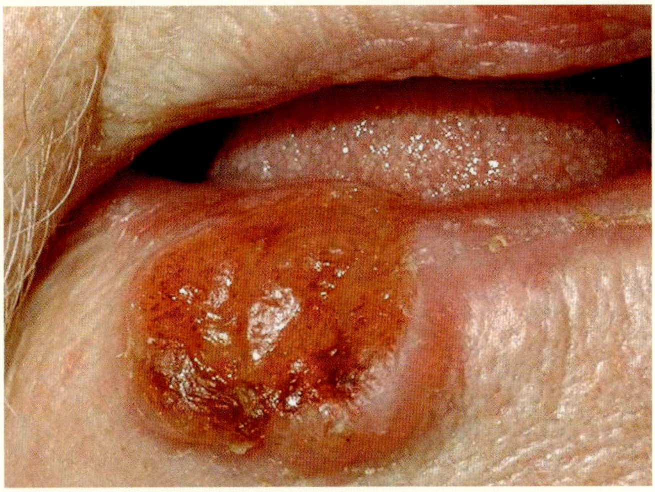

Fig. 8.5 Squamous cell carcinoma of the lip of a smoker.

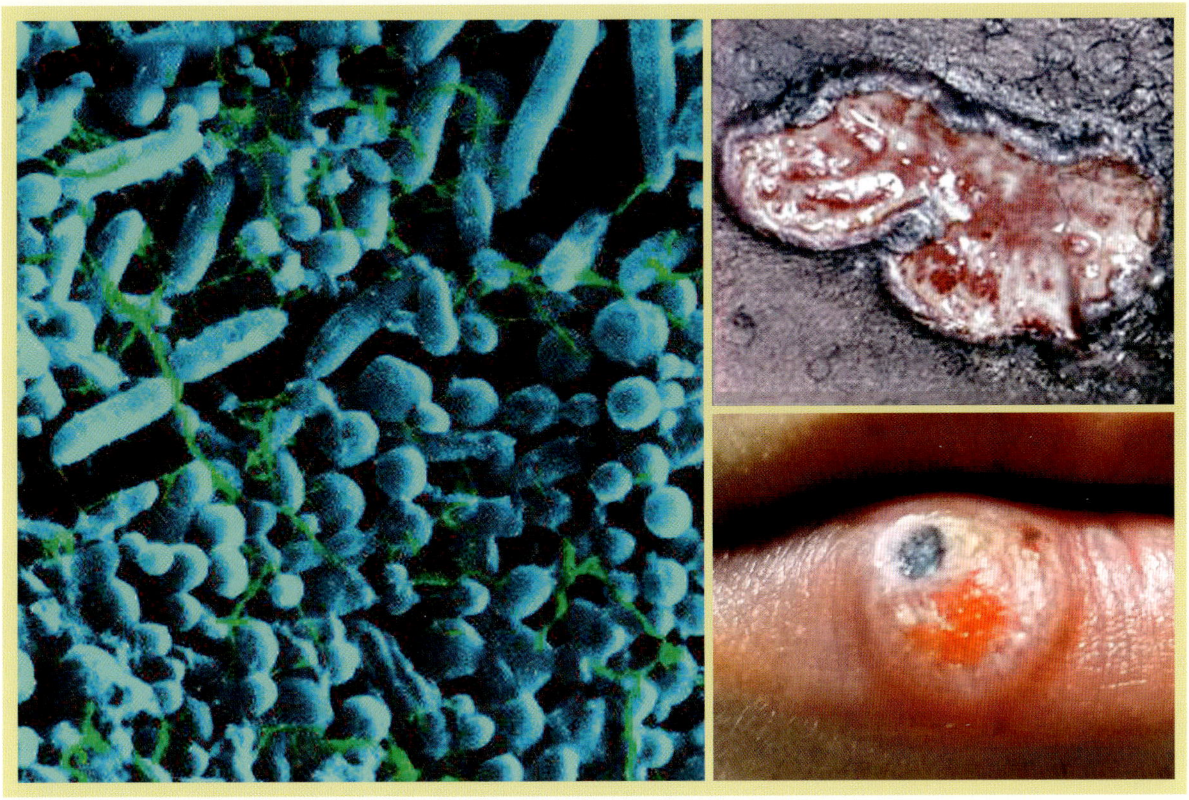

Fig. 8.6 Chancroid of the lip and the mouth. (*Photo credit to WebMD.*)

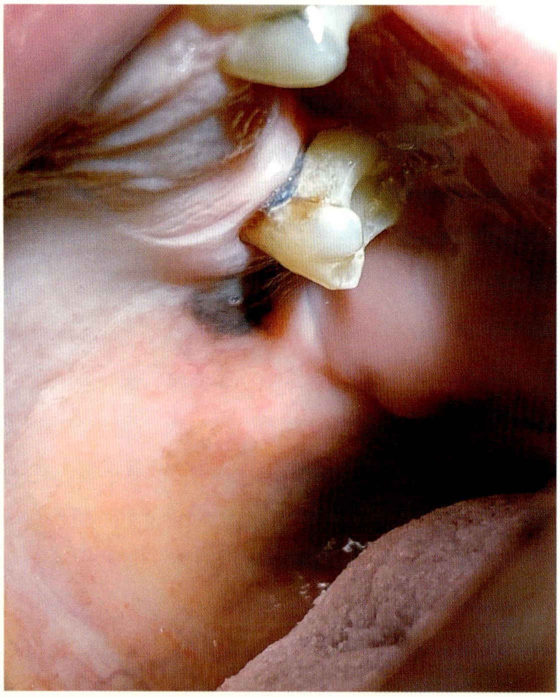

Fig. 8.7 The lesion on the posterior palate of an 80-year-old woman could be any of the following issues: bruising from oral sex, a blood dyscrasia, a syphilitic lesion, an amalgam tattoo, or a spreading type of melanoma. Biopsy is in order here.[6]

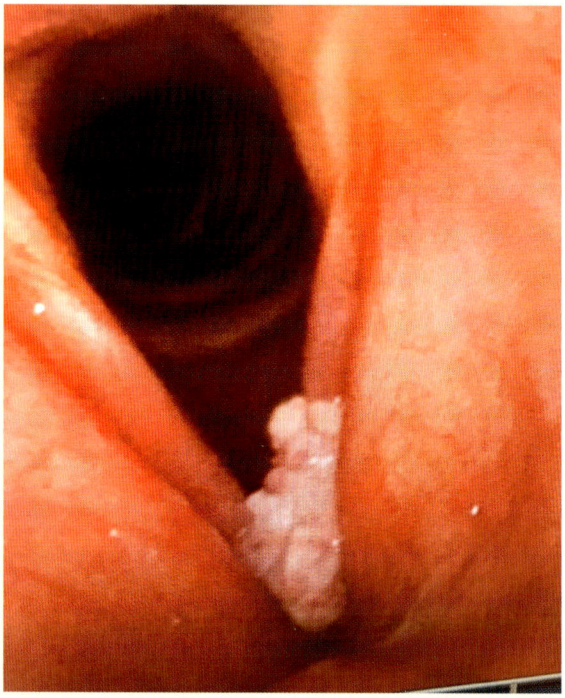

Fig. 8.8 Oral laryngeal verrucous carcinoma just under the epiglottis and most probably caused by HPV. (*Courtesy of Dr. Irwin Cohen, DPM.*)

There has been a drastic increase in HIV infection in older Americans with nearly 39,000 people diagnosed in 2017, but 17% of them were over 50 years of age![7] A big concern at present is that the older population is not educated about these sexually transmitted infections, how they are caught, how to test for them and how to protect themselves before they get this type of disease in the first place. This means that this cohort of individuals from 55 years and above could already have experienced major damage to their immune system with respect to being infected without knowing it. It is a sad statement altogether. This is information the dental practitioner needs to know about their patients.

8.3 What Can the Dental Practitioner Do to Assist the Older, Compromised Patient Affected by Oral-Sexual Disease?

Being a dental practitioner means not just being a person who "fixes" multiple issues with a patient's teeth or gingiva and the oral cavity in general. It means that we are teachers as well and, for us to get a treatment plan accepted, we must teach our patients about themselves and why it is necessary to do the things that we are recommending to them.

I once had a young mother bring her 7-8-year-old daughter in for an examination. She was a new patient to my office, and I did not know her at all. During the examination, I noted that this young girl had ground her teeth down substantially enough to almost expose the pulps of all her teeth. I asked the mother if the young girl was having difficulty in school or with friends, but she was unsure and appeared evasive, not really wanting to answer my questions. I then asked if there were problems at home and explained my observation about her daughter's teeth and how this could be related to stress or something physical that was causing her anxiety. The mother immediately got extremely angry and said, "We are leaving now! I want a dentist to fix my child's teeth, not a 'shrink' to tell me my kid has emotional problems". I then knew what part of the issue was... a domineering and strict mother and perhaps abusive as well. The mother's defensiveness was a key sign of her anxiety about the issue at hand. They got up and immediately left.

I never felt bad about my findings and discussion questions with the mother of this child, but I did feel uncomfortable about this mother internalizing what I was saying and perhaps feeling guilty about her relationship with her daughter. We learn from experience and now when I see an older adult, who may be compromised either physically or mentally or both, I take my time, gather my clinical information and then inform the patient of my findings; then again, I ask questions to the answers I do not have, whose answers I need to know. I have found that older people are usually accepting of being asked questions and answering them directly. I have been interviewing many older adults of all kinds from all walks of life and ethnic backgrounds, religions and diverse backgrounds and professions for a book I am also writing about *Sex after 60*. Most of the people talk freely about their sex lives and a lot of their comments are good learning information for my future and many are humorous yet honest statements about true life experiences. One gray-haired older women, in her late 70's, who was a pie maker in a fishing camp in Alaska, told me when I asked her about her sex life, "that just because there is 'snow' on the mountain top doesn't mean there isn't any fire in the belly!". She had waited 30 some years to meet the man of her dreams to finally have sex again, but not before he married her. So, I ask about a patient's social history and part of that is asking about an active sex life, etc. If I find that the patient (male usually) is taking an erectile dysfunction (ED) medication, I will then pose more questions about who, what, how, why and when. I want to know if they have had any sexually transmitted diseases recently or in the past and oral-sexually transmitted disease as well, and if there were any infections recently. I ask about their personal habits and protecting themselves as well. From this point, should they answer "Yes" to my questions, I then ask permission to discuss my thoughts with them and inform them how some habits can harm them long-term and how we need to treat the oral cavity in the meantime. I usually get an exceptionally good response. This is one way we can assist our older patients with sexually transmitted disease infections to their bodies and oral cavities and mouth tissues.

Another way is to have pamphlets in the reception room that discuss these types of diseases so that the patient can be free to pick one or several out at the dental office. These are available through the local public health office or at any hospital and numerous physicians' offices as well. A third way is to inform your patients, who may be afflicted with an STI or STD, the name of a physician that they can see for examination and treatment prior to your treatment starting. If they have a family doctor they can talk to and trust, they can see that person whom they trust and have a long-term relationship with.

The difficult part of all this is working with dementia patients or cognitively impaired older patients who cannot answer these questions (Fig. 8.9); therefore, one must ask their family member, guardian, or caregiver. There is the privacy act, so when there is a third party involved and they sign a consent form and tell us they have the power of attor-

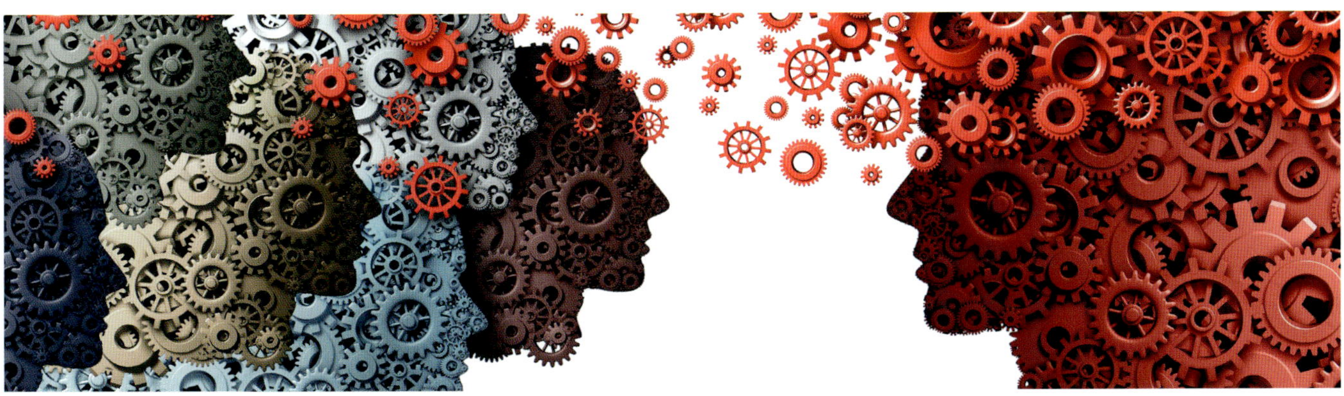

Fig. 8.9 Dementia and the loss of self. (*Photo from Shutterstock.*)

ney, it is alright to discuss the treatment findings and ask for assistance with these questions, should the patient still have an active sex life with a wife, husband, or significant other that they know about.

In most assisted living/memory care facilities there is an "open door" policy. In many states, such as California, the law prohibits locking patients in their rooms or prohibiting them from roaming the facility, at least in the section that they live in. In these communities there is a lot of "hanky panky" going on between men (of which there are very few due to women statistically living longer) and women who live there. My mother lived in one of those facilities prior to her death and was always having men and women coming to bother her and touch her; however, she was a feisty woman and fended them off in the middle of the night while sleeping, not being as advanced with her dementia as they were. Several times, she was awakened in the middle of the night to find a man sleeping on her floor just inside her door and this startled her to no end. When this happens, one knows that there are not enough caregivers to inhabitant's ratio to watch the residents 24/7 and things do happen.

In another facility, I had a patient who decided he would take another inhabitant, a woman, about the same age, 85 or so, and marry her. First off, they smiled at each other and then moved to holding hands. After they did this for a few weeks, they were spending their nights together in his or her room. And then apparently it progressed to foreplay and then finally sex of some kind (I was not privy to that information). The gentleman's son decided to hold a faux wedding for them using an impersonator priest and a fake marriage license, due to logistical complications of insurance, trusts and inheritance issues, etc. that would complicate the relationship and the families dealing with this scenario. The son bought a pair of simple rings and used them for the ceremony. The woman passed away about 6 months later, followed by the husband about 4 months after that, probably due to a broken heart. Neither of them knew or remembered each other's names, but they were ecstatically happy at the end of their lives for they had found each other in a sea of mental confusion and managed to block it out with their love for each other.

8.4 Host Immune Response in Patients with STDs Having Dental Treatment

When any disease entity occurs within the human body, a host immune response begins. Inflammation is a part of the innate defense mechanism of the body against infectious or noninfectious etiologies. Inflammatory cells are alerted and go to the area of infection. C-reactive protein is elevated and is a marker for infection and inflammation in the body, but it is not specific for the disease that is causing the issue. One can test for it clinically through a blood test to determine the degree of infection. White blood cells are increased, as are cytokines and other chemicals that cause and fight inflammation and alert the body of their presence (Fig. 8.10).

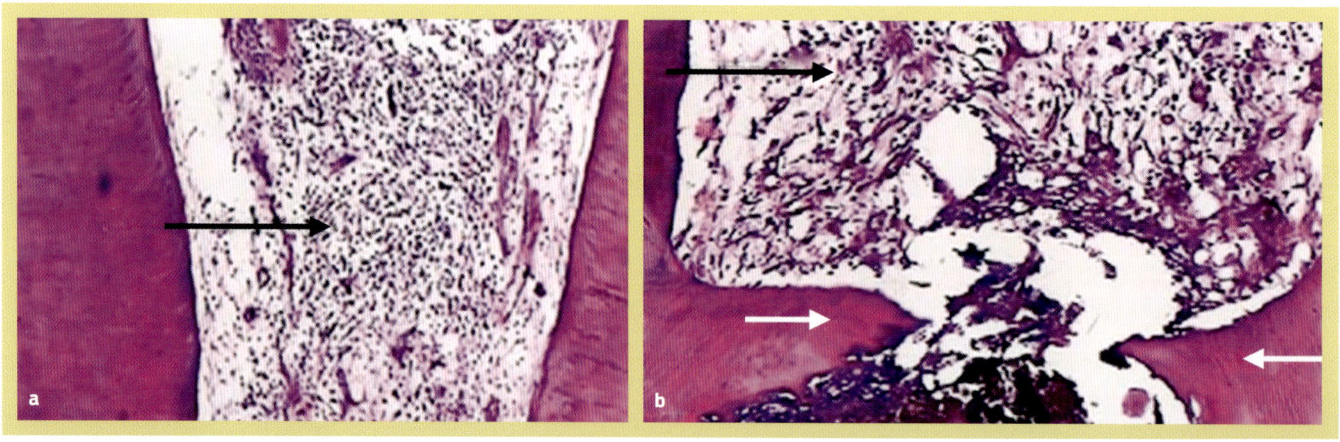

Fig. 8.10 **(a, b)** Inflammatory infiltrate in skin. (*From the archives of Robert Goldstein, MD, Ob-Gyn. Procured with permission.*)

Clinically, infection in the mouth is seen in the signs of redness (rubor), swelling (tumor), heat (calor), pain (dolar), blanching (pallor), loss of function (functio laesa), as well as bleeding, ulcerations, suppuration, and growths of one kind or another. The four cardinal signs of inflammation can be explained by the behavior of the underlying tissue. This response consists of physiologic processes triggered by the release of pharmacologically active substances such as histamine and heparin. These activate acute inflammation which is released by mast cells that are scattered about in connective tissue and react to tissue damage or other modalities causing a change or disturbance.[8]

Should the practitioner do an examination and find these signs and symptoms, they should think the presence of "disease" first and investigate thoroughly. Taking tissue samples of lesions of unknown etiology is recommended for biopsy or cytology or both. It is important to measure all lesions, take photos and chart the position of the lesion, should a biopsy subsequently wipe-out any reference to the primary lesion, resulting in the loss of references to where the original lesion initiated. If the lesion was a carcinoma, then a surgeon might have to go back and do a wider excision, but without a reference point, more destruction from a more involved surgical biopsy might occur without the reference and coordinates to the original lesion.

Of course, diagnostic instruments such as *Velscope*® (Fig. 8.11) or *ViziLite*® or other similar light systems can be used to visualize any lesions in the mouth or direct staining with the Toluidine blue stain method as well. This method, Toluidine blue, I used for many years, and it was most effective. To use Toluidine blue, first clean the lesion with sterile water, followed by bathing the area with a diluted vinegar (1% acetic acid) solution for 20 seconds. Then rinsing with sterile water, after which the stain is placed over the affected area with a Q-tip. Then reduce the area with a diluted vinegar (1% acetic acid) solution for 20 seconds and rinse with sterile water again. Anything left around the lesion or affected area that remains "blue in color" points to a possible abnormality to be determined by biopsy and microscopic examination. It is a simple treatment and usually gets good results. You can procure the stain from a pharmacy or dental school pathology lab. The *ViziLite*® or *Velscope*® diagnostic tests (see Fig. 8.11) have their own system and techniques. It is quite accurate and can afford us the ability to see lesions and pre-malignancies that we could not see with our naked eyes. The cost of the equipment is worth it when one considers the cost of not finding something detrimental to your patients' overall health and long-term welfare.

Studies have shown that HPV is more prevalent in younger women, however, older women are at a higher risk between the ages of 57-85, especially those with multiple partners, who are sexually active, smoke and have their uterus intact. Current marital and smoking status, frequency of sexual activity, history of cancer and hysterectomy were all associated with high-risk HPV positivity. One in 16 women in a representative population aged 57-85 were found to have a higher risk for HPV, with this prevalence being stable across older age groups. Women aged 65 and older will comprise 21.7% of the population by 2030, allowing for more frequent infection in a larger cohort of people.[9]

I suggest to all my older female patients that if they do not have regular visits to an OB-GYN, that they consider doing so, to make sure that they do not have any issues with HPV, cancer, and the like. I refer my older male patients to a Urologist for testing and treatment as well. Sexually transmitted diseases know no boundaries and do affect the oral cavity, subsequently causing cancer as well. With the onset of dementia, and an increase in indiscrim-

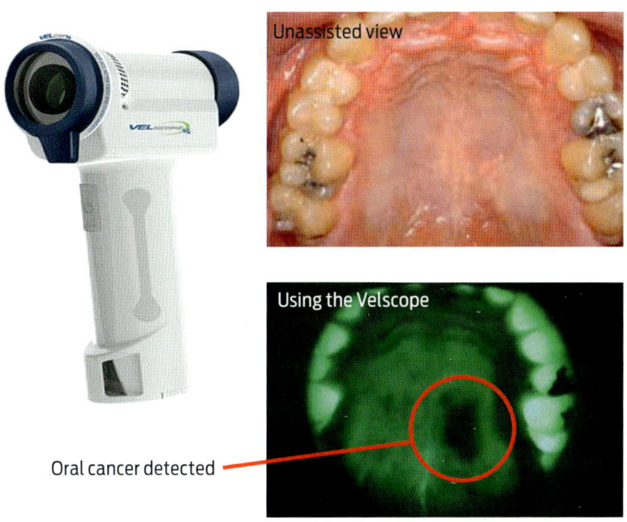

Fig. 8.11 *Velscope*® oral cancer screening instrument. (*Courtesy of Velscope*®.)

inate sexual activity with multiple partners, finds disease rates in both older men and women at an extremely high titer among the population. Being a dental practitioner and having purview of the head and neck areas and the oral cavity, as well as taking a general medical and social history, allows us to guide the patient into respecting their overall health. Again, "attached to every tooth is a person". This allows the dental practitioner to be a leading "change agent" when it comes to total body health, especially for our older patients.

"It is in your moments of decision that your destiny is shaped."

Tony Robbins

We, as dental practitioners working with the older segment of our Society, will find a plethora of disease states, if we look for them. It behooves us to learn as much as we can about sexually transmitted diseases and infections and how these are inherently in higher frequencies among the older segment of our population and on the rise, especially with the population aging at a more rapid rate and with people living longer.

Many of my older male patients are taking ED (erectile dysfunction) medication so that they can be active sexually when with a partner. Because the mind-set is such, that older women are beyond having children, they go unprotected, without condoms more that not. Older women are also taking chances with unprotected oral and other sexual practices. *Going without knowing* is an issue that needs "***Sex Education 101***" again. We need to be able to educate our older patients about the risks they take when they are sporting multiple partners and not thinking of the ramifications of what they are risking.

I have given numerous lectures on *Sex 101 and Oral Disease*, as well as *the History of Sex and Sexually Transmitted diseases* over the last 10 years. The lecture halls are filled to the brim with older individuals who show a nascent curiosity for many reasons, I am sure. But the over-riding raising of hands to ask questions is proof that the lack of knowledge about the spread of disease through sexual contact or any kind of lovemaking is overwhelmingly present and on the minds of these people after they hear me speak and see my slide show. So be curious with forethought during your initial dental examinations and do not hesitate to investigate this avenue of life with your older patients. You could save someone a lot of grief and prolong their life at the same time.

References

1. Kumar T, Puri G, Aravinda K, Arora N, Patil D, Gupta R. *Oral sex and oral health: An enigma in itself.* Indian J Sex Transm Dis AIDS. 2015 Jul-Dec;36(2):129-32.
2. Percentage increase in average rate of STDs by Age group (2014-2018) Chart. Accessed online 05-20-21. https://www.theseniorlist.com
3. Centers for Disease Control and Prevention, *STD Risk and Oral Sex-CDC Fact Sheet.* Accessed online 05-24-21 https://www.cdc.gov-std-healthcomm-stdfact-stdris.
4. Centers for Disease Control and Prevention. *Older Adult Oral Health. Fact Sheet.* Accessed online 05-24-21: https://www.cdc.gov/oral-health/basics/adult-oral-health/adult_older.htm.
5. Griffin SO, Jones JA, Brunson D, Griffin PM, Bailey WD. *Burden of oral disease among older adults and implications for public health priorities.* Am J Public Health. 2012 Mar;102(3):411-8.
6. de Andrade RS, de Freitas EM, Rocha BA, Gusmão ES, Filho MR, Júnior HM. *Oral findings in secondary syphilis.* Med Oral Patol Oral Cir Bucal. 2018 Mar 1;23(2):e138-e143.
7. Historic High Rates of STIs Among Older Americans. Accessed online 05-25-21. https://www.forbes.com/sites/claryestes/2020/02/26/historic-high-rates-of-stis-among-older-americans/.
8. Hannodee, Sally, Nasur Uddin. *Acute Inflammatory Response.* STAT Pearls Publishing; 2021 January. Accessed online 05-30-21. https://www.ncbi.nim.nih.gov/books/NBK 556083/.
9. Lindau ST, Drum ML, Gaumer E, Surawska H, Jordan JA. *Prevalence of high-risk human papillomavirus among older women.* Obstet Gynecol. 2008 Nov;112(5):979-89.

Chapter 9

Habits and Other Factors that Lead to Oral Disease in the Older Population

"God grant me the serenity to accept the things I cannot change, the courage to change the things I can, and the wisdom to know the difference."

The Serenity Prayer

9.1 Habits

We live in a visually oriented society. This makes us vulnerable, as Humans, to the things we see other people doing and achieving on a daily basis. Some of these things affect our psyche more than others and when our brains sense that we are excited about the things we may notice directly or subliminally, making us think that we need to copy those actions, we want to feel just as important or as famous as the person whose actions made us feel important inside; so, we try to emulate these actions to make ourselves more important in the scheme of things. Some of these things that are observed are the "habits" of other persons, which may be bad habits such as using drugs, smoking, vaping, having unprotected sexual relations, spending excessive monies on wearing expensive clothing or eating certain calorie rich and sugary foods. Other processes in our brains may bring to the forefront of our minds, things we have rejected in the past as children, having been influenced by our parents, our clergy, our peers and teachers. Actions that become repetitious over time have a propensity for becoming habits. Good habits assist us in a positive way and bad habits do the opposite, even though we may not know that what we are doing is bad for us, especially if it makes us feel good in a physical and/or emotional way.

I have personally quoted the following quote by the great Mahatma Gandhi (Fig. 9.1) many times over my 50 years of teaching, because his philosophy was able to penetrate the actions of our inner psyche with respect to visualizing our outer actions and the consequences of these actions. Without awareness that there is an inner system at work which defines our basic sense of self, our attitudes, certain needs and actions in Society, we would continuously be in the dark... lost in the mire we call

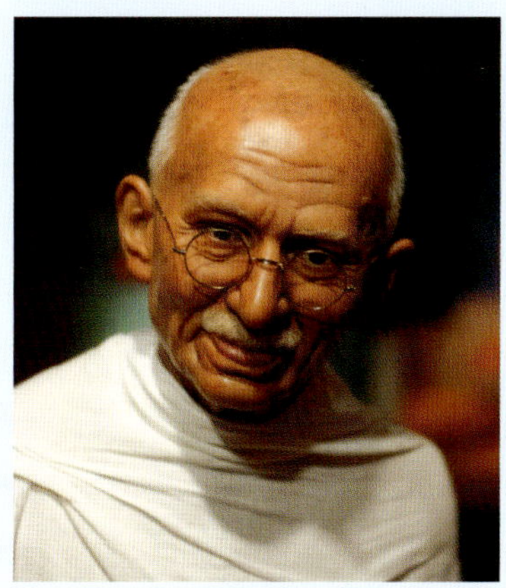

Your **beliefs** become your '**thoughts**',
Your **thoughts** become your '**words**',
Your **words** become your '**actions**',
Your **actions** become your '**habits**',
Your **habits** become your '**values**', and
Your **values** become your '**destiny**'.

Fig. 9.1 Mahatma Gandhi.

our World, seeking the light from both within and without... Our Destiny, one might call it.

The question to ask oneself then is "Where do these initial beliefs branch from and how can they be so strong as to change the actions of a person who may eventually harm themselves in some way or rather change the world in some positive light?".

Where did this desire to practice a "habit" emanate from and was it voluntary or was it forced upon someone or both? To gain answers and insight about someone and their habit(s) takes study, questions to be answered in an honest and open way and personal introspection on the part of the person exhibiting the habit being exercised. It may be an intrusive act to ask about why a person is possessed so that the habit stays with them, which in turn, may meet with rejection. An open-minded and honest person would probably meet this challenge with reflection, in an effort to make themselves a better person.

The innate knowledge we gain about people's habits can be used to help us break down the defenses of the specific behaviors supporting their habit, thereby causing the habit to slowly dissolve into oblivion, out of sight and mind of the person it inhabited.

9.2 Specific Habits that Cause Oral Disease

9.2.1 Smoking

Typically, a habit which for some unknown reason becomes so, resulting in a myriad of deleterious physical entities that can and do shorten one's overall lifespan and can cause hypertension; heart disease; stroke; pulmonary disease, including COPD (Chronic Obstructive Pulmonary Disease); emphysema; bronchitis and asthma; lung cancer; loss of appetite; cervical cancer; wrinkly skin; problems with pregnancy and newborns; increased risk of blood dyscrasias; creates yellow fingers and body odor; increases high cholesterol and triglycerides in the system making long-chain fatty acids that cause plaque in one's vessels; lowers immune system defenses; can cause infertility and erectile dysfunction; causes anxiety and irritability; complicates diabetes type 1 and 2; can increase blood clotting; causes early menopause; poor vision; dulls the sense of smell, as well as taste; promotes oral cancer; initiates periodontal disease and subsequent loss of teeth; spawns halitosis; creates darker teeth due to extrinsic and intrinsic staining, and initiates a dark or stained tongue, in turn, causing a change in taste coupled with xerostomia, and burning mouth syndrome.

Smoking can stem from an oral fixation in childhood, whereby the baby was not suckled for any length of time by its mother. It can be from boredom and nothing else to do to pass the time away, literally, under any situation at all. Or it is a learned response from childhood because it was a behavior copied from family, friends, co-workers or other kids who had more stature than oneself; thus, doing it for power, stature, feeling important and doing it repeatedly until it becomes habit, despite the side-effects of the nicotine, tars and the threat of unknown disease. Smoking tobacco is believed to be common among patients with psychiatric disorders like anxiety, depression, schizophrenia and affective disorders.[1] Nicotine is an addictive chemical and causes most of the addiction besides or in concert with the other psychological reasons

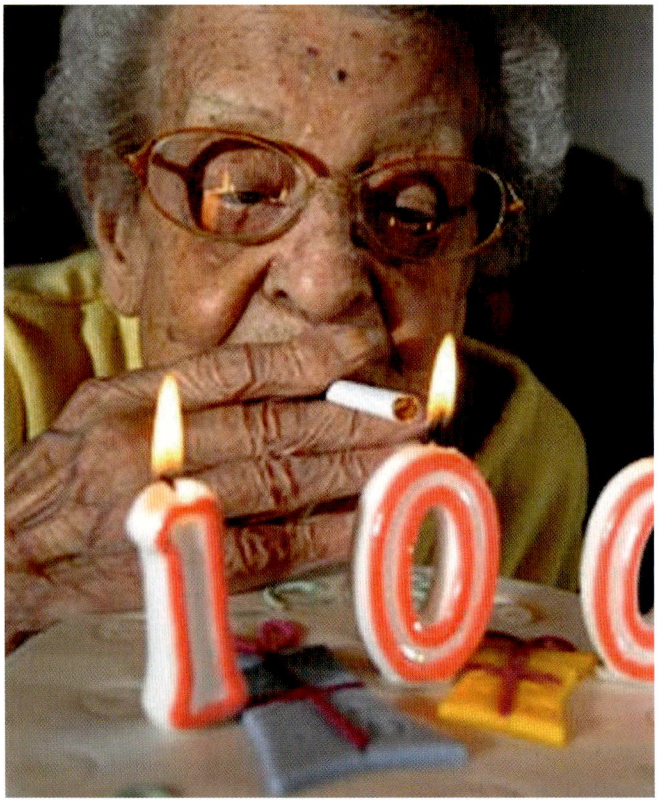

Fig. 9.2 Photo taken in a senior facility.

that spawns one to try smoking in the first place. Anyone who starts using tobacco can become addicted to nicotine, as it is a drug that naturally occurs in tobacco and thought to be as addictive as heroin or cocaine.[2]

According to the Surgeon General in a report dated 2014, nearly 9 out of 10 adults who smoke started before the age of 18, and nearly all started by age 26. The report estimates that about 3 out of 4 high school smokers will become adult smokers, even if they intend to quit in a few years.[2] These statistics have increased exponentially based on the coming of vaping and its deleterious side effects.

9.2.2 Chewing Tobacco

This is a habit mostly seen in men. Sports, like professional baseball, apparently made this a "fad" which caught on with younger people and continued into older age. The effects of nicotine are the same with this type of tobacco product, especially addiction. The oral disease that "Chew", as it is called, is devastating and oral cancer is the largest issue of concern. The tobacco is taken from a pouch, rolled into a wad and pressed into the buccal fold area of the mucosa, usually in the maxillary and mandibular anterior or side areas of the mouth. Recession of the gingiva around the teeth in the area the "chew" is placed is common, necessitating gingival grafting in those areas to prevent subsequent periodontal disease and possible tooth loss. The irritation from the juices of this type of tobacco can and does affect the oral mucosa, the pharynx, the stomach, the intestines (colon and rectum) causing inflammation, cancers and organ diseases. Chew is a dirty and unsanitary habit because the "chewer" must spit the excess juice out wherever they are at the time, unless they choose to swallow it, which most users do not do as it will make them ill.

9.2.3 Vaping (E-Cigarettes)

Recently made popular to attract those who want or need to smoke, but do not want the attributes of smoking cigarettes, as well as those who want to quit smoking, thinking that this will do the trick... However, this device that contains a mixture of "flavored" chemicals and nicotine is addictive and very harmful, causing an increase in people wanting to smoke cigarettes or increase the amount of nicotine one gets in an e-cigarette by buying extra-strength refills. It has attracted mostly younger children and teens but is gaining ground in older adults as well.

Seeing a person get out of a vehicle in a cloud of smoke is disheartening and scary. One would think they were on fire. However, both youths and older adults find that the lack of smoke is appealing and with the lack of smell, e-cigarettes reduce the stigma of smoking. Vaping is dangerous, no matter what age one may be. The mixtures inside do the same damage as smoking cigarettes and more, as well as having an instrument that can and periodically does explode leaving people burned and maimed and injured for life. I have not seen too many older people vaping, as it has been marketed to attract younger people who have a wish to smoke for the first time, but who are looking for a "safer" alternative. This is pure ignorance in my estimation.

Regardless of age, those who choose to use e-cigarettes are subjecting themselves to the same list of disease processes as those who smoke cigarettes and possibly more. The added flavoring makes this entity more desirable and smoking increases, leading to the heightened prospect of subsequent disease.[3]

9.2.4 Alcohol

This "drug" has been in existence for a long time and has been extensively used by people both socially and personally. The effects of alcohol (EtOH) have been found in both social and abusive uses. Many people who have started drinking EtOH when they were in their youth have become addicted to it and sustained their habits of having a daily constitutional once or twice or three times a day for life. It has been used as a relaxant, stimulant, sedative and for pain relief, both physical and psychological. My mother told me to place some Brandy on a washcloth and rub it on my teething baby's gingiva! As a local anesthetic, it did a good job, topically, for teething. I do not drink alcohol, but if I had, I would have probably taken a shot or two all those nights of rocking my crying baby to sleep.

Coupled with other medication, especially alcohol-interactive (AI) drugs, EtOH itself can be very deleterious to one's overall health. In a study done in 2005, encompassing some 83,321 participants, it was noted that 77% of all prescription drug users

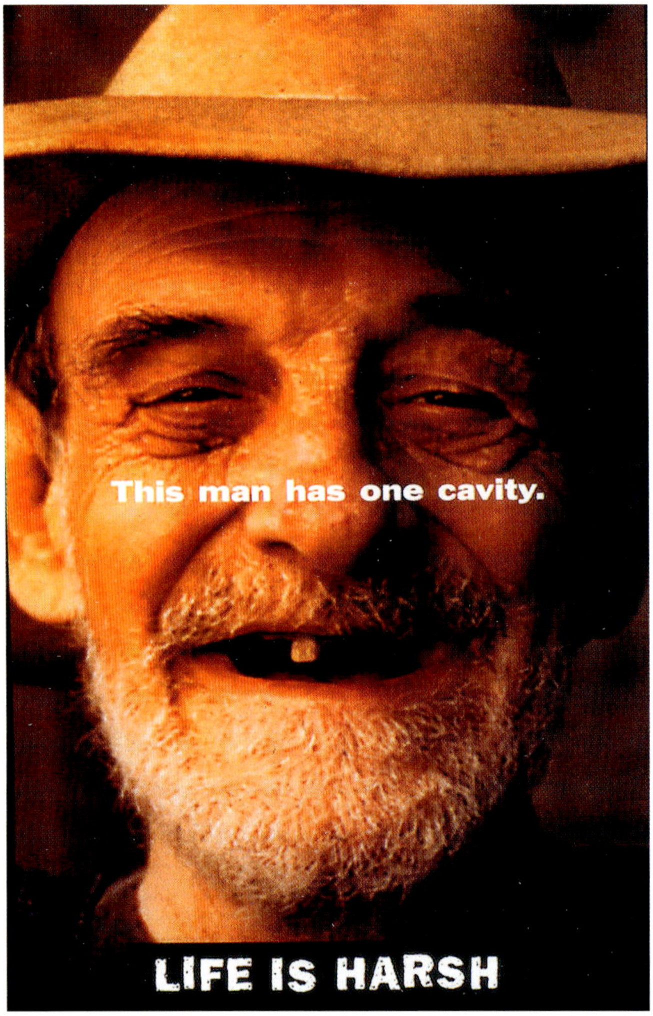

Fig. 9.3 Effects of alcohol abuse.

were exposed to AI medications, with significant variation in exposure and concomitant alcohol use.[4] This is extremely dangerous and risky for those that take both prescription medicines and drink alcohol in a clandestine manner. Taking a medical history then should illuminate this type of history in case dental prescriptions should be given out and if a surgical procedure needs to be done. It is important to know if a patient consumes alcohol, what type and how much. Alcohol thins the blood and can cause bleeding during and after a surgical procedure, and it can delay healing. I have seen it firsthand. Commingling pain medicine with alcohol is dangerous, to say the least. One might find that older patients take more prescription medications than the norm and may also clandestinely drink alcohol as well, possibly placing themselves in a dangerous and life-threatening situation.

As evidenced by Figure 9.3, people who abuse alcohol coupled with medication perhaps, lose their inhibitions, their sense of self and maintain a lack of self-efficacy. Typical findings, especially among older, habitual drinkers are tooth loss, lack of homecare with evidence of chronic geriatric periodontal disease, as well as acute chronic gingivitis, dental caries and gross oral infections of all types, and cognitive impairment. This patient photo is of the extreme, exhibiting a multi-vector concomitant mix of disease processes subjecting this person to systemic disease and ultimate tooth loss due to oral disease findings.

Beer, liquor and mixed drinks have high sugar content and high acidity, causing a breakdown in tooth enamel that leads to decay and periodontal disease as well. Most people who suffer from alcohol abuse forget to brush their teeth and may not care at all about doing good oral hygiene. The cumulative effects of drinking EtOH leads to dry mouth, or xerostomia, which in turn sets the teeth up for decay and the oral tissues up for mucositis, fungal infections and other diseases that affect the oral cavity, such as Burning Mouth Syndrome. The dehydrating effect of alcohol inhibits the production of ADH (Anti-Diuretic Hormone), which regulates the amount of urine one may excrete. The kidneys, therefore, expel more water than they normally do, causing a general dehydration of the mouth and entire body. Xerostomia is a perfect nidus for higher incidences of gingival diseases, as well as having been linked to a higher prevalence and risk of cancer.[5] A study was done in 2015 and published in the Journal of Periodontology[6] that demonstrated the negative effects that alcohol had on the gingiva, which assessed a sample of 542 non-drinkers, occasional drinkers, and regular users of alcohol some of whom had periodontal disease and some not.

The findings of this study concluded the following:

- Users of alcohol on a regular basis without signs of periodontal disease showed more bleeding gingiva than non-drinkers.
- Users of alcohol with existing periodontal disease had their condition slowly decline on a regular basis with the increase in alcohol use.

- Those drinkers with no evidence of gingivitis or periodontitis had more plaque than non-drinkers.
- Alcohol users with no evidence of previous gingival disease presented with periodontal pockets of 4 mm or larger more frequently than non-drinkers.

The Centers for Disease Control have defined moderate alcohol consumption as one drink per day for women and no more than two drinks a day for men. This being in a single day and not multiple days.[7]

A one-drink equivalent has been calculated as 14 g or 0.6 fluid ounces of pure alcohol. Social drinking amongst older individuals needs to be investigated thoroughly on a regular basis. We need to replenish the water we lose by drinking water more during the day. How do we know if we have had enough water to drink? Look at your urine and if it is clear, you have done a good job; otherwise, keep drinking water in increments throughout the day. All too often, as a practitioner, I can smell the alcohol in a drinker because it is absorbed by the lungs and expressed in one's exhaled breath. It is incumbent upon me to ask questions to which the answers can assist me in protecting the older patient from themselves. Sometimes, the patient is dishonest and answers, "No, I have not had a drink for some time" when I know they have. If I must intervene surgically or endodontically in some way that might cause possible bleeding and hemorrhage, I need to know this kind of information beforehand. History taking is important and we must delve into our questions and insist upon answers that we know will be important in the scheme of things and our subsequent treatment, as well as having answers that will protect both the practitioner and the patient to be treated in the end.

9.2.5 Nutrition

We are in a fast paced, fast food, highly technological advanced Society. We are supposed to be smart about living life, but it does not always happen that we think before we act. Skipping a meal, catching a quick bite at a fast-food restaurant or a donut and our morning coffee, repeating this activity within a short lunch span and dinner can be harmful to us over a long period of time, especially if we are in the habit of doing this day-in and day-out. Eating is something we must do in order to stay alive. It is what we eat that needs to be looked at in the sense of maintaining good bodily functions and a low BMI (Basal Metabolism Index). High carbohydrate diets will add weight to our bodies and raise the BMI. I had a professor once in medicine who informed us that for every pound of fat in our bodies, we are collectively shunting blood through a mile of extra blood vessels that takes blood away from the heart. The heart must subsequently pump faster and harder to get that blood into the adipose tissue that we have put on our bodies. Thus, our blood pressure becomes elevated in the process. Over time, this can cause atherosclerotic plaque build-up in our arterioles and essentially "squeezing" the blood through a smaller and smaller lumen in the vessels affects an increase in its speed (the Bernoulli Principle) and again our blood pressure is elevated in the process. All of this can fatigue the heart over time, causing it to fail, leading to a stroke or heart attack which may occur with imminent death as a result.

We are what we eat, so to speak. Eating healthy means staying healthy, but then we have genetics involved too. Being predisposed to cardiac disease, diabetes, cancer and the like are things that we really do not have control over, but we do have control over trying to keep these diseases at bay. About 70% of our make-up is controlled genetically and 30% controls how ***we*** deal with the other 70%. I believe that we can override some of the negative effects our genes predispose us to and prolong our lives through diet, regular exercise, good self-efficacy on all levels, and train of thought. What we eat and do, in essence, is the nidus for our continued efforts to maintain healthy lives.

Taking adequate histories on our patients and their dietary habits clarifies their habits, function and diseases, if any. Most older people have complex medical histories and a list of medical issues that hopefully are controlled.

I remember in dental school our being taught to do diet analyses on all our patients. This is a good thing to do with our older patients and to challenge them to eat healthy and to log what they eat for every meal. Then ask them to bring the log in for a consultation visit to go over their menus and habits with either a trained dental hygienist in your office, an outside nutritionist you can refer to or yourself, the practitioner, who is supposed to know about these things as part of doing dental health education with their patients. This type of exercise is a great tool for one's Kinesthetic patients.

Diet influences the development and onset of the oral cavity. The mouth and oral pharynx are influenced by what we place in it and what we eat. Diets rich in acids, coupled with poor homecare, low self-efficacy, high fruit intake, chronic use of fruit juices, soda, carbonated drinks and vinegar can cause erosion of both the enamel and underlying dentin, known as dental erosion. A good majority of older persons who present for dental treatment suffer from this condition. If people live long enough, they should show some signs of this malady. It is also attributed to attrition due to chronic bruxism, and poor brushing habits.

If I see this type of symptom (Fig. 9.4) during an oral exam with an older individual, I think not only oral habits, but diet related as well.

An insufficient supply of proteins, lipids and carbohydrates during development can significantly alter the development of the oral cavity. Once formed, a shortage of vitamins and minerals, and a balanced diet, can cause continued oral disease based upon this poor development, a low immune response coupled with a high plaque index, poor homecare, low dental IQ and a multifactorial mix of these entities, which in turn destroys or sets the mouth up for tooth loss, oral mucosal diseases and the possible onset of systemic disease as a result of this mixture of factors (Fig. 9.5).

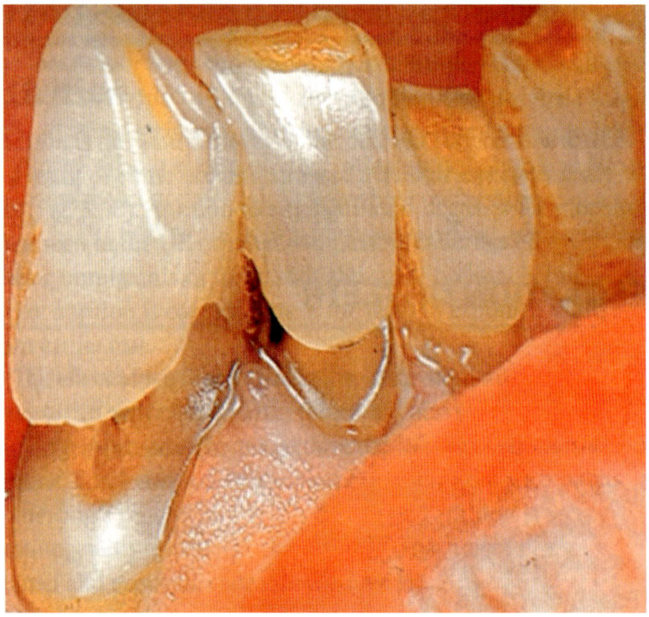

Fig. 9.4 Dental erosion. (*Photo from Scardina and Messina.*)[8]

9.2.6 Cancer

Cancer is a serious disease that presents itself in over three hundred thousand new cases a year worldwide. The greatest incidence, as I have mentioned, is in persons who smoke, chew tobacco, vape and consume alcoholic products. Unlike this mechanism of disease preponderance, a lack of vitamins in a diet that can cause oral cancer exists with respect to vitamins C, A, E, and beta carotene, which all have antioxidant type properties. These vitamins do the following:

- They can neutralize metabolic products.
- They interfere with the activation of procarcinogens.
- They inhibit chromosomal aberration.
- They potentially inhibit the growth of malignant lesions (leukoplakia) (Fig. 9.6).[8]

An imbalanced diet depletes antioxidants. One can find these antioxidants in all kinds of fresh berries (Acai berries, Blueberries, Blackberries, Olallieberries, Raspberries, and more), Coenzyme Q10 (CoQ10) supplements, carrots and other fruits and vegetables. Older persons on fixed budgets may have a difficult time procuring these food stuffs. Malnutrition interferes negatively with cell formation and tissue repair. It can alter the way medication is metabolized and interfere with significant medical treatment for oncological treatment. It can cause or accelerate heart disease and cancer in the oropharyngeal area.[8] So, we need to try and assist the older more infirm patients with this dilemma, whereby with assistance and sociological care we can ultimately protect them from systemic and oral harm.

The National Cancer Institute and the American Cancer Society have established some prudent dietary recommendations:

1. Maintain a desirable body weight.
2. Eat a varied diet.
3. Include a new variety of fruits and vegetables in the daily diet.

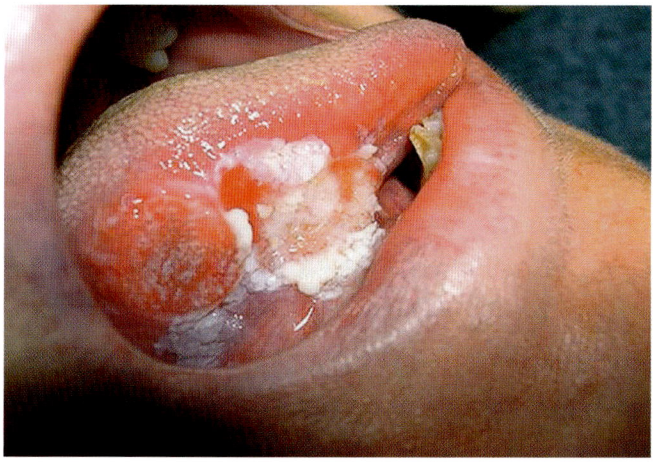

Fig. 9.5 Oral cancer. (*Photo from Scardina and Messina.*)[8]

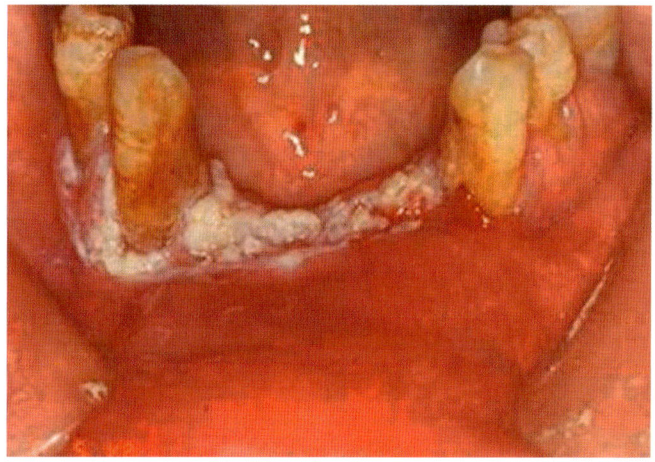

Fig. 9.6 Oral leukoplakia in an older patient. (*Photo from Scardina and Messina.*)[8]

4. Consume a greater quantity of foods rich in fiber.
5. Decrease the total intake of fats (to less than 30% of the total calories).
6. Limit the consumption of alcohol.
7. Limit the consumption of salted foods or food preserved with nitrates.[8-10]

Oral candidiasis, a fungal condition that affects the mucosa, gingiva and oral tissues in general, as well as the angular creases of the lips, can be caused by lack of homecare, malnutrition, alcoholism, an overabundance of plaque in the oral cavity as well as evidence that points to the lack of iron, folic acid, vitamin A, B1, B2, C, K, as well as minerals like zinc and a diet that is balanced and contains adequate carbohydrates. Additional nutritional deficiencies can bring about glossodynia (painful tongue), Burning Mouth Syndrome, irreversible systemic and neurologic damage, angular cheilitis and cheilosis (chronic), recurrent aphthous ulcers, oral candidiasis, diffuse erythematous mucositis and Plummer Vinson syndrome.[8] Diseases such as Scurvy, a vitamin C deficiency, and Rickets, a vitamin D deficiency, have been around for years and are most treatable. Scurvy runs havoc with the breakdown of the oral tissues, as vitamin C is an intermediary in the process of making collagen and connective tissue, the fabric of gingiva. Vitamin D plays an important role in the formation of bone in conjunction with calcium metabolism and the parathyroid glands. Healthy bone support is affected by Rickets and in effect, periodontal disease and tooth loss can be attributed to this disease as well.

Nutrition is an especially important entity to learn about, by having your patient give you their related information about this important "piece of their puzzle". The patients' nutritional habits can tell you much more about his or her health, future possibility of disease, success of your projected treatment and any validity in your ability to continue treating this person without first trying to eliminate any cause of diseases in the present or those that might occur in the future, which, in turn, may come to "bite" you where it hurts should a patient blame you for not informing them before you performed treatment on them, for something other than a looming issue that could and can affect their total overall health.

9.2.7 Sugars

Organic substances that are labelled "-ose" at the end of the word are considered sugars. For example, sucrose, fructose, lactose, galactose, maltose, ribose, cellulose, dextrose, xylose, mannose, malto-dextrose, amylose, arabinose to name a few. There are 56 varieties of sugar (mostly six-carbon) that are cariogenic in nature. Xylitol is a five-carbon sugar that is non-cariogenic. Stevia from a natural leaf is a sugar substitute that is non-cariogenic. Some sugar substitutes have been known to be carcinogenic and those I am not listing here. The one thing that all the "ose's" have in common, except for xylose or xylitol, is that they are cariogenic

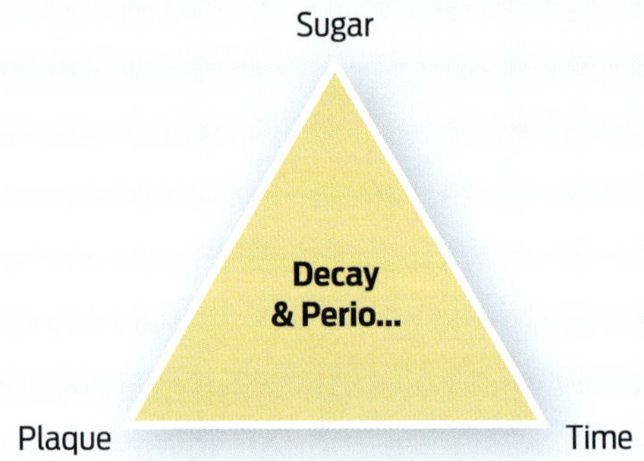

Fig. 9.7 Depiction of *The Caries Triangle.*

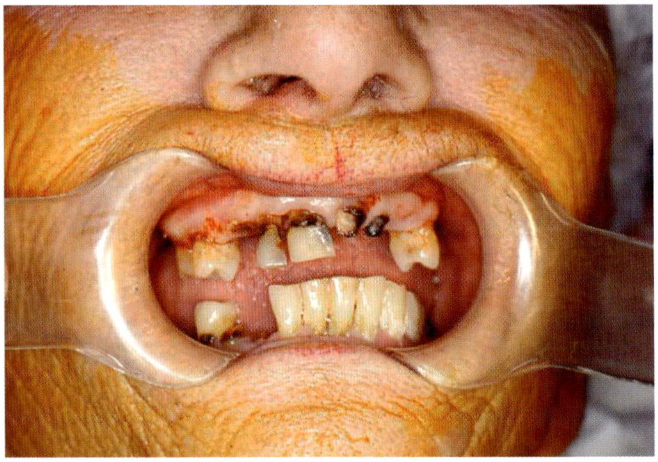

Fig. 9.8 Uncontrolled diabetes, poor homecare and oral disease.

and contribute to the major cause of dental disease that being dental caries, periodontal disease, and other systemic diseases such as diabetes (the most common), cardiac disease, pancreatitis, liver disease, generalized hereditary metabolic disorder, and obesity. The *Global Burden of Disease Study 2017* estimated that oral diseases affect close to 3.5 billion people worldwide, with caries of permanent teeth being the most common condition. Globally, it is estimated that 2.3 billion people suffer from caries of permanent teeth and more than 530 million children suffer from cares of primary teeth.[11] Dental caries result when dental plaque converts free sugars, as well as naturally occurring sugars present in foodstuffs like honey, syrups, fruit juices, soft drinks, candy and even some vegetables (carbohydrates) and the like, to acid, which, over time destroys tooth structure.

Most oral diseases and systemic conditions share unpredictable and modifiable risk factors. Unhealthy diets are a big part of this triangle (Fig. 9.7) with respect to the noncommunicable diseases: cardiovascular disease, cancer, chronic respiratory disease, and diabetes. In turn, diabetes has been linked to the development and progression of periodontal disease, due to the high consumption of sugar in the diet, as well as in the system that cannot process it effectively due to insulin resistance.[11]

Insulin resistance is a major factor in metabolizing sugars. When the Islet cells in the Pancreas are unable to process sugar effectively, it is shunted into all parts of the body and can cause one harm. Older persons who may or may not suffer from a compromised immune system, can be systemically compromised by high blood sugar concentrations. It is important to find out whether the older patient can metabolize sugars normally or whether they are compromised with either diabetes type 1 or diabetes type 2. They should then be treated accordingly if they are diabetic, with pre- and post-treatment antibiotics for surgical or invasive treatment procedures (Fig. 9.8). Medical clearance is always advisable under these circumstances with this type of systemic disease.

It is advisable for all older, medically compromised patients to have a medical clearance before any invasive treatment is initiated. Without this clearance, and with the risk of doing harm to the patient, a lawsuit might be forth coming. Be a "Boy Scout" and **be prepared** and **be aware!**

9.2.8 Bruxism

Is a common finding among older people along with what might appear to be bruxism in the form of attrition, or severe wear patterns on teeth (Fig. 9.9). It can happen unconsciously when one is awake or while sleeping. It is insidious, long-lasting unless treated and can be associated to various sleep or nervous disorders as well.

As one continues to brux in the night while sleeping or while awake at work in a stressful or demanding job, bruxism will take its toll as time goes on and no treatment occurs to nullify the cause(s). The longer one lives, the more wear one accumu-

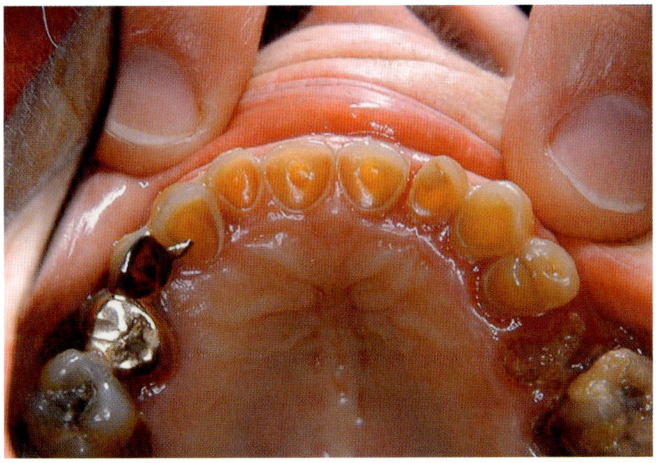

Fig. 9.9 Extreme attrition from bruxism.

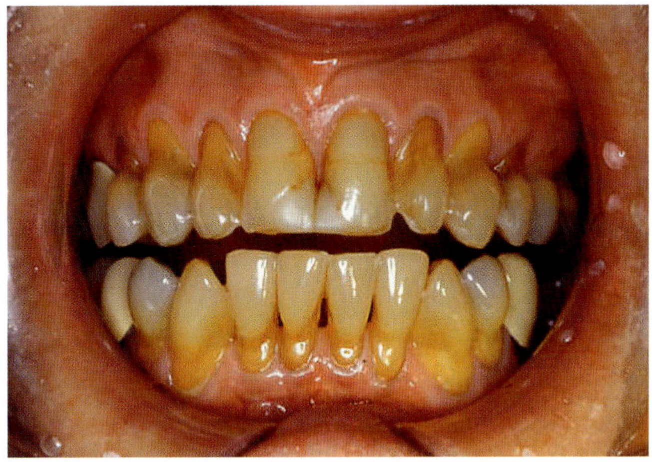

Fig. 9.10 Deceased 85-year-old bruxer with attrition and erosion.

lates over time that can be indicative of underlying stress, emotional issues, neurological conditions, dementia, systemic diseases such as Parkinson's disease or Multiple Sclerosis, complex psychological issues like obsessive compulsive disorders and Bipolar disease or gastroesophageal reflux disorders that mimic wear patterns of bruxism.

The signs and symptoms can easily be picked up at the intraoral and extraoral routine dental exam. One can see the wear patterns on the incisal surfaces of the front teeth especially, as well as broken or chipped teeth and the large tender masseter muscles of the cheeks that are enlarged, firm and give one a "swollen" looking appearance. Other damage can be evident looking at recession of the gingiva and looking at intraoral radiographs that can show bone loss around severely damaged teeth that are worn down to the pulp of the tooth. The difficult part in all of this is trying to figure out the exact root of the cause once the practitioner picks up the cues from the damaged teeth.

Ear pain may be a sign of bruxism and clenching habits, as well as an underlying major sleep disorder.[12] These entities can be followed up on if symptoms persist by referring to an ENT specialist or a Sleep Medicine physician or dentist who can do a sleep test to determine the extent of the issues at hand.

In Figure 9.10, an 85-year-old women patient of mine shows much gingival destruction and some incisal destruction with posterior occlusal wear as well. This woman was a "shut-in" and refused to go out because of her looks. She was very vain and concerned about her looks and troubled by not being able to cope with the loss of her beauty as she aged (in her own mind). She had a difficult time sleeping and was probably using alcohol to relax her, but at the same time it was doing just the opposite. Her daughter wanted to move her into an assisted-living facility in order to provide her an environment that was more social and with persons who were similar in age. I had spoken to this patient several times about restoring her gum line erosion and brushing defects with composites, but it did no good. But finally, when her daughter told her mother that she was going to move her into a facility with other people, did the mother make an appointment with me to make her smile more pleasant, hence increasing her self-esteem and beauty (Fig. 9.11). Being alone, she had no one to look at her and there was no need for her to do anything to make herself more attractive or acceptable to anyone else.

The patient had her upper teeth restored and decided not to do the lower anterior teeth because of finances and because she thought that others would not be able to see them with her lip covering the cervical portions of her teeth. She apparently was a "social butterfly" at her new facility, and this helped her relax, gave her time to talk while being social with others in her new facility and in her interactions with others, especially those whom she made friends with after she moved there. In retrospect, the restorative that she had completed extended her life and happiness until she died in her sleep of heart failure about a year after her move.

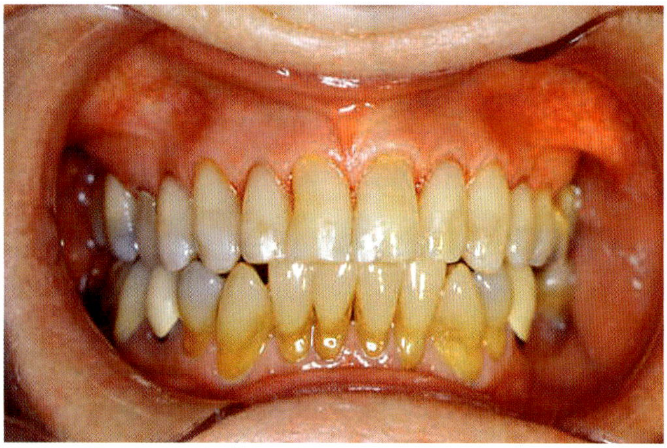

Fig. 9.11 Post-composite treatment on the maxillary arch.

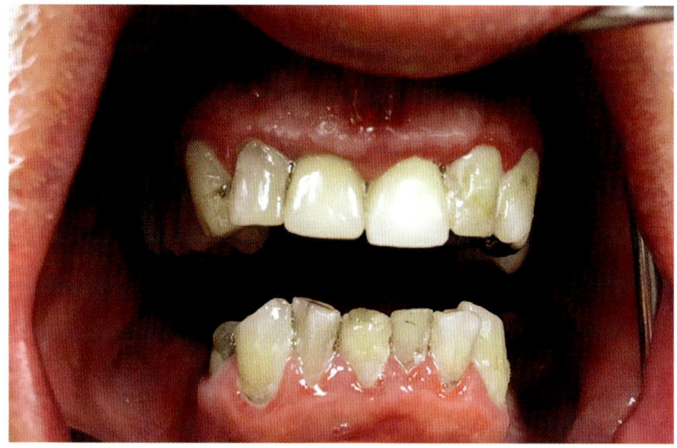

Fig. 9.12 Deceased 80-year-old Parkinson's patient with dementia, no self-efficacy and worn teeth.

Parafunctional habits in older people can be very deleterious to their health and hidden from them by their lack of knowledge and taking these habits for granted (Fig. 9.12). Parafunctional activity is also recognized as muscle hyperactivity and can be coupled with generalized wear on teeth and teeth that cause damage to other teeth once they are impaired in the first place by grinding or clenching activity. Apparently, there is no single factor that is attributed to bruxism and no single treatment that is effective for reducing or eliminating the habit itself.[13] If your teeth are touching at rest, then you are clenching. Be aware of your hidden habits and teach your patients.

A combination of treatment modalities can be recommended such as a bruxism appliance of one kind or another or reconstruction of the bite by opening the vertical dimension and restoring the missing occlusal anatomy and the like, but this type of treatment is somewhat radical to older individuals unless they have some positive motive to urge them into committing to doing this type of full mouth rehabilitation. Biofeedback exercises are also good for conditioning patients to keep their teeth apart when resting. The "KISS" method of treatment is in order here, especially for people in their 8th, 9th, and 10th decades of life. That is "Keep it Simple Stupid" in treatment design. It is best to essentially keep all bruxism treatment as easy as possible for cognitively impaired individuals. Having an appliance to wear and a schedule in which to wear it in is a difficult thing to adhere to and a treatment that is doomed to failure, unless there are teeth that one can either cement, bond or clasp to that will hold the appliance in place to protect whatever remaining teeth are left in one's dentition of this category of patient.

9.2.9 Sleep Apnea

Is a condition characterized by an abnormal breathing pattern during sleep that exhibits multiple extended interruptions or pauses in sleep, with the tendency of periodically waking up and gasping for air. This is due to hypoxia and the lack of oxygen and CO_2. Snoring is usually involved in this sleep activity as is agitation, movement, being over-weight, having lung disease or not, enlarged tonsils, which constrict the airway, and a high, narrow palatal vault. These findings, in part or collectively, may lead to a higher classification of the Mallampati configuration of the oropharynx (Fig. 9.13) from Class I to IV indicating a restricted airway of some form.

The more obscured the posterior soft palate becomes, the higher the classification, meaning the more restricted the airway.

Obstructive sleep apnea can occur in any age group, but has a prevalence for middle-aged and especially the older male individual. It is a serious ailment that can cause the demise of the person who exhibits it if not treated in a timely manner. Most people who have this malady tend to snore loudly and frequently, with periods of silence when airflow is reduced or blocked. Choking noise may be heard or snorting and gasping sounds when their airway reopens.[14]

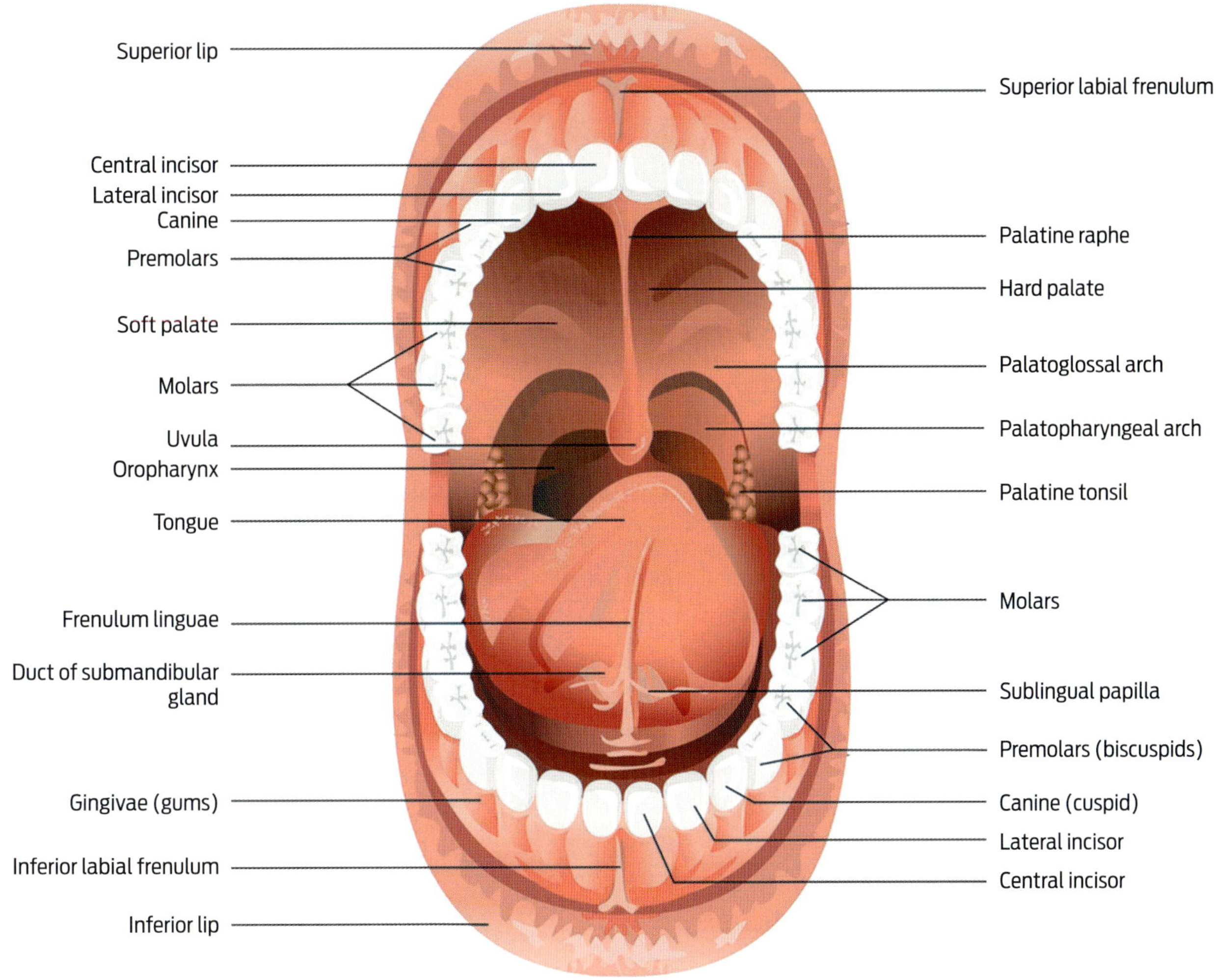

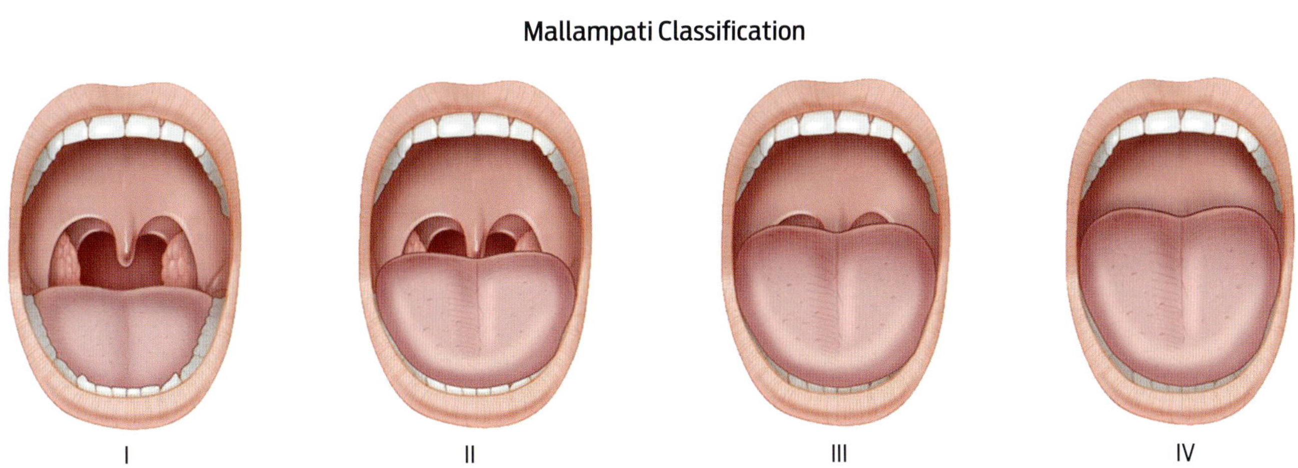

Fig. 9.13 Mallampati scoring system. (*From the Airway and Sleep Group.*)

Risk groups include:

1. Those individuals who are overweight or obese with a body mass index of 30 or above.
2. Men and women with large neck sizes (17 inches or more for men and 16 inches or more for women).
3. Middle-aged and older men and post-menopausal women.
4. Ethnic minorities.
5. People with anatomical abnormalities of bone and soft tissue around the head and neck area.
6. Down's syndrome patients (who usually have large, wide tongues that can block their oral airway when they are in a supine position).
7. People with large tonsils and adenoids, especially when they are chronically inflamed.
8. People who have a genetic propensity towards OSA in their families.
9. Persons with endocrine abnormalities.
10. Smokers and vapists, especially with chronic lung or breathing diseases such as COPD and asthma.
11. Persons prone to severe allergies affecting the nose, nasal cavities with congestion, especially when laying down, who may have abnormal sinuses, narrowed nasal passages, history of broken noses and deviated septum; all of which can and do affect proper breathing.[14]

The effects of these risks involve the following:

- Mood swings, both anxiety and depression.
- Chronic elevation in daytime blood pressure.
- Increased risk of stroke and TIA.
- Increased heart rate, in general leading to an increase in blood pressure.
- Death due to heart attack.
- Varied blood oxygen levels in any one period of the day.
- Increased blood glucose and insulin resistance in conjunction with diabetes.
- Falling asleep at the wheel and accidents leading to death.
- Disturbed sleep of a bed partner and oneself.[14]

All patients, but especially older individuals who fall into these categories, should be considered for a sleep apnea work-up prior to any kind of involved dental treatment. Taking measurements for Mallampati classifications (see Fig. 9.13), oral architecture analysis, systemic issues from the medical and observed examination studies coupled into a diagnosis for OSA should be referred for a sleep study and subsequent treatment. Treatment may consist of an oral appliance and/or a CPAP machine to sleep with, surgical intervention if need be, to correct an oral architectural defect that inhibits proper breathing, nasal surgery to open the airway, physical therapy to correct postural positions, changing habits of sleep and positioning, strips (*Breathe Right®*) to widen the nasal airway by pulling out the nares giving the airway more room and elevating the head while sleeping with several pillows or a bed that one can raise on its own are viable methods of treating this disorder.

Sleep deprivations due to OSA or other reasons can be dangerous and full of symptomology that the dental practitioner needs to become familiar with in doing routine Head and Neck examinations and oral physical examinations. The effects of the lack of sleep are deleterious to ones overall physical as well as mental health (see Fig. 9.14). Being able to observe the entire patient from the time they walk into your office, to the taking of their histories, to the actual consultation and discussion of your findings will allow you to follow-up on any symptomology that you may uncover along the process. Once discovered, a discussion should ensue to make the patient aware of their issues which they may be unaware of at that time. Enlightenment will commence with the hopeful willingness of the patient to want to do something to rectify his or her maladies for the better.

"I started counting sheep so I could sleep but that got boring, so I started talking to the shepherd..."

Anonymous

9.2.10 Xerostomia

Dry mouth is not a habit, it is a symptom and can be attributed to various habits and medical conditions that cause a decrease in the salivary flow of the mouth. Aging can bring on a decrease in salivary flow by itself due to atrophic salivary glands and lack of function due to the aging process itself. It is

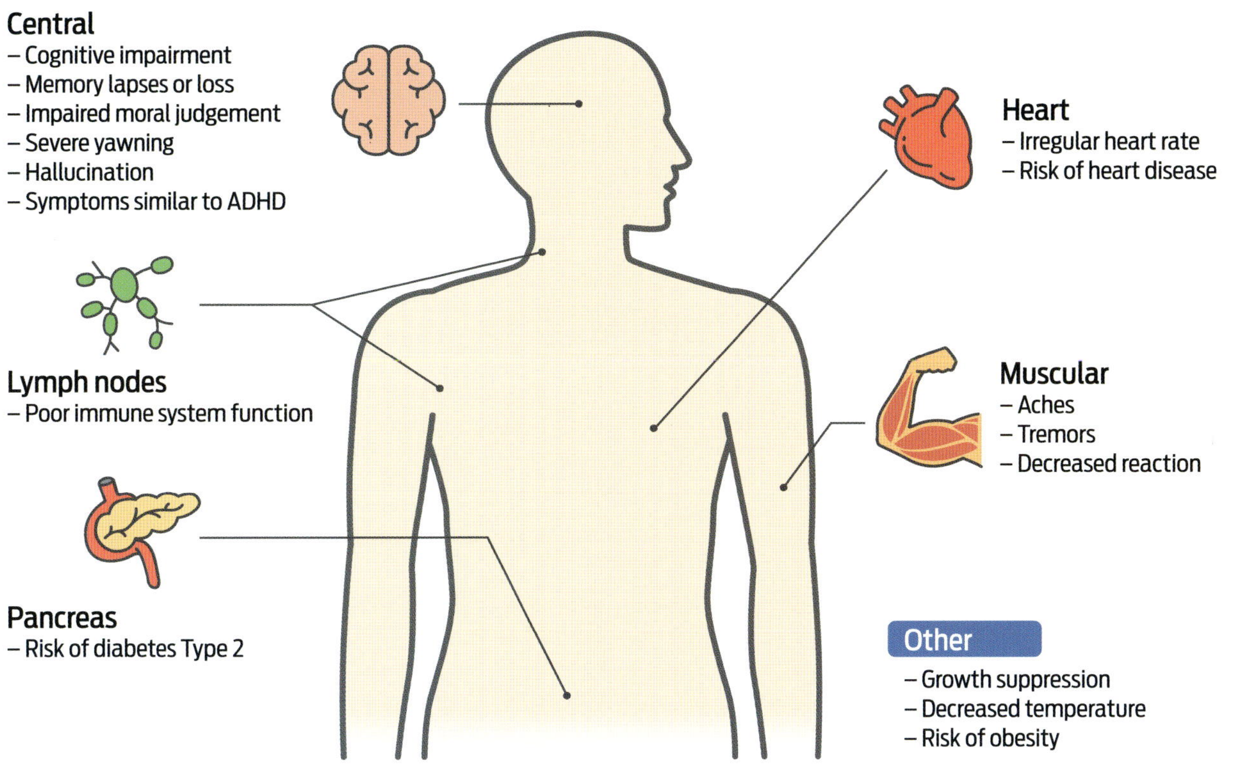

Fig. 9.14 Effects of sleep deprivation.

something to look for and test when doing an oral examination on older people and it can give the practitioner insight into the overall health of the older individual. Saliva helps keep the oral tissues and teeth healthy. It cleanses the mouth through the various enzymes it contains and the moisture it possesses. Without saliva one may manifest some of the following symptoms:

- Halitosis. Bad breath is a sure sign of too many bacteria in the mouth and the lack of saliva can cause this, as well as diet related foodstuffs and poor homecare.
- Discomfort in the form of pain and/or burning of the oral tissues and tongue.
- Poor oral hygienic conditions causing increased plaque build-up, increased calculus, increased periodontal disease and chronic gingivitis conditions and dental caries.
- Older persons who wear dentures would have a difficult time maintaining their denture stability in the mouth without a salivary interface and this, in turn, would cause emotional trauma for the patient.
- Trouble with speech and especially swallowing food and in general.
- Sore throat.
- Difficulty speaking and being hoarse when one speaks.
- Difficulty in tasting food or drink.
- Sjögren's syndrome can couple dry mouth with dry eyes and skin.
- Skin rashes.
- Joint pain.

Those older individuals who take specific medications that cause xerostomia would be considered "causing dry mouth through habitual use" of these drugs. Especially those who have year-round allergies and would need daily antihistamines and decongestant medication. Other medications that can cause xerostomia include:

- Antianxiety drugs and antidepressants.
- Anticholinergic medication, used to treat COPD, urinary tract conditions, such as incontinence, overactive bladders sometimes coupled with infection.

- Certain hypertensive drugs can cause dry mouth.
- Medication for Parkinson's disease.
- Chemotherapeutic medication.

Avoiding alcohol, caffeine and carbonated drinks, which our Society has become accustomed to imbibing on a regular basis to the point of considering these drinks an addictive habit, causes dry mouth. Avoiding spicy, salty and dry sugary foods and beverages, which we as a culture have become addicted to, should be avoided, or at least minimized for the most part as well. Mouthwashes that contain alcohol should be avoided because of the drying nature of the ingredient of alcohol itself. It is a desiccant.

Many older adults with arthritis have difficulty holding a toothbrush and find it painful. Approximately 60 million adults have some form of arthritis in the United States and 49.6% of those individuals are above the age of 65 years of age.[15] Due to the difficulty in holding a toothbrush in an effective manner, hence causing a decrease or lack of proper oral hygiene, these individuals use mouthwash to "mask" the plaque and retained food product odors that are consistent with not doing proper hygiene. If these patients are not reading labels and only looking at price when they make their decisions to buy mouthwash type products, then they may be subject to low-cost mouthwashes which contain high percentages of alcohol as a major ingredient and, therefore, suffering from the side-effects of xerostomia.

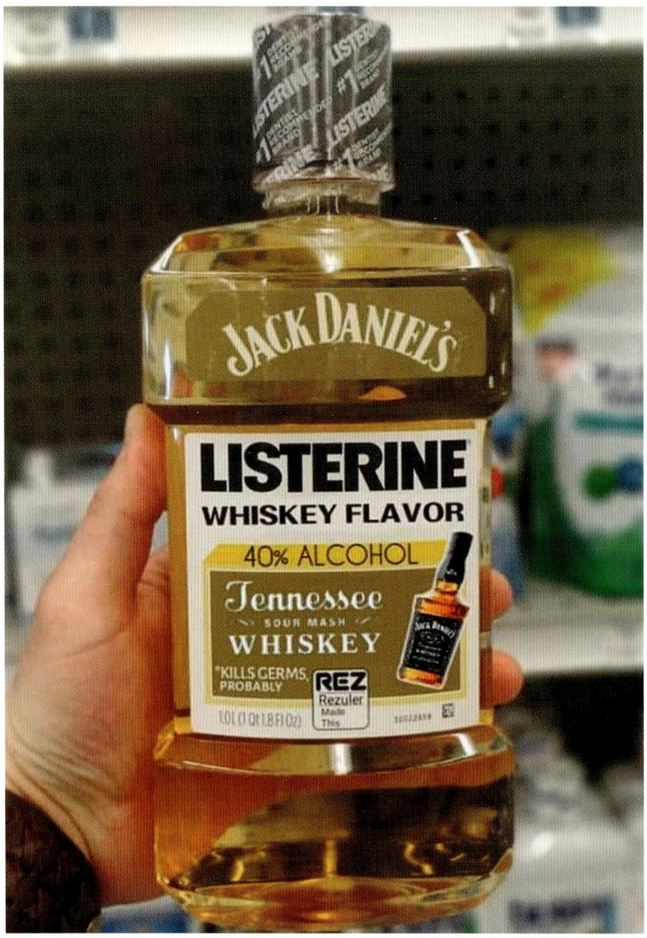

Fig. 9.15 *(Photo from Pinterest.)*

Counseling these patients in our offices should be rote and without question. Although, I must admit that many older people are "set" in their ways and may not want to listen to information about how they can better their oral health conditions. Many times, in treating patients like this, I find myself "knocking" my head against the wall in trying to get them to understand that this is one habit they need to change for the betterment of their overall health. It is only a matter of finding a mouthwash without alcohol in it and not giving up using a mouthwash itself. There are many non-alcoholic mouthwashes on the market today. As an aside, I have even had those older patients who rinse, gargle, and then swallow the mouthwash to get a "buzz" out of it in the process (Fig. 9.15). This type of habit is a difficult one to break, to say the least.

9.2.11 Lack of Oral Care

This act, oral care, above all is responsible for a major portion of the oral ailments of our older patients. It is not enough to think that someone is brushing and flossing daily, but not doing it all. It is not enough to think that an older, maybe compromised patient, is going to his or her dentist for regular care every three to four months, but not at all. It is not enough to think that someone's self-efficacy is compromised by depression, drug abuse, alcohol abuse, dementia and cognitive impairment, severe rheumatoid arthritis, Parkinson's disease or multiple sclerosis and ALS, and not able to help themselves, considering possibly not having the wear-with-all and finances to have a caregiver or family member who can provide the care they need in one way or another. It is truly disheartening.

9.2.12 Self-Efficacy

Self-efficacy in the frail elderly is tied into many factors. Some of which can be related to the following: being social and competent; having stamina; memory; perceived health including exercise; efforts to attain goals both individually and in cooperation with others; making long-term plans, as well as trying to achieve them.[16] In a study done in 2016 by Doba N. et al., the authors have indicated that the three parameters, stamina (physical strength), power (spiritual) and memory (cognition), showed significant correlations with the cluster of self-efficacies in the overall population that was studied. Males seemed to fair better than females in this select study of 257 elderly people in Japan with a mean age of 82.3.[16] One can infer from the information at hand that in this population, men do better at self-efficacy than women, but this is not true in other parts of the world.

Especially in the United States, where women seem to live longer than men with the main reason being that they are more socially inclined. Living longer and having self-efficacy with regards to oral care may be a factor related to peer pressure or the type of care the person gets on a personal basis overall. There are many questions to ask and factors to consider that still need to be investigated in relation to continued oral care into the 8th, 9th and 10th decades of life. The fact that we are living longer means that men and women need to be aware of taking care of their entire health system with an emphasis on a healthy oral cavity. Part of this responsibility lies in the hands of the dental office personnel and the dental practitioner to make sure there is adequate follow-up and less time between routine examinations and hygiene recall. Being responsible for the care of our patients means that we, as health practitioners, allow the patient to choose their care, but with prompting from us in a direction that will keep them healthy in all respects. I even go so far as to reduce the fee for service so that my elderly patients have some incentive to return at least three to four times a year. If we do not see them, we call them to assist them in making and keeping this routine.

Figure 9.16 shows a patient who has little to no self-efficacy in oral homecare or continuous periodic hygiene recall prior to coming to see me. Part of the issue here was the low dental IQ of the caregivers at hand (more than one), the lack of follow-up by this person's family members and/or guardian and the patient's own inability to care for herself with respect to her age, frailty, lack of dental knowledge, lack of strength, priorities and cognitive decline. Her oral condition exhibited poor homecare, chronic geriatric periodontal disease, heavy plaque, and calculus (a nidus for both oral and systemic disease), dental caries, missing teeth, mobile teeth, and malnutrition as seen in her oral tissues with flaccidity, xerostomia, Burning Tongue Syndrome, difficulty eating due to trouble in swallowing and difficulty speaking as well. Patients like this are our "silent sufferers", and are at the whim of those who are supposed to care for them daily in all respects; then again, they are not monitored closely enough to ensure that oral care is high on their list of things to manage. After observing my own mother in her last year of life, living in an assisted living memory care facility, the ratio of caregivers to patients went from one caregiver for every 3-4 inhabitants to one caregiver for every 10 inhabitants in a two-year span. This was obviously not enough personnel to make sure that each person being cared for had all that they needed and that all aspects of their ADLs (Activities of Daily Living), such as brushing and flossing, etc., were cared for regularly, let alone personal hygiene in all ways daily. As my mother's son and guardian, I made a concerted effort to make sure that she had dental cleanings every two to three months and all her medical appointments made and followed-up on regularly. I made sure her dental supplies were handy and instructed her in her care. Without me,

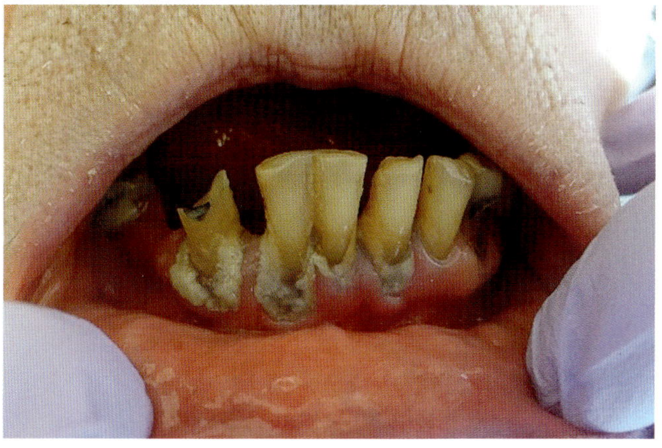

Fig. 9.16 Deceased 89-year-old patient lacking self-efficacy.

she would have been severely neglected and lost all her teeth. I realize that not everyone has this type of "bird-dogging" to watch over their parent(s) in a situation like this, but I knew if I did not take the responsibility, she would not have lived as long as she did. She died in August of 2020 at the age of 97.

With respect to my mother's care, I am reminded of a lecture I was giving years ago on geriatric dentistry for our state dental society, where a dentist in the audience asked me if I was going to speak on homecare in a long-term care facility, apparently one like where his mother was staying at that time. I told him that I was speaking on geriatric dentistry in an office setting but asked him what it was he specifically wanted to know. He was angry that his mother was not getting cared for and that no one was brushing her teeth for her. I did not know his mother, nor did I know her condition, but obviously this dentist was angry and chose to take his anger out on me. His wife was a dentist as well, sitting right next to him. He wanted to know why staff in these facilities did not care for their patients' oral health. I told him I thought it was because no one like himself, who had a vested interest in this facility, mainly his mother, went in there to teach the staff what they needed to know about and how to do it. It was obvious to me, he was making me the scapegoat for his lack of self-efficacy in terms of his mother's care. I told him I thought it was a perfect time for him and his wife to teach the staff in this facility how to maintain not only his mother's oral health, but the other people who lived there as well. He retorted it was not his responsibility! This is the mindset of most of the private caregivers and guardians responsible for their loved one's care... "Let someone else do it, because I pay you to do it as part of my monthly fees to the facility". Not realizing that there is a shortage of people working in these facilities, places a burden on them to carry out everything that is needed all the time for their tenants. I told him that I would be happy to speak to him on how to educate people on this type of care, but he did not want to hear it. He wanted to make an example out of me for his own inequities because he thought I should be addressing the subject in my lecture that day, which I was not slated to do per se. I did touch on it, but not in detail, and not to his satisfaction I am afraid.

I think it is necessary for all of us to take part in going to these places and educating staff on how to care for their patients there. It is a practice builder for new practitioners as well as for seasoned practitioners. There are people that work and live there that need a dentist. Teaching in these facilities builds character and allows others to see that we must all take responsibility for the space we occupy in life by sharing our knowledge for the betterment of others, no matter whether we get remunerated or not for our efforts. This is food for thought on the space we all occupy and how we conduct our business, our profession, and our lives in assisting others who can not assist themselves because of the lack of knowledge and inability to do what needs to be done.

9.2.13 Accidents

Falls are the number three cause of death in the United States included as an "unintentional injury". Overall, the rate of deaths from unintentional injuries rose 40% between 1999 and 2017 and from 35.3 to 49.4 deaths per 100,000 standard population in 2019. In 2021, falls rank at about 40,000 deaths or more per year over the last three years of calculations by the Centers for Disease Control and Prevention (Fig. 9.17).[17]

Falls for the older generation who are frail, cognitively impaired, and medically compromised are and can be lethal. Dental practitioners should take special precautions to ensure that "safety" measures are in place for fall risks and for things that can cause all patients, especially older patients, to possibly not see something and fall in our offices.

A podiatrist friend of mine had an office with three steps leading up to the front door and no handrail. One rainy day, an elderly patient of his was hobbling up the steps in the rain and slipped and fell and broke her foot. She had a foot issue before, but now she had an even bigger foot issue and so did the practitioner, who ultimately got sued for not ensuring safety measures outside his front door. He was not the landlord. He was the tenant and responsible for the safety of his patients.

"An ounce of prevention is worth a pound of cure."

Benjamin Franklin

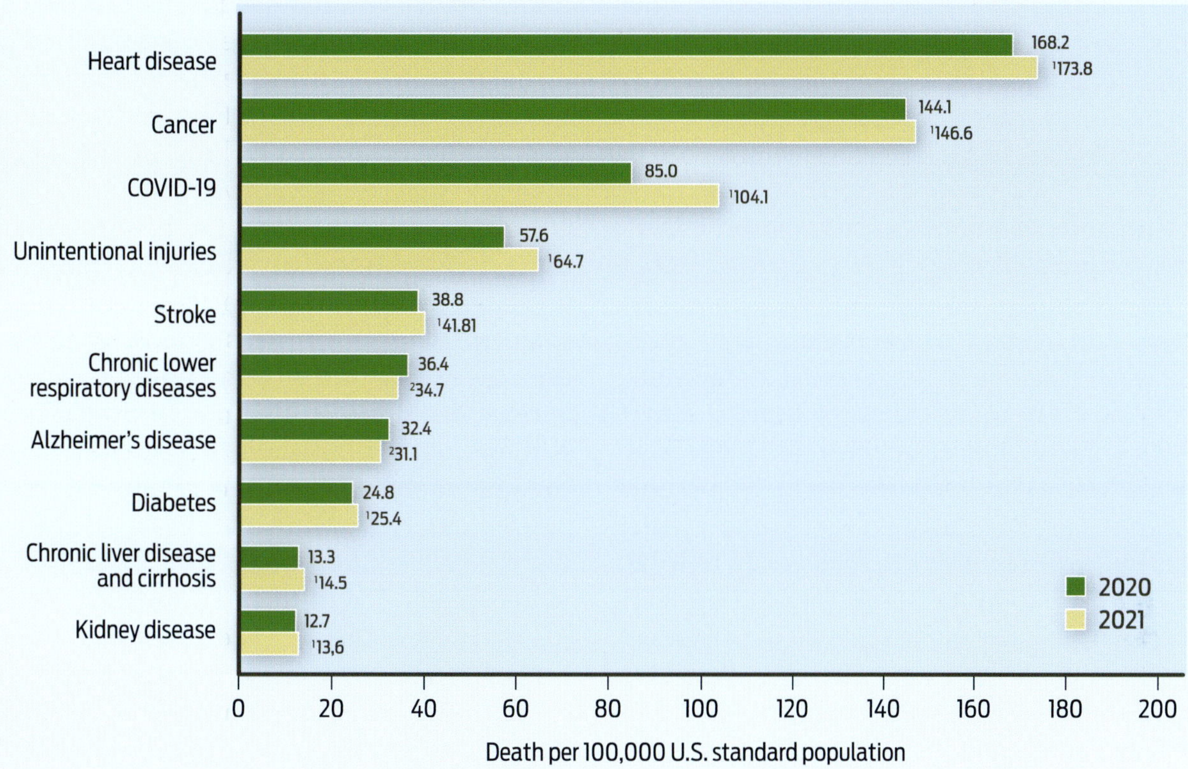

[1] Statistically significant increase from 2020 to 2021 ($p < 0.05$). [2] Statistically significant decrease from 2020 to 2021 ($p < 0.05$).
Notes: A total of 3,464,231 resident deaths were registeres in the United States in 2021. The 10 leading causes of death accounted for 74.5% of all U.S. deaths in 2021. Causes of death are ranked according to number of deaths. Rankings for 2020 data are not shown. Data table for Figure includes the number of deaths for leading causes and the percentage of total deaths.
Source: National Center for Health Statistics, National Vital Statistics System, Mortality.

Fig. 9.17 Age-adjusted death rate for the 10 leading causes of death in 2021; United States, 2020 and 2021 (CDC 2021).

I have had older patients, who make a living by habitually falling for one reason or another and suing the establishment where they fell, claiming neglect. It behooves us to be aware of whether our older patients are fall prone, have had accidents of one kind or another and who for one broken bone or another, cannot use their hands or arms because they were injured and again, neglecting their oral care in the process. Who is going to pay? Our insurance companies and us. Make sure your medical and dental histories ask this question and look at the eyes of the patient when they answer. Depending upon which direction they look when answering, they could be prevaricating about not falling or having perpetual accidents, but they do. Practice defensive dentistry and you will be alright in the end.

I am not saying that falling is a normal habit. I have patients that present with alcohol on their breath, and I know that they have been drinking. I have patients with Alzheimer's disease, Parkinson's disease, Down's syndrome, multiple sclerosis and the like who need personal attention when they walk into the office, go to the restroom and when they leave-always accompanied by someone. This is to make sure that they do not fall. Hand holds should be placed in the office bathrooms, non-slip mats if any, and good lighting are imperative. Patients with generalized weakness due to old age and/or their failing physical condition, should be watched and accompanied, no matter their ages. "It is better to be safe, than sorry", as I always allude to my staff and my family.

Here is a photo (see Fig. 9.18) of one of my Centenarian patients who tripped and fell on a door mat of some kind. She had most all her teeth at the time and a porcelain bridge from #4-6 that had broken off in the fall fracturing the root on tooth #4 and #6. Teeth #7, 8 and 9 were mobile and with these teeth she had pierced through her lower lip into the underlying mucosa requiring debridement and suturing. Her upper lip was also damaged from the fall itself and was cut up. Her hands, arms, legs and knees were also injured. She came to the dental office first because she always took pride in her teeth and smile and wanted everything "put back" like it used to be. A tall order from a little old lady. I did the best I could for her on a temporary basis, but I wanted her to go to either her personal physician or the emergency room to get checked out thoroughly. She obliged me only after I temporized her upper cuspid, placed a temporary crown on #4 and sutured her lip as well as cleaned up her face and other facial wounds. She was totally cognitive.

No one is immune to falling, but it is the elderly who usually receive bad wounds when they do have an accident because they are somewhat infirm physically and their teeth, in this case, are brittle due to calcified roots, which fracture easily when hit. I was amazed that at 100 years of age, she did not have more facial or oral issues to deal with. I suspect that there were a few more underlying issues I could not see and that is why I wanted her to follow up with her MD or an ER to have the appropriate head X-rays and perhaps an MRI and/or CAT scan of her head and face. I placed all my history in my notes for that day as well as documentation with photos and radiographs and a copy of my referral. She ended up okay with no further issues, only the ones I had to restore eventually.

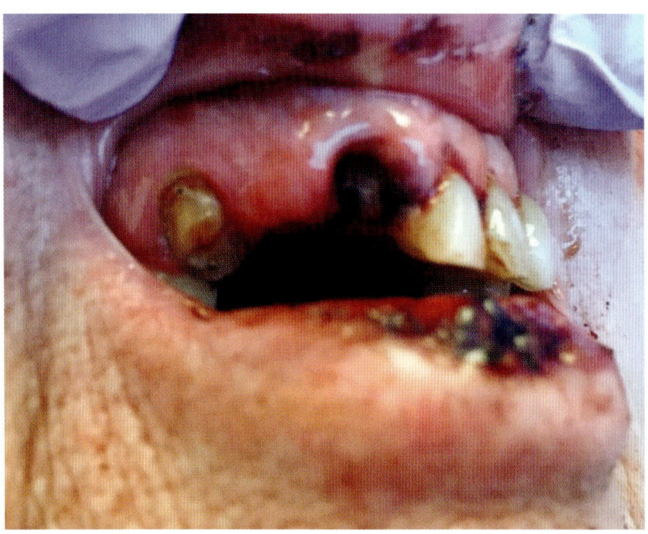

Fig. 9.18 Deceased 100-year-old woman with an oral fall injury.

Age 65 is commonly used as a default age to define an "elderly" or "geriatric" patient.

However, the prospect of an older person having preexisting conditions and comorbidities may perhaps be a better predictor of long-term complications secondary to trauma such as falling.[18] It is these underlying medical conditions, polypharmacy and the many medications one may take at an older age that compound injuries from falls and make it more difficult for a patient of this ilk to recover or compensate for their injuries in the long-term. It is these comorbidities that make this cohort of individuals more susceptible to injury in the first place. Research has shown that elderly patients, older than 65 years old, have about a 27% chance of falling each year.[18]

Internal bleeding, which I was concerned about in my 100-year-old fall patient, is a more prominent issue due to the frailty of the patient, the progressive brain atrophy that leaves more space for subdural hematomas in older individuals to collect blood, delay in treatment due to the patient thinking they are alright in conjunction with cognitive decline and dementia of one kind or another that may give the patient a false sense of security and being alright after a fall or accident of some sort. But an internal head bleed is nothing to scoff at and can lead to blindness, loss of consciousness and ultimately death.

The patient in Figure 9.19 was a 96-year-old woman (my mother), who woke up in the middle of the night, neglected to turn on a nightstand light, got disoriented and fell against the door of her room hitting her nose and face and then again, falling to the floor. She suffered from vascular dementia, diminished hearing, generalized muscle weakness and loss of strength, lack of balance and had a habit of thinking that she could do things that she could not really do and was a definite fall risk. She sustained a broken nose and internal bleeding from this fall. She was on blood thinners. She also

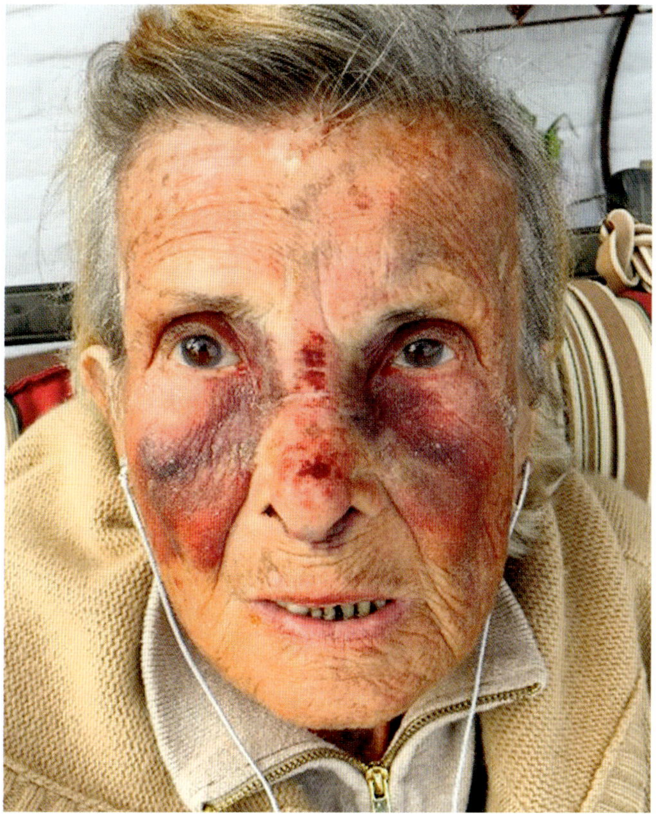

Fig. 9.19 Deceased 96-year-old woman, B. Shapira. Results of a fall with cuts, a fractured nose and subepithelial and subdermal bleeding.

fractured several teeth on her upper denture at the same time. She had a habit of waking up in the middle of the night and wandering around the room. What she was looking for, I am not sure? But then she would return to bed and fall asleep, until she did this behavior again. She was somewhat obsessive compulsive about her actions and never stopped fidgeting or moving. It was nerve wracking to be around her for any length of time. She also used to pick at her fingers and move her hands constantly. I made it a "habit" to sit next to her and hold her hands to get her to relax, whereby, her fidgeting and picking usually stopped. I think the reward for her was the attention she got from me and her allowing herself to stop this negative habit for the time being. However, getting up in the middle of the night and not turning on a light may be pure forgetfulness and part of her dementia process. The habit worsened over time and in her memory facility, when she moved there, they would not place gates or sides on her bed to keep her in bed. It was against the law and their policy to do so.

9.3 Conclusion

As stated before, actions that become repetitious over time have a propensity for becoming habits. A habit is a settled or regular tendency or practice, especially one that is difficult to give up. It is a behavior that starts as a choice and then becomes a nearly unconscious pattern with respect to some hidden psychological reward. Every habit, no matter how simple or complex in its make-up, has the same structure with respect to being called a "habit loop." Habits tend to "loop": around from one moment to the next circling from remission to activation and back again until the cycle can be broken through therapy or hard-core action on the part of the person involved with the particular habit. There is a cue, and then a trigger that tells the brain to go into action on automatic mode and then the satisfaction of getting the act over with to achieve the goal. Most people do not think about their habits in a conscious way, for them "It's just the way it is". I know that I am in the habit of cleaning my teeth in a specific regimen daily. When I accomplish what I set out to do, I feel good. If I am in a hurry and skip a step in the process, I feel incomplete and know that at some point, when I return home and before I go to sleep, I will need to start this ritual all over again until I can reassure myself that my teeth are relatively free of debris and plaque and that my smile looks good along with my mouth feeling healthy. This is my reward, and also in knowing that I may keep my teeth for a lifetime, barring that I do not get into a bar room type of bash or have an accident of some kind that will cause my possible tooth loss. Habits must have a pay-off for the person who possesses these rituals. As a practitioner of the head and neck, teeth and gingiva, we need to find out what people's "pay-offs" are in terms of both coming to our offices for routine maintenance and propagating their own self-efficacy in taking care of themselves; both causing an increase in the patient's longevity and limiting their contracting a debilitating disease of some kind in the process. When we find out what this reward is, we need to nurture it in our patient's behavior with praise and positive feedback, even going so far as to have this patient share their secrets with others who need a positive motivation

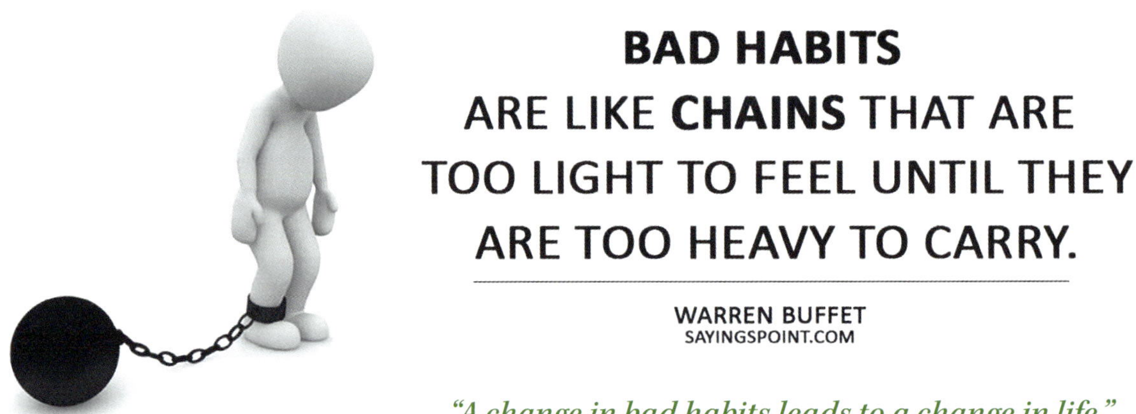

"A change in bad habits leads to a change in life."

Anonymous

to do the same action. Negative habits are the ones that we do not want to nurture and then, in turn, we need to honor and reward the positive actions of our patients continuously for a desired result.

It is difficult to break a bad habit because the chemicals in the brain that are "turned on" during this process tend to amplify the specific persons' actions and reinforce the habit altogether.

Chemicals, such as endorphins and epinephrine, act like stimulants and are a powerful force of nature. The person with the habit, whether good or bad, basically feels a "high" from their actions and this feeds into every part of their body and mind. It is difficult to erase the habit because the reward is so powerful sometimes and prevents us from overcoming the "bad" habit and giving into normalcy. It takes a lot of positive feedback and possibly referring the patient for therapy of one kind or another to assist in this quest.

We can look back in history to see the power behind all the good and the bad habits notorious men and women have displayed over their lifetimes. History does repeat itself unless positive stopgaps are placed in the way of negative habits that create a larger reward than the negative actions creating the natural "high" in the first place. This must be a learned response that comes from someone of authority, like a health practitioner, such as a dentist, who can show someone how to keep their teeth in a healthy condition for a lifetime and how important it is to do so. However, there are some people in the myriad of patients we come to meet in our professional lifetimes, that cannot or will not be influenced by any of the positive things we as dentists can assist them with. It's all about choices... So, we need to be prepared for this in our minds and take stock in the fact that we tried our best to positively influence our patients in a better and more productive direction. I have found in my years of practice that we cannot save everyone who passes our way. But that does not mean we should not try.

References

1. Gülsen A, Uygur B. *Psychological Features of Smokers.* Respir Care. 2018 Dec;63(12):1492-1497.
2. American Cancer Society Fact Sheet. Why People Start Smoking and Why It's Hard to Stop. Accessed online 06-03-21. https://www.cancer.org/health/stay-away-from-tobacco/why-people-start-using-tobacco.html
3. Blaha, Michael, Joseph, M.D., M.P.H. Health: 5 Vaping Facts you need to know. Johns Hopkins Medical Fact Sheet. Accessed online 06-06-21. https://www.hopkinsmedicine.org/health/wellness-and-prevention/5-truths-you-need-to-know-about-vaping.
4. Pringle KE, Ahern FM, Heller DA, Gold CH, Brown TV. *Potential for alcohol and prescription drug interactions in older people.* J Am Geriatr Soc. 2005 Nov;53(11):1930-6.
5. The Surprising Truth About Alcohol and Oral Health. Alcohol and Oral Health, Public Health pamphlet. Penn Dental medicine. Accessed 06-09-21. http://penndentalmedicine.org/alcohol-and-oral-health/
6. Lages EJ, Costa FO, Cortelli SC, Cortelli JR, Cota LO, Cyrino RM, Lages EM, Nobre-Franco GC, Brito JA, Gomez RS. *Alcohol Consumption and Periodontitis: Quantification of Periodontal Pathogens and Cytokines.* J Periodontol. 2015 Sep;86(9):1058-68.
7. U.S. Department of Health and Human Services and U.S. Department of Agriculture. 2015 – 2020 Dietary Guidelines for Americans. 8th Edition. December 2015. Accessed online 05-12-23 https://health.gov/our-work/food-nutrition/previous-dietary-guidelines/2015.
8. Scardina GA, Messina P. *Good oral health and diet.* J Biomed Biotechnol. 2012;2012:720692.
9. National Institute of Health: National Cancer Institute- Nutrition in Cancer Care- An Overview. Accessed online 06-12-21. https://www.cancer.gov/about-cancer/treatment/side-effects/appetite-loss/nutrition-pdq
10. American Cancer Society: American Cancer Society Guideline for Diet and Physical Activity. A Cancer Journal for Clinicians at: https://acsjournals.onlinelibrary.wiley.com/doi/full/10.3322/caac.21591Accessed online 06-12-21. https//www.cancer.org/healthy/eat-healthy-get-active/acs-guidelines-nutrition-physical-activity-cancer-prevention/guidelines.html
11. World Health Organization: Fact Sheet on Oral Health. Accessed online 06-12-21. https://www.who.int/newsroom/fact-sheets/detail/oral-health
12. Mayo Clinic Patient Care & Health Information. Bruxism (teeth grinding). Access online 06-19-21. Mayoclinic.org/diseases-conditions/bruxism/diagnosis-treatment/drc-20356100
13. Reddy SV, Kumar MP, Sravanthi D, Mohsin AH, Anuhya V. *Bruxism: a literature review.* J Int Oral Health. 2014 Nov-Dec;6(6):105-9
14. American Academy of Sleep Medicine Patient Information Fact Sheet. Obstructive Sleep Apnea. Accessed online 06-20-21. aasm.org/resources/factsheets/sleepapnea.pdf
15. CDC: Centers for Disease Control and Prevention. Arthritis-Related Statistics. Accessed online on 06-22-21. cdc.gov/arthritis/data-statistics/arthritis-related-stats-htm
16. Doba N, Tokuda Y, Saiki K, Kushiro T, Hirano M, Matsubara Y, Hinohara S. *Assessment of Self-Efficacy and its Relationship with Frailty in the Elderly.* Intern Med. 2016;55(19):2785-2792.
17. CDC: Centers for Disease Control and Prevention. Fact Sheet: accidents or Unintentional Injuries. Data for the U.S. Accessed online 06-22-21. cdc.gov/nchs/fastats/Accidental-injury.htm
18. Yee, Garrett, Jain, Ashika. Geriatric Head Injury. 07 January 2021 Update. NCBI Bookshelf. National Library of Medicine, National Institutes of Health. Accessed online 06-23-21. https://www.ncbi.nim.nih.gov/books/NBK553101/

Chapter 10

Case Construction and Presentation: It Is Not All That You Say... It Is How You Say It. It Is Not What You Bring, It is How You Show It...

"When you reach the end of what you should know, you will be at the beginning of what you should sense."
Khalil Gibran

10.1 What Do We Need to Present Our Findings to Our Patients?

The great baseball player and sometime philosopher, Yogi Berra, once said "That if you don't know where you are going, any road will take you there!". Being prepared, having a somewhat standard operating procedure and being able to demonstrate what you want to tell the patient is a good start. Everyone is different in how they approach an examination and treatment plan presentation. In respect of these facts, I think it behooves you, the practitioner, to keep an open mind and a "bag" full of options that you can use when you do your workups for new or existing patients. When I fully examine a first-time patient for matriculating into my practice, I have a set systematic method of acquiring clinical information, after which I go through my list of questions regarding the various histories of the patient: medical, dental, social, familial and economic. This allows me to get a good mental picture of who I am working with and what the challenges of treatment might be for me and my staff, as well as the patient.

To begin with, one needs the forms for which the patient will write the appropriate informational responses down that are requested by the office. Financial information forms, such as dental insurance or other means of paying for the treatment rendered is a must. But before any of this, one should have a form that explains the office policies, informs the patient about who you are and what kind of dentistry the office does and does not do, as well as listing the staff names, positions and duties (possibly an insert due to constant changes), allowing the prospective patient the knowledge about who everyone is that works in the office and where to go should they need something specific. The office information packet or brochure should include the materials listed in the Box 10.1 (from my own practice).

Should one not "Think Ahead" about these informational materials for a new or existing patient, then it becomes a one-sided issue: you know about the patient after reading their materials presented to you, but they know truly little about you, except, perhaps, what they have heard from people outside your practice. This is an unknown and can be detrimental to your relationship with the patient. Always try to remember when speaking or listening to another person that **communication is a "process" that involves a two-way simultaneous transmission of thoughts, information and feelings**, that will "hopefully" create **mutual understanding and common meaning** between two parties. Having to try and remember all these factors at the onset of a meeting with a new patient, or even an existing patient is difficult, to say the least, and it takes a lot of time. So, put it all out front and in the open, allowing yourself to be transparent and known to the patient before they endeavor to see you and your staff.

BOX 10.1

Think Ahead

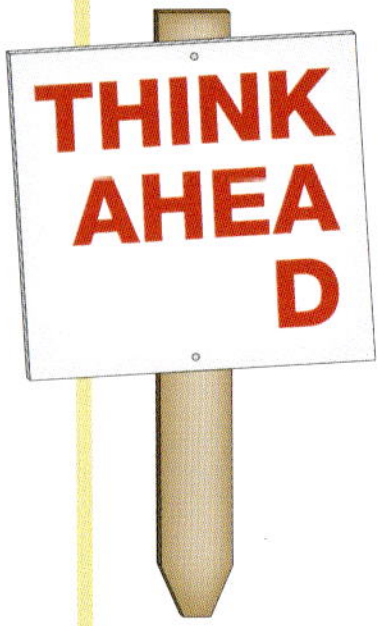

1. Information on cleanliness and sterilization techniques used in the office.
2. Information about dental procedures available, as well as clerical (insurance filing referrals and letters to insurance companies, etc.).
3. Information about sedation available, if any. This should include a travelling on-call dental anesthesiologist that might be available should someone need or want to have general anesthesia for their treatment due to anxiety, dementia and dental phobias.
4. Information about emergency preparedness. (A schematic map of the office layout and the exits can be included).
5. Information about the kinds of materials the office uses to restore teeth, including the benefits and alternatives, as well as the Material Safety Data sheets that are available on request for the materials used in the office.
6. Information about special needs patients and care and the ability to treat them in comfort and safety, or not.
7. Information about geriatric patients and their needs and comfort and safety.
8. A diagram schematic of the office showing the restrooms and exits.
9. A sheet for the patient to write down any questions they may have that has not been answered by the information sheet(s).
10. A form to fill out to place in an office suggestion box that requires no signature as to be anonymous for any positive or negative feedback.
11. A sheet that defines the Mission Statement of the practice, the Vision Statement and any other information that can educate the patient about the practitioner and practice that you want them to know.
12. Lastly, periodically inform your patients about the new innovations in dentistry that you have learned, that you are studying to become an expert in and the newest in sterilization equipment and other equipment that will keep the office free of "germs and viruses" for their protection and up to date with modern technology.

10.2 What Clinical Records Are Important to Have at the Onset of Treatment?

I like to have the following information as part of my initial examination:

- **Intraoral:** A full charting of the mouth and existing teeth with restorations and caries that are visible; Classification of occlusion, malocclusion and position of teeth; Measurements of overbite, overjet and protrusive; Anatomy; Probing depths; Recession measurements around the teeth; Missing teeth; Extra teeth; Caries on teeth; Existing restorations on teeth; Amount of attached gingiva; Bleeding on probing and position on the tooth, i.e., position, surface and amount; Abnormalities in tooth structure or gingiva; Pigment location and measurement of same on soft and hard tissue; Salivary gland function; Varicosities; Tonsils; Cheek biting lines (Linea alba); Hyperkeratosis position and amount; Mallampati classification of the oropharynx; Intraoral scars and position; Palatal vault shape and height-high or flat, shallow, narrow or wide; Floor depth and shape; Tori on the maxillary arch and mandibular arch; Speech patterns; Smile line (positive or negative); Breath (halitosis or not); Stain (amount and position); Calculus classification, location, and plaque amounts.

- **Extraoral:** Information on the palpation of the lymph nodes of the head and neck areas (soft versus firm, moveable versus non-moveable, pain versus non-painful); Charting of nevi position with color and size; Scar position and size; Piercings (number and position); Color of the eyes; Eyelid mucosa color (usually lower lid); Movement of the eyes following a finger moving in front of them, from one side to the other to show astigmatism and whether there are any cataract surgeries with new lenses that can reflect in the light across a moving eye; Arcus senilis around the outside of the iris of the eye showing aging and possible elevated lipids in the body; Hearing in each ear by whispering to each ear; Thyroid palpation for size, stones, lumps, bumps and granules; Palpation of the subclavicular space or notch for nodes and abnormalities; Blood pressure and Oxygen levels using a pulse oximeter meter. (See the examination sheets in the Appendix, Figs. 4 to 11.)

Once these entities are charted one has a fairly good idea of the existing complexity of the oral and extraoral anatomy that the patient brings with them. If no radiographs are brought with the patient, it is prudent to take what is needed: perhaps a full set of radiographs or four bitewings, two to four periapical films and a Panographic film will work as well for screening. Other films may be needed, after the fact, and further evaluation, which can be taken as needed. If the patient is needing extensive treatment, I always take impressions or a scan of the mouth so that I can duplicate these in study model form. When I speak to the patient during a consultation visit, I will have all this information and models of the patients' mouth for them to see and visualize, as I am discussing what I feel are their dental needs for treatment. I do this at a separate visit to make sure they are "fresh" and alert and able to listen, as well as to ask pertinent questions.

Should implants be part of the treatment plan, I will have a referral form for a CBCT (Cone Beam Computerized Tomography) film of the area, from which I can have an implant surgical guide made. If I need to look further at the TMJ, I will recommend a set of open and closed mouth tomograms as well. I always take photographs of every mouth that I treat for the before and after results and the change in smiles after treatment. These are all legal records and can assist the practitioner in not only treating the patient, but in referrals and for any legal issues that may arise.

Currently, it is not without saying that dental X-ray companies are making owning a CBCT machine more financially reasonable and easier to obtain. It might prove unbelievably valuable to have this type of informational equipment in one's office, considering older people's teeth become more brittle and subject to fracturing as they age and there is usually more pathology to be found that one can pick up in people of all ages, not just geriatric individuals.

The CBCT machine (Fig. 10.1) is small but still needs space to keep it. Many Panographic machines can be adapted to CBCT as well should the Panorex be adaptable. As you can see from the film below, the CBCT can and does provide a three-dimensional picture of the jaws and teeth unlike the normal dental X-ray film. It is quite accurate and immensely helpful in diagnosing anatomical landmarks, abnormalities, size and shape of the boney ridges, fractured teeth and most pathology in the oral cavity.

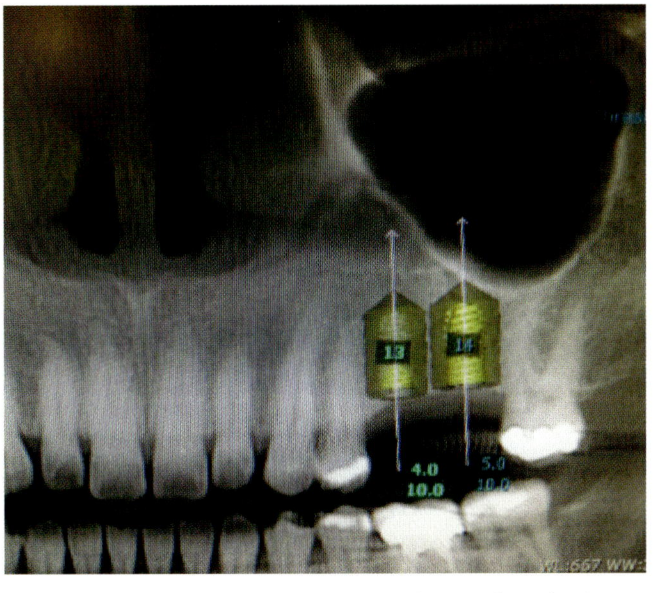

Fig. 10.1 CBCT Film showing the ability to place implants by the size and the space available. The CBCT can also determine the size of the implant being used in the appropriate space with the type and make of the implant system at hand.

10.3 The Importance of Study Models

Since we are in a visually oriented Society, as I have mentioned before, it is more prudent to be able to show the patient a tangible model of their mouth to not only visualize what their mouths look like, but to explain why it needs attention. A deceased philosopher patient of mine, Dr. Heinz von Forrester, once said to me: "We don't know what we don't know, and we don't see what we don't see". After ruminating on this comment for many years, I realize how germane it is to be teaching my dental patients about themselves using models of their own mouths. The adage, "seeing is believing" kind of hits me when I think of Dr. von Forrester's quote. We, as practitioners, can talk until we are "blue" in the face, but if the patient is not cued into listening or even comprehending what it is we are saying, we are out of luck. On the other hand, if we couple what we say with what we can show the patient about themselves, we are likely to succeed in having them understand what it is "we" think they need and hopefully this will push their "want" button into an acceptance of these visual facts, which, in turn will allow them the opportunity to discuss what was said and hopefully accept the treatment proposal.

I use a lot of different types of models for discussion with patients. When I speak of dental implants, I have models to show the patient about what an implant looks like, how it works and the rationale behind the model. The same goes for periodontal disease and the like. **The older the patient, the more important it is to use visual models** in explaining what the treatment consists of and how it can be managed.

10.3.1 The Importance of Mounted Study Models

I am an advocate for using an articulator with my study models (Fig. 10.2) rather than hand holding them. It is a more accurate way of illustrating to the patient how their mouth moves with respect to wear patterns, broken teeth and misaligned teeth. This way the patient can visualize their mouths in a more accurate duplication of the way their teeth function together.

On another note, using commercially made study models to explain disease states, such as periodontal disease (Fig. 10.3) and its progression, is an invaluable tool to teach and show your patients. Older patients especially "take stock" in seeing a model of a disease state that they can relate to, rather than a dentist pointing to a radiograph and showing them their bone loss without the visual views of the plaque, calculus and red, swollen tissues around the teeth on the model that emulates their own oral situation. Geriatric patients tend to be somewhat suspicious and stand-offish about accepting anything without fully understanding why they should do something that is costly, even if is very harmful for them not to do what is recom-

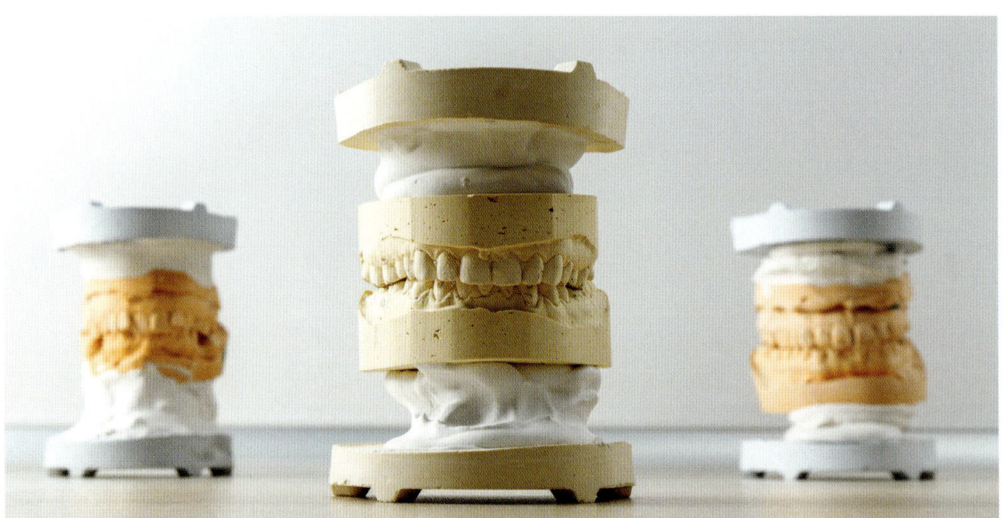

Fig. 10.2 Mounted models off the articulator for demonstration.

mended. The validity of seeing not only their own study models, but both ideal models of a dentition and models that show procedures and disease processes as well, comes to light when they finally "get it." Models allow for understanding and understanding allows for decision making with respect to treatment.

The periodontal study model (Fig. 10.3) is invaluable in teaching older, more cognitively impaired patients about their periodontal disease state. Being able to understand a discussion about treatment is often met with a "stare" or eyes that look away from the practitioner. Determining if it is lack of interest, not being able to understand what is being said needs to be determined before the practitioner can advance in discussing treatment. Having this kind of model or the like, will help in one's discussion with these types of patients. My pointer in hand and the patient's eyes on the model can follow my pointer and hear the explanation. Patience is needed as well as extra time to discuss treatment with the older patient. Therefore, I always appoint for a separate visit for the consultation. I never charge for this appointment, as some practitioners do, because I feel that it is an investment in the relationship I have with the specific patient and an investment in my gaining a consent to treatment in the end. Spending added time with the patient shows that you share concern for them, understand where they are coming from and respect them for who they are. You can not buy this anywhere. It must be earned.

10.4 Appropriate Medical Testing

It is not too often that I will ask for a medical test of one kind or another for something that a patient brings in with them, but I do refer for testing when I feel it is necessary. With older patients one can expect to refer a good deal of the time since they are subject to lower immune responses and to more disease and complex bodily issues than the norm. Performing a simple visual inspection of the patient can allow one to entertain a perception of the possibility of a medical issue, a disease perhaps not mentioned in a history form or a symptomatic visual problem such a jaundice, exophthalmia, "pea" rolling of the fingers as in Parkinson's disease, difficulty breathing or orthopnea consistent with heart disease.[1] Being cognizant of these kinds of issues, I will consider sending the patient to a cardiologist for an ECG.

Should I see a great deal of gingival inflammation in someone's mouth, I may send them for a C-reactive protein blood test. In most instances, with respect to doing an involved and somewhat invasive treatment regimen, I will send an older patient back to their primary care physician for a medical release before starting my treatment with them, just to be on the safe side for both of us. Periodically, I will send a swab of plaque or have my hygienist do this, to a lab for a genetic test on the type of harmful bacteria in the mouth, so we know how better to chemically and pharmacologically treat the patient's periodontal issues. I will periodically

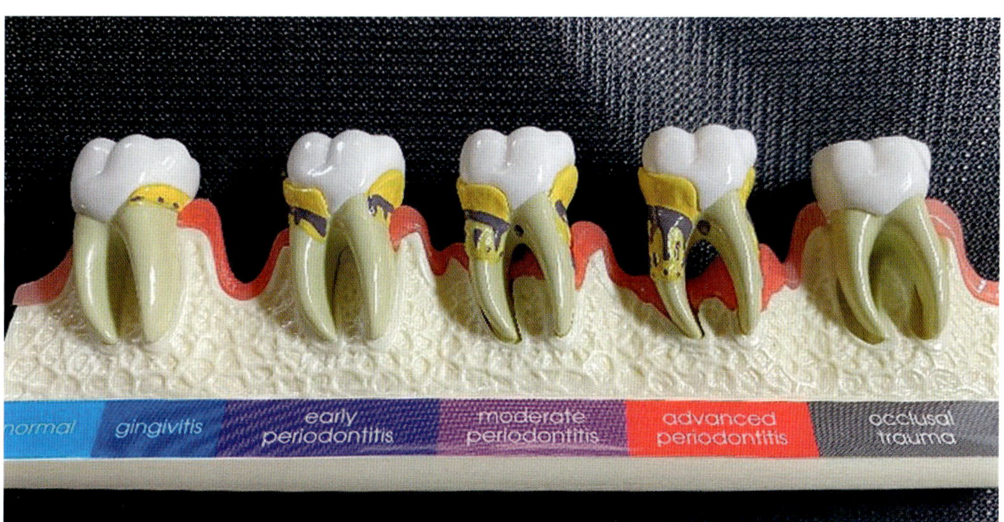

Fig. 10.3 Periodontal disease progression model from Kilgore International, Inc. Photo by Dr. Eric Z. Shapira.

send a patient out on a referral for an allergy test, especially when they tell me that they are allergic to some type of dental material, such as amalgam, composite, or acrylic.

If I suspect an older patient has a breathing problem, an elevated blood pressure, or any other physical issue that presents itself to me before, during or after treatment that could lead to an emergency for them, I will most definitely refer them back to their medical doctor for a work-up or to the emergency room, before there is an emergency in my office with them. One cannot be too careful in practicing this type of care but watching that you do not carry it to the extreme for fear of scaring off the patient forever. Most older individuals I have taken this kind of action with end up thanking me and respecting more than they would have otherwise. Most of them have referred their families and friends to me for treatment, because they know that I care about them and that I know what I am doing.

Many years ago, I had an older woman for a patient in her late 80's. She was from England, and she had a son who was an emergency room physician in a local hospital in my community. He was also a "sometime patient" of mine as well. One day she came into my office for an appointment in a cheery mood, a smiling face, but pale looking to me out of the ordinary. I asked her if she was alright as she sat back in the chair and she said she felt a little dizzy. I immediately laid the dental chair back, gave her oxygen, took her blood pressure and then called a "*STAT*", my office emergency code, when I noticed that she was not speaking very well when I returned to her from being on the phone. The paramedics came within minutes to my office in response to our calling them and the patient's son showed up as well, as he was on call in the ER at the local hospital and one of our staff people called him in the interim, being the next of kin. The moment he stepped into the operatory, he started questioning me about "what I injected into his mother or did to her". I did nothing to her except take care of her based upon her symptoms. I told him, but he was enraged and threatened to sue me for negligence. At that point I asked him to leave and totally lost respect for him, as I felt he, being a physician, should understand that what I did was appropriate care under the circumstances.

I followed up with the ER sometime after the incident and they told me that my English patient was alright. They informed me that she possibly had a TIA (Transient Ischemic Attack) or small stroke and that I had saved her life with my actions. Much to my chagrin, her son came back to my office several days later and apologized in person, as he had heard from his mother that all she did was sit in my dental chair and the rest was history. He was so embarrassed by his acting-out in the office under duress that he never returned as a patient. His loss....

We have covered emergencies in the dental office in an earlier chapter, but I felt it prudent to bring this story to light for several reasons:

- Early recognition of emergencies begins at the first observable signs or symptoms.[2]
- It is important for the entire dental team to be prepared for any emergency that can happen in the dental office at any time.
- CPR classes must be taken **yearly** even though the certificate is good for two years, as I advocate that "practice makes permanence."
- Each office employee needs to have a specific function for an emergency in or outside the office. One person is to take copious notes of every observable action and conversation. This action is important to record the care, the event, the people present and to protect us all from false accusations and an eventual suit against us in any respects.
- Patient charts need to be reviewed prior to the patient coming into the office so that the staff can be apprised of any medical issues or ongoing medical problems that can be affected by the upcoming dental treatment and be prepared.
- All staff must be prepared to give treatment based upon the orders of the dentist.

The most notable requirement in dealing with medical issues in the office, especially emergency management, is the updated knowledge of the doctor that aids in the early diagnosis and management of the issues at hand.[3] It is also prudent to always have the necessary equipment in the office, such as an emergency kit with useable and up-to-date drugs, including an ammonia inhalant at the chair for syncope; an IV set-up with either D5W or Normal saline solution; an emergency defibrillator and oxygen readily available to name a few.

"Be prepared at all times" for everything and anything, as one never can predict the unpredictable.

10.5 What to Look for in Your Examination of the Older Patient

Examination of an older patient brings with it a myriad of surprises, laughter, tears, anger, and the entire gamut of emotions, even silence from those who suffer from advanced dementia of one sort or another, as well as anger or depression related silence. It is up to us, the practitioner, to figure out all parts of the "puzzle" the patient brings with them to solve.

"The pessimist sees difficulty in every opportunity. The optimist sees the opportunity in every difficulty."

Winston Churchill

I quoted Sir Winston Churchill here because of his salient comment as it relates to many practitioners who examine an older, sometimes compromised patient, the same way they do everyone else. The important thing here is to remember that older individuals have had many years of experience under their belts, so to speak, and thus bring more "baggage" with them to the dental office; for example, with the declining years comes not only more experience, but more medical issues. The frailty that accompanies us all as we age, the physical and mental pain due to the loss of many things including, but not limited to family, friends, function, and fun cause us irreparable changes in who we are and how we deal with these things in the time we have left to confront them. Loss brings grief and unresolved grief brings anxiety, guilt and depression, with the ultimate loss of self-esteem.

Our functionality is different. Our anatomy changes compared to our youth. Our brains slow down, for the most part and our memories can be affected in the process and slowdown too, especially our short-term memories. Our abilities to cope with change and our physical and emotional strength diminish as well. Our physiology changes and our abilities to cope with stress, which dental treatment can create for this ilk, is limited. So, it behooves all practitioners to consider the differences in our examination techniques in working with the older, infirm, or older patients with special needs and mentally compromised individuals, subsequently treating each person as an individual in a specialized way (Fig. 10.4). **The examination for this cohort should be respectful, gentle, slow, thoughtful, involved, exacting and detailed, recorded, informative, and efficiently discussed during the process like a roadmap giving direct information of a location to a desired destination.**

In Box 10.2 you can see what one should look for in this exam process (Figs. 10.5-10.25).

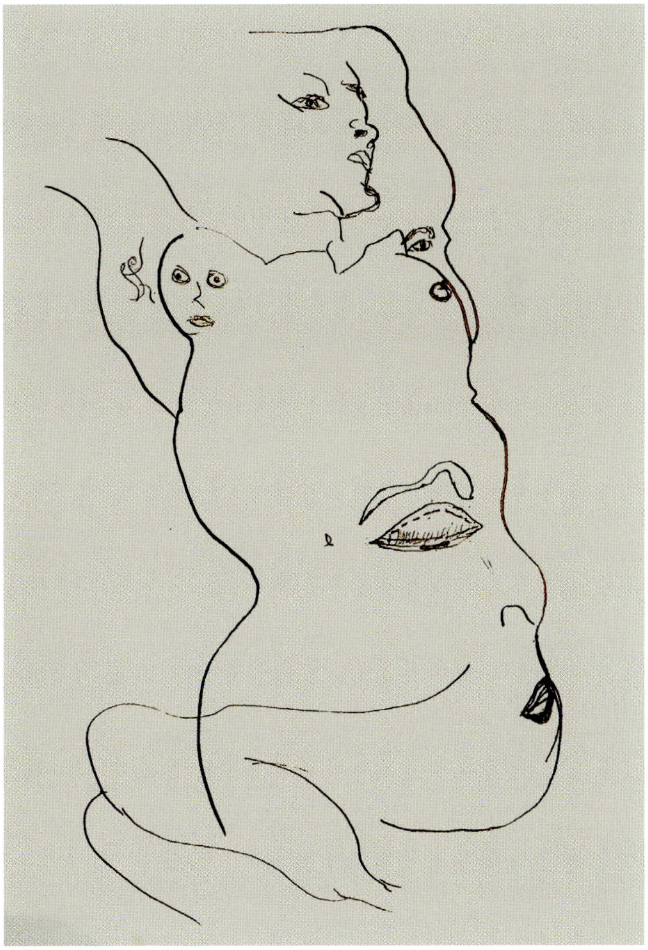

Fig. 10.4 Ink Illustration to remind the viewer that when examining a patient there is more than meets the eye. Art by Dr. Eric Z. Shapira, 1970. The Woman of Many Faces.

BOX 10.2 What We Should Observe in the Neck and Head Exam

It is especially important to have a baseline measurement of the function of the teeth as well as an initial record of the existing facial and intraoral anatomy. We need to know what exists, what has been damaged, what changes from the ideal exist and what we think the patient needs in conjunction with his or her initial concerns. Should we find abnormalities during our exam, we need to record them in writing, drawings and photos. I have even gone so far as to take impressions of a palatal abnormality or floor of the mouth abnormality. Today, we can scan the tissues and have models made rather than take direct impressions. We can use an intraoral camera for record taking as well. It never hurts to have too much information. Once we change what is there in the first place, our undeniable "footprints", so to speak, have already sunk into the sand. We have made our mark and there is no turning back. We need the initial record of what the patient brought with them in order to compare them with the changes in the future.

Learning takes a lot of practice. The more we do something, repetition, the more proficient we are at it, until it is rote... we can do it with our eyes closed, at least it seems that way, but we cannot. We need eyes wide-open. The anatomy is different for all of us, even though we have been blessed with the same "equipment", so to speak. Our equipment breaks down with repeated use, has accidents, gets damaged from personal abuse and changes shape and condition due to force in terms of bruxing, clenching, grinding, eating habits, self-afflicted wounds, smoking, drugs, alcohol, accidents and disease. This is a good enough reason to document a baseline for each person you examine.

There is more to look at when one sees an illustration of the anatomy (Box 10.3, Figs. 10.26-10.31) we need to examine. Looking at the tongue, there is the papillae, the texture, shape, color, movement, frenae, vessels, surface markings, scars, width, length and size.

The Face

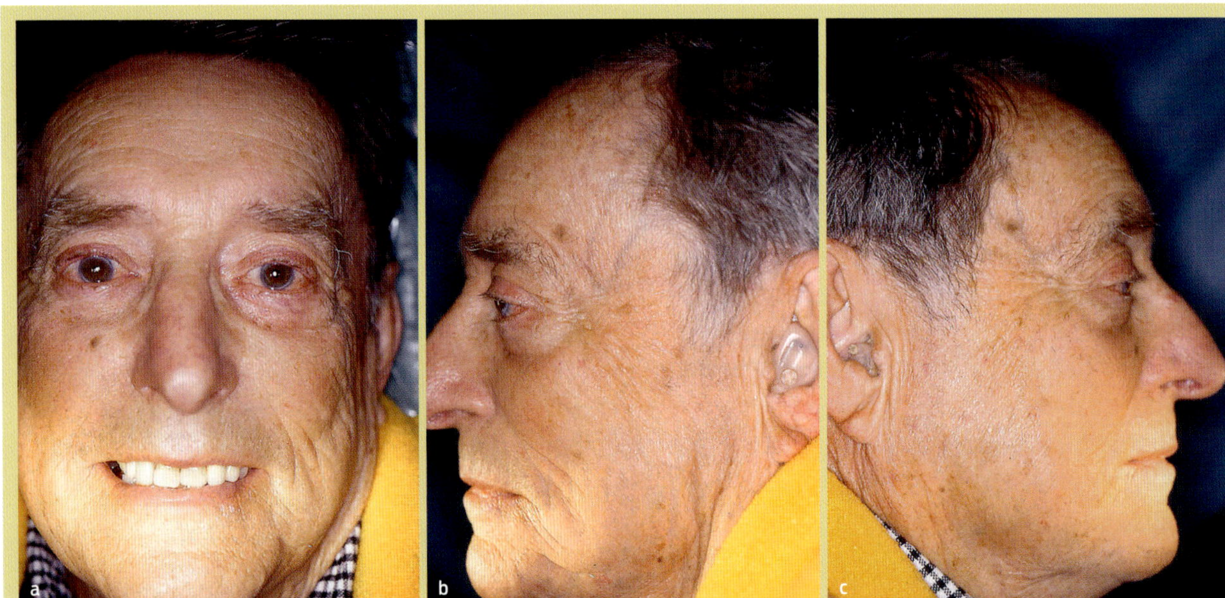

Fig. 10.5 (a-c) Deceased 90-year-old patient. Note the facial anatomy and hearing devices present. There are bilateral arcus senilis of the eyes, multiple pigmentations on the face and forehead, thinning lips and a loss of vertical dimension.

The Neck

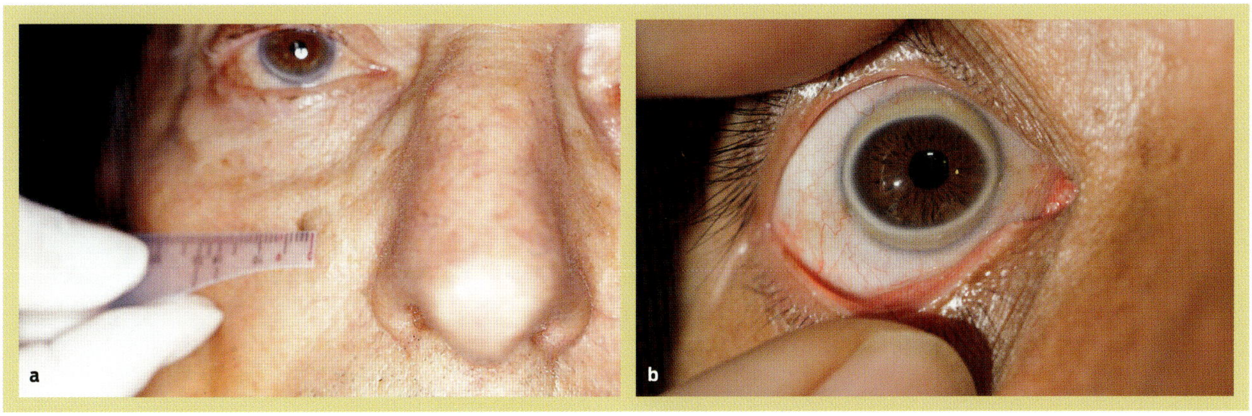

Fig. 10.6 **(a)** The nevus is measured and charted in position. Note the right eye and the white arcus senilis around the iris. **(b)** Arcus senilis is a collection of fat in a circular ring-like pattern around the outside of the iris and it can invade the cornea. It is significant to diagnose this condition during the dental exam and refer the patient to an MD for a blood work-up, as the Arcus signifies an issue with high cholesterol and triglycerides, essentially fat metabolism. If unchecked, this can lead to possible cardiac issues such as myocardial infarction and stroke. Having identified this during your dental exam, you can possibly save a life by your action of referral. This is medicine and not usually taught in dental school. It is something I learned in my Dental/Medical residency in a hospital many years ago. I do not believe many dental practitioners know to diagnose this condition, it is found in 50% of people over the age of 60 years. Socrates stated, "The eyes are the windows to the soul". In this case they are a receptacle of knowledge about the Human body they are attached to in perpetuity.

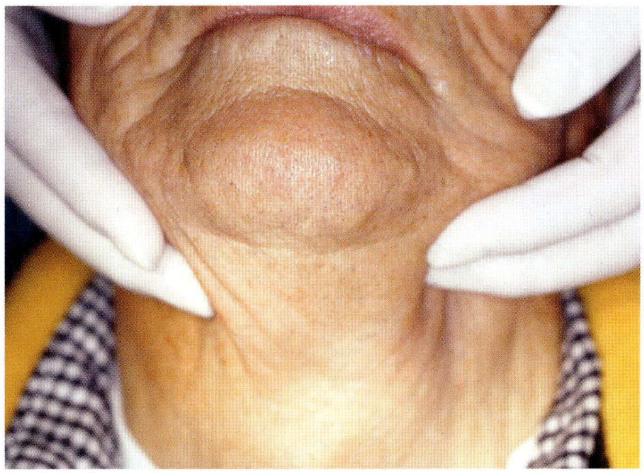

Fig. 10.7 Submandibular and cervical lymph node palpation.

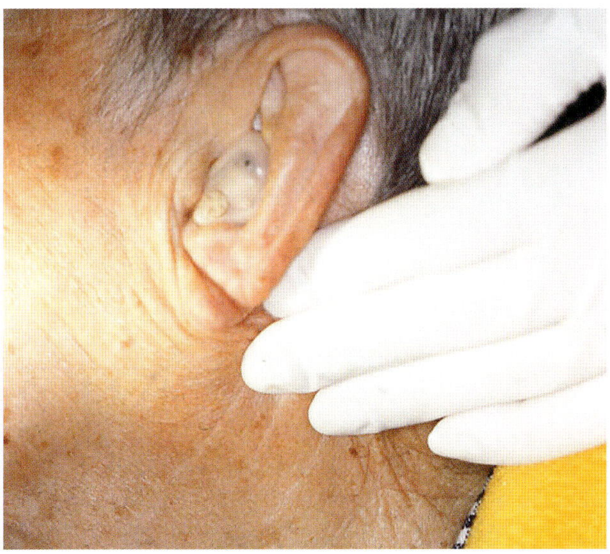

Fig. 10.8 Posterior auricular lymph nodes charted and hearing tested.

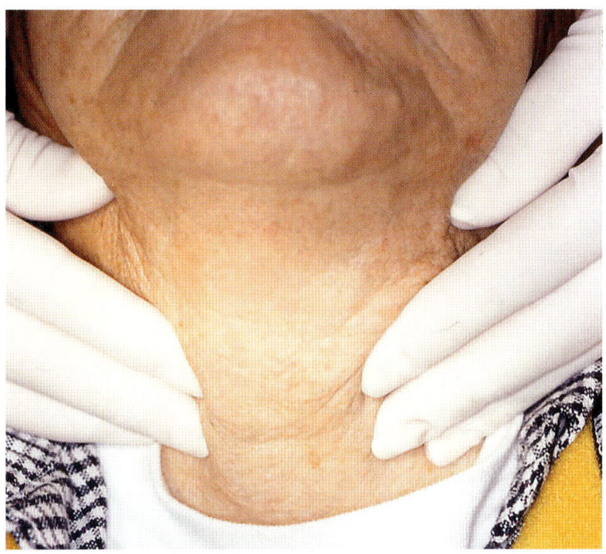

Fig. 10.9 Palpation of the thyroid glands, anterior triangle and cervical anatomy.

The Oral Cavity

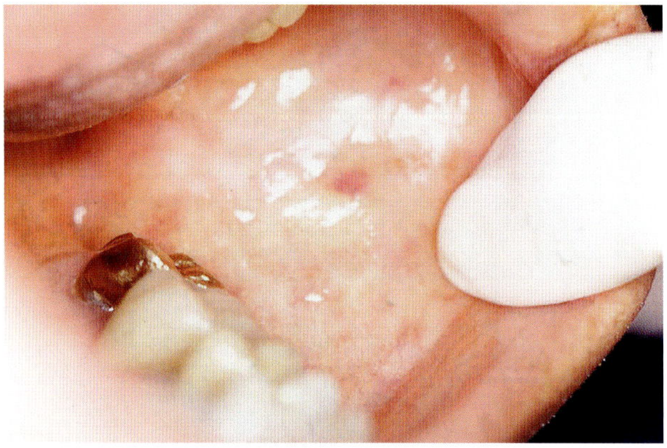

Fig. 10.10 Left cheek mucosa, Stenson's salivary duct.

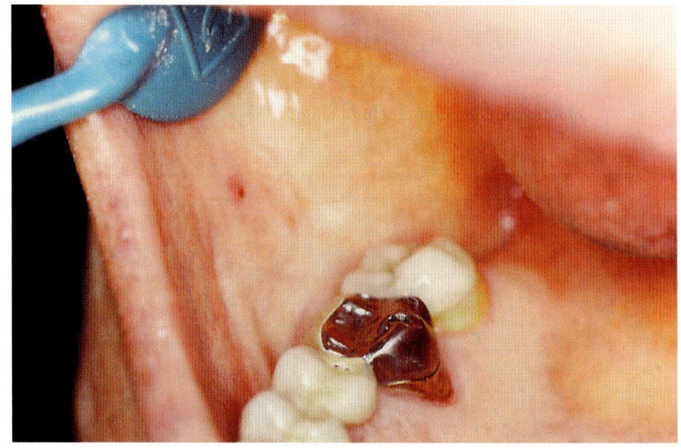

Fig. 10.11 Right cheek and anatomy as well as lingual root recession and stain on tooth #30 root.

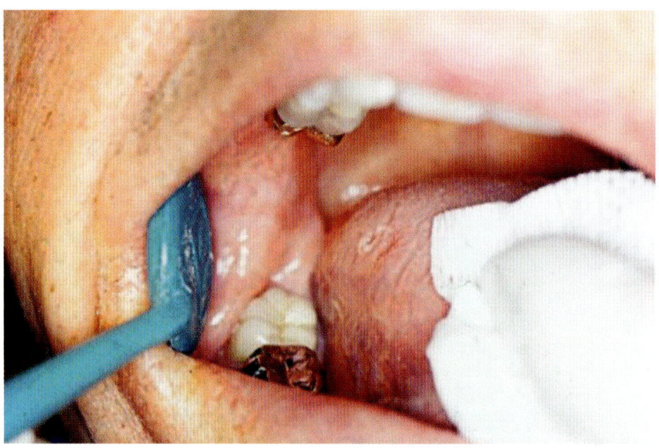

Fig. 10.12 Lateral border of the tongue and floor of the mouth right side.

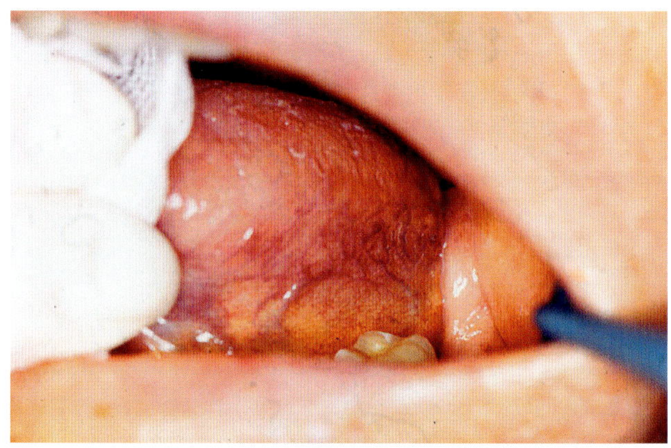

Fig. 10.13 Left border of the tongue with varicosities.

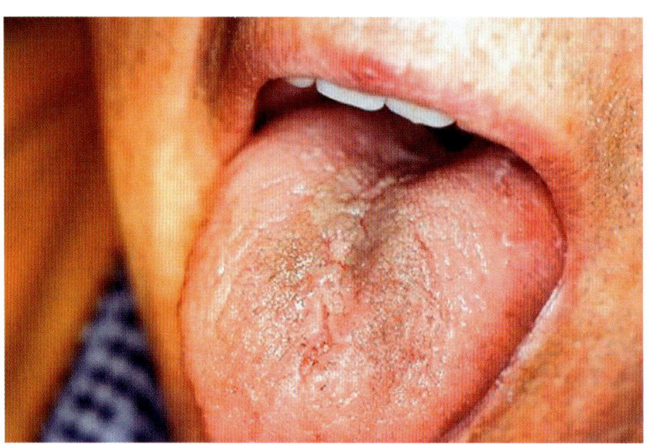

Fig. 10.14 The dorsum of the tongue with black coloration on the surface as well as fissures.

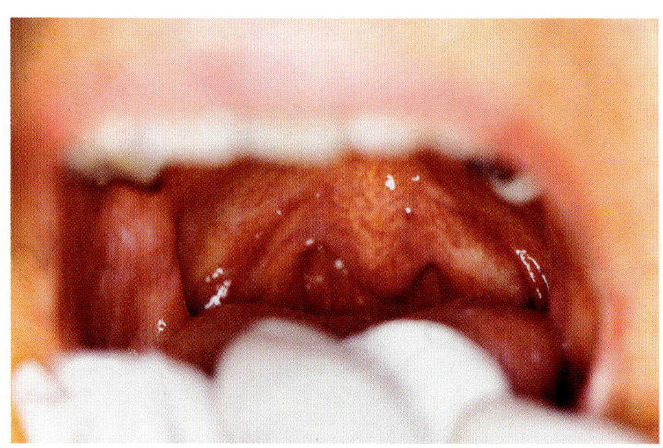

Fig. 10.15 The oropharynx, tonsillar pillars, uvula and posterior access to the airway.

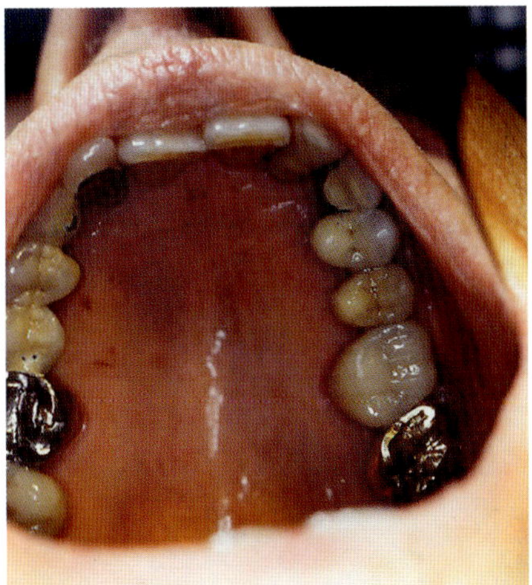

Fig. 10.16 The palate and maxillary arch form with teeth.

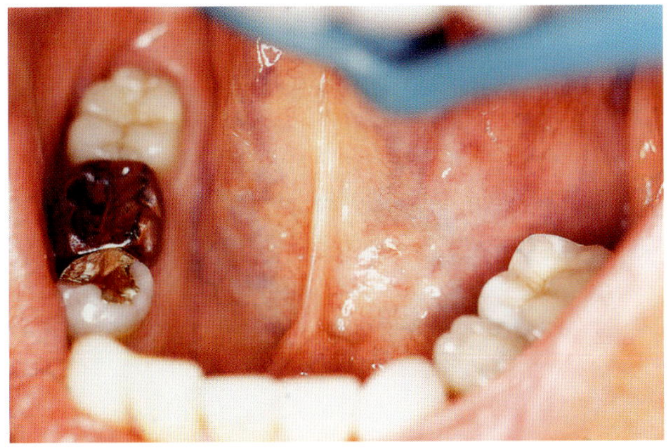

Fig. 10.17 The floor of the mouth, sublingual salivary glands and mandibular teeth.

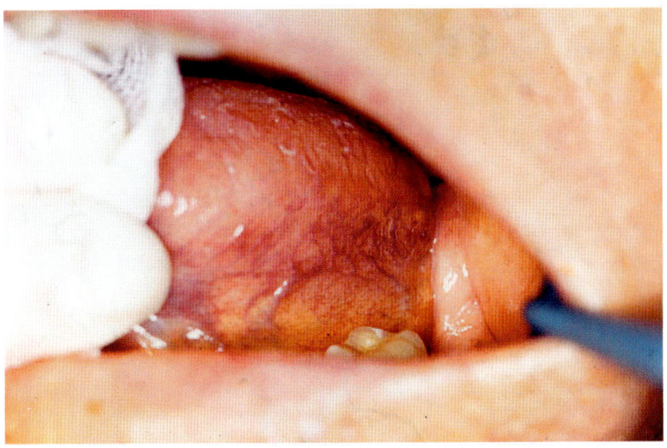

Fig. 10.18 The lingual surface of the tongue, varicosities, salivary glands and teeth.

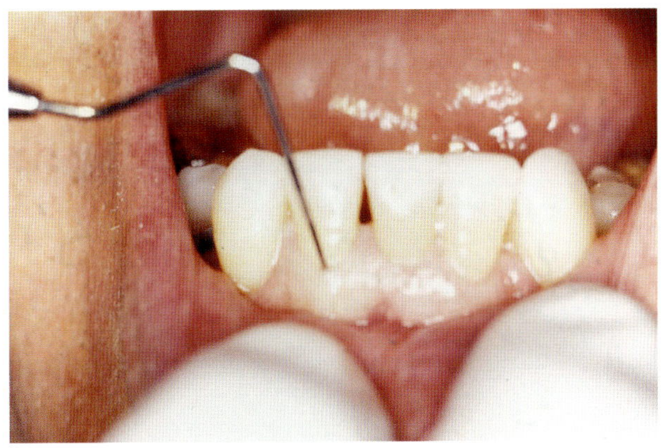

Fig. 10.19 Recording periodontal probing depths, recession and bleeding.

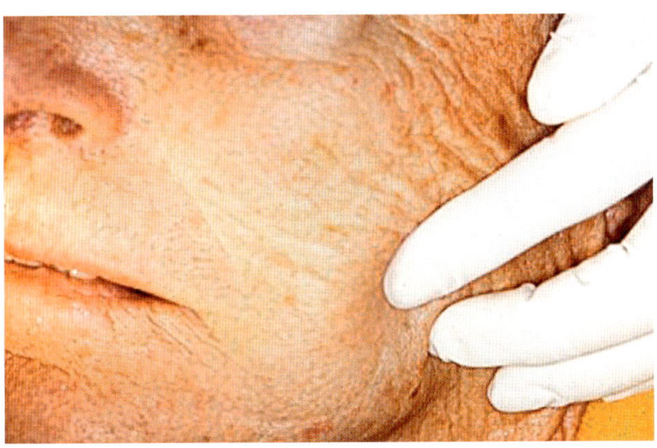

Fig. 10.20 Checking the masseter muscle, TMJ and looking for joint sounds and movement.

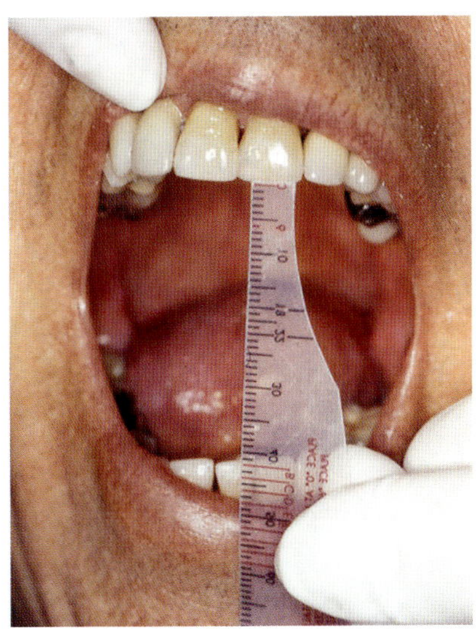

Fig. 10.21 Measuring maximum opening.

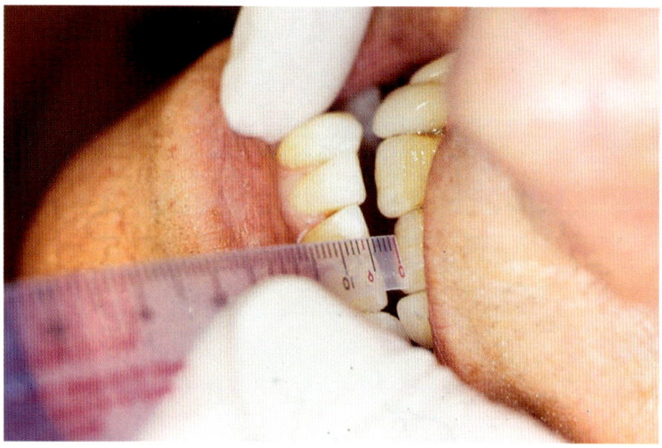

Fig. 10.22 Measuring protrusive movement.

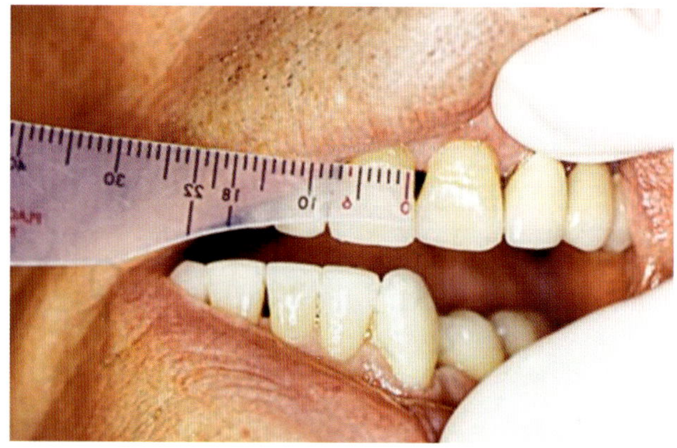

Fig. 10.23 Measuring right lateral side-shift.

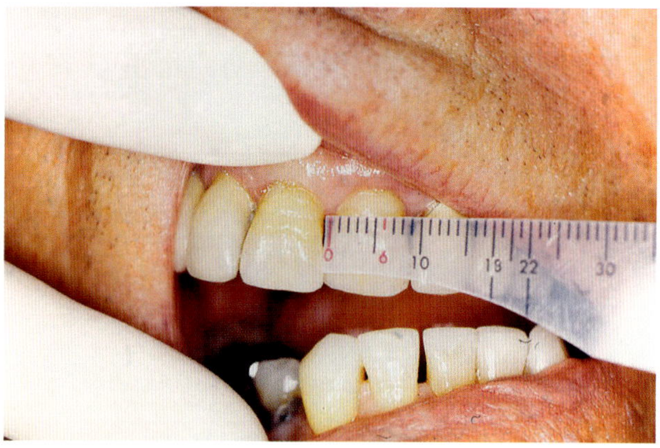

Fig. 10.24 Measuring left lateral side-shift.

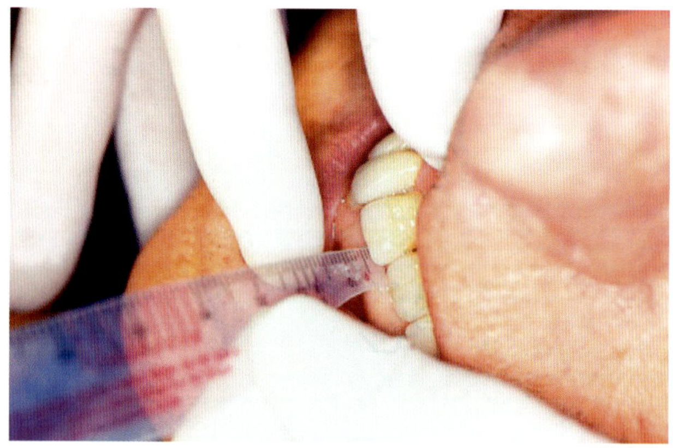

Fig. 10.25 Measuring overjet and overbite.

BOX 10.3 Anatomical Illustrations

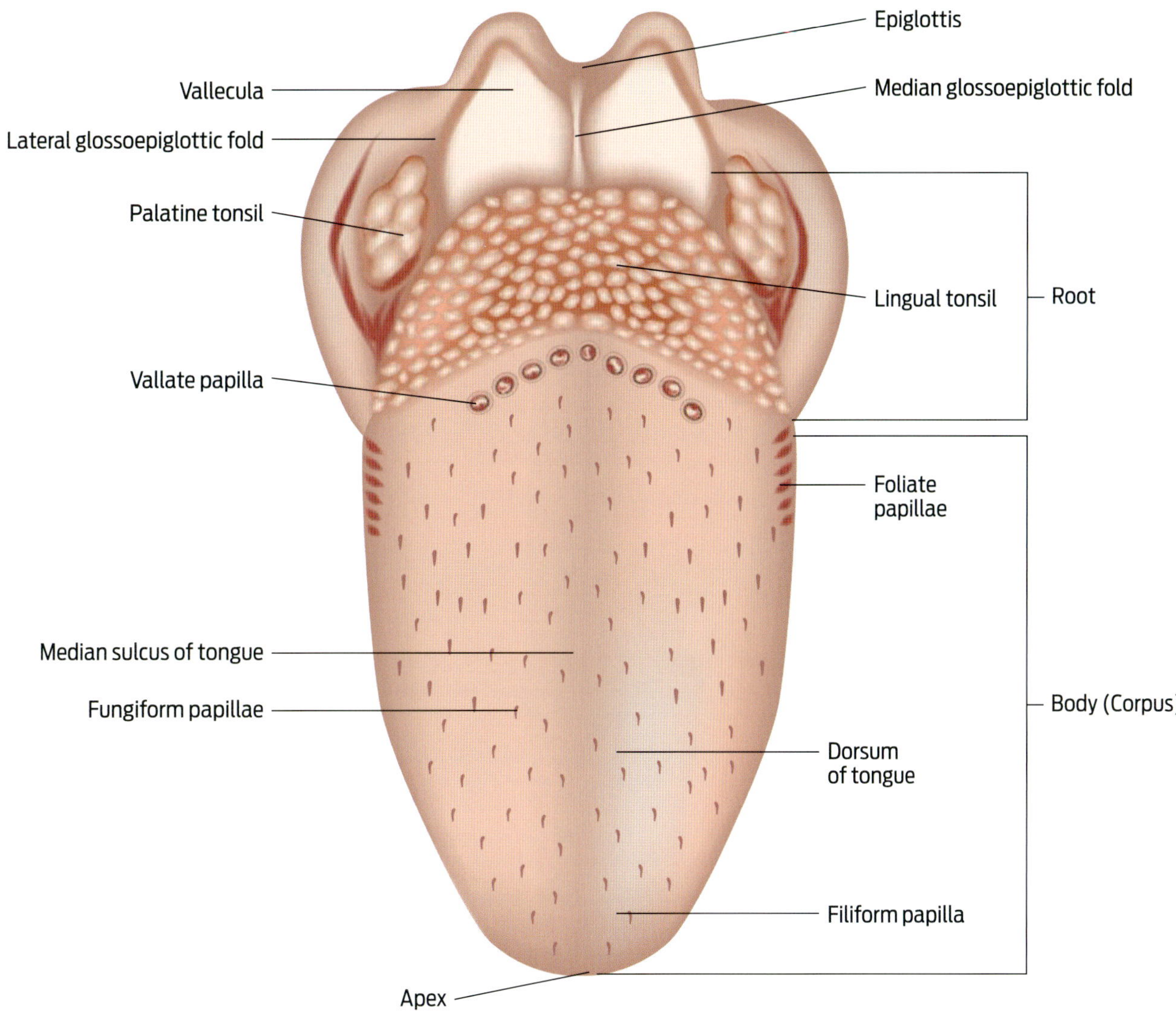

Fig. 10.26 Reference for Identification of landmarks on and around the tongue.

(continued)

(continued)

LIP

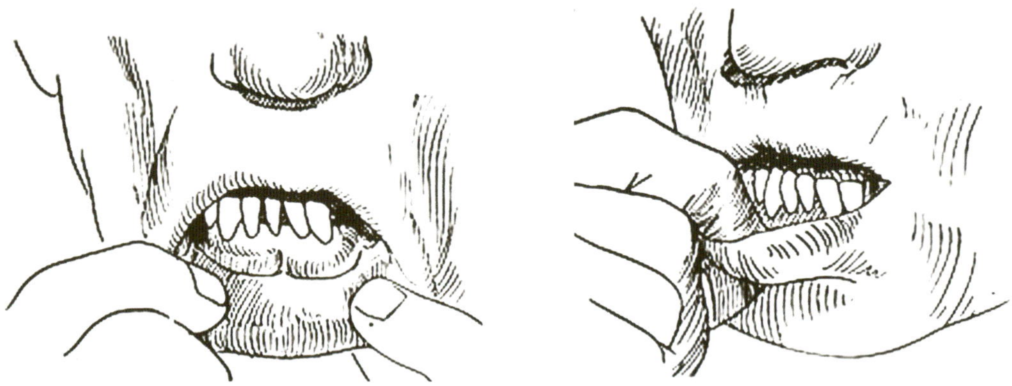

LOOK FOR... Color changes (red, white, or blue)
Scab or crack
Swelling
Bleeding

FEEL FOR... Sore spot or bump
Swelling
Numbness
Thickening

Fig. 10.27 We want to feel, bimanually palpate and look at the tissue.

CHEEK

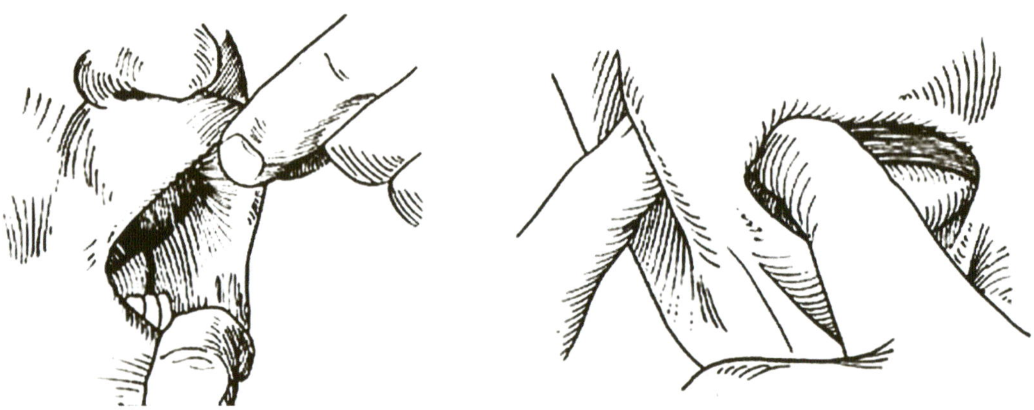

LOOK FOR... White patches or soft velvety-red spots
Ulcers

FEEL FOR... Bumps or lumps
Swelling
Painful area

Fig. 10.28 We want to bimanually palpate the cheeks, check the salivary glands and mucosa.

(continued)

(continued)

TONGUE

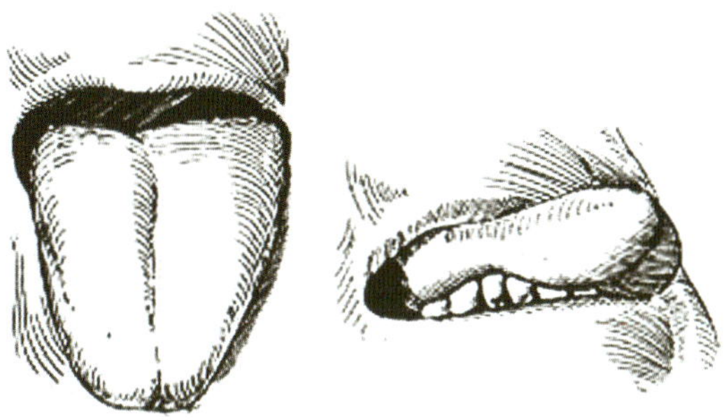

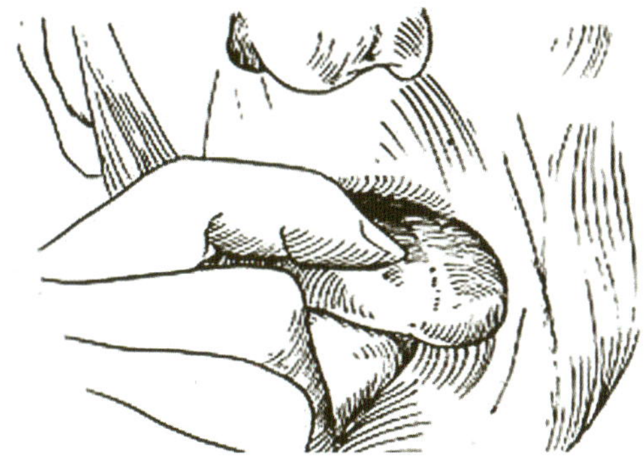

LOOK FOR... White patches or soft velvety-red spots
Swellings
Ulcers
Red edges and tip

FEEL FOR... Lumps or bumps
Sore spots
Lack of movement

Fig. 10.29 Examine all sides of the tongue and bimanually palpate it.

ROOF OF MOUTH

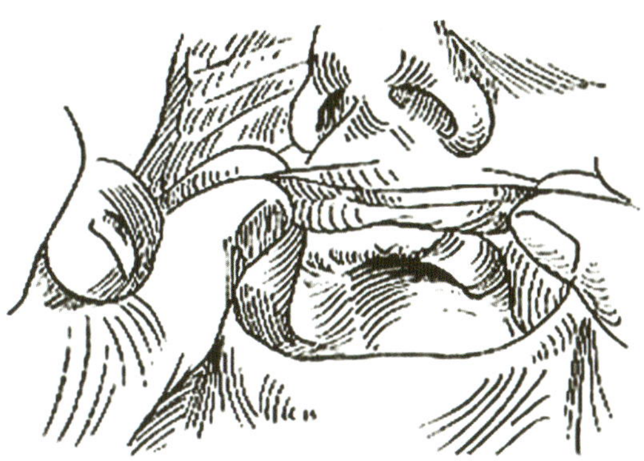

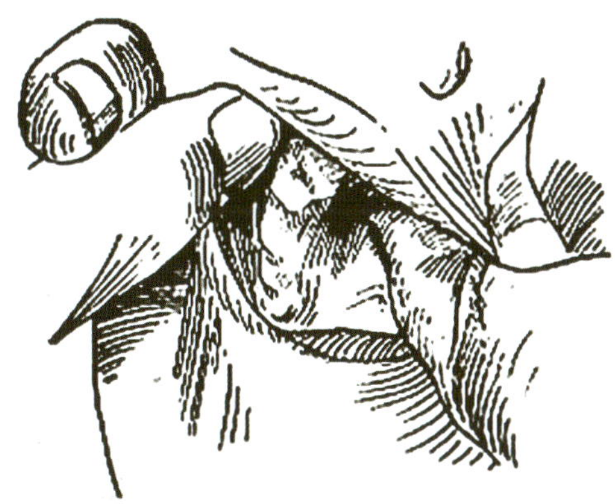

LOOK FOR... Bluish color or white patches
Ulcer

FEEL FOR... Lumps or bumps
Soft swelling

Fig. 10.30 The palate, both hard and soft, should be palpated and examined for changes.

(continued)

(continued)

FLOOR OF MOUTH

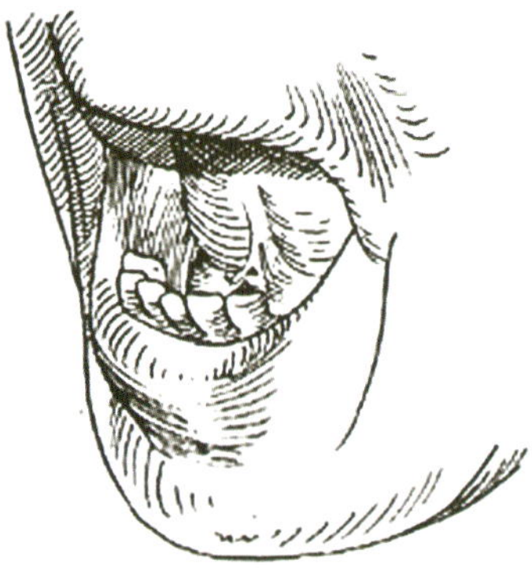

LOOK FOR... White patches or soft velvety-red spots
Bluish swellings

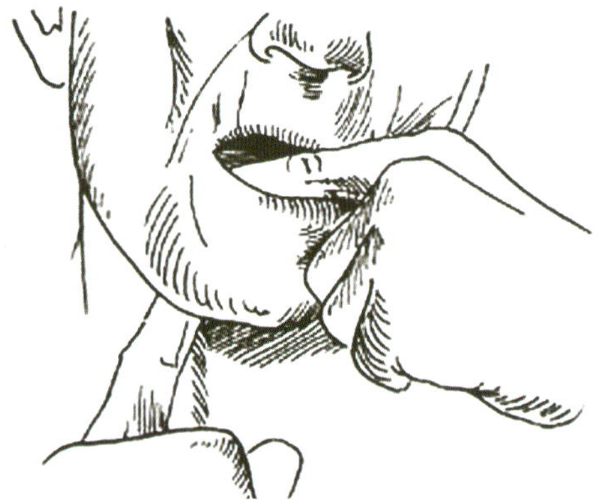

FEEL FOR... Lumps, swelling or soreness along side and far back

Fig. 10.31 Feel the floor of the mouth bimanually as well as the salivary glands. Look for changes in color and size. Look for varicosities, salivary stones and frenum pull.

Case Study 1

A Patient Scenario

An older patient came to see me in an office I worked in for someone else. I was an associate dentist. The owner of the practice wanted me to see the patient because of my experience. The patient was in her early 60's, a retired dental assistant frought with dental issues, which she was fixated on. From her dental and medical history I found out that she had fallen several years before in a dental office she had worked in and damaged her body and her teeth. The doctor she worked for restored her like a "movie star" before the fall. He had her photo of "his" smile makeover of her placed on a City magazine cover. This patient wanted to look like that again thinking that her workman's comp insurance would pay for the treatment. She presented on this visit with a fractured upper right bicuspid below the gingiva, leaving a space (Black Hole) that she could not tolerate.

Doing a full examination, which she did not want me to do, was difficult. She was a smoker, a coffee addict, an alcoholic, addicted to narcotics, a chronic pain patient and obcessed with her looking like the cover of the magazine she was on some years before. I should have stopped before I did anything because this seemed like a no-win situation, which I felt in my gut. But remembering Sir Winston's quote, I seized the moment and made her a temporary bridge to "fill the space of the fractured tooth". After that she wanted me to do all her treatment. This temporary treatment alone took over four hours, with her continued stopping to drink a large coffee she brought with her from the 7-11 store and then getting up, almost falling, due to the drugs she had previously put in her body that morning, to use the restroom at least five to six times.

I eventually did my examination and found rampant root caries, chronic geriatric periodontal disease, mobility, no posterior occlusion per se and other missing teeth. She was a disaster, to say the least. Her tissues were bright red, her teeth were mobile, brown in color on the linguals due to chronic smoking and fully caked up with calculus and plaque.

> She told me that she brushed her teeth three to four times a day, as well as had her teeth cleaned on a "regular" basis. I am just wondering what the practitioners reading this are thinking at this moment in time. Would you treat her?
>
> After months of trying to get her weaned off her *Oxycontin*®, she told me that she did not take it anymore and that she was in a program at a local hospital to learn how to stop her habits. I later found out that she was in a smoking cessation group, which did not work for her and that she switched from *Oxycontin*® to 90 mg of morphine sulfate two to three times a day. Who was she fooling?
>
> This treatment, which I diagnosed, was for upper full extractions of the teeth she had left and an implant supported denture. She did not want to wear an immediate denture after implant surgery and she refused to wear a denture over implants. I did the initial work-up and then told her that I was referring her to an oral surgeon for treatment due to the complexity of it all and that the staff I worked with in the present office were not trained enough to assist me in this endeavor, which was the truth. The owner wanted to do the restorative, after the fact, because she was motivated by the money and she wanted to keep the patient in her practice. The woman's husband was an ex-sheriff and threatened me if I did not see his wife, whom he filed for divorce from soon after this conversation with him, admonishing me that he had more than 100 guns at home (a subtle non-explanatory underhanded threat to me if I did not treat his soon-to-be ex-wife). Needless to say, there are limits to working with some patients and we need to remember that we cannot help everyone and we also have the right to dismiss patients should things not pan out. Documentation is required why we dismissed our patient from our practice, or in this case, my practice. For this particular patient, her rejecting my doing a full examination and then trying to modify what I thought was in her best interest qualified for a dismissal in my estimation. She was not happy about it, did not accept it and her husband made things even worse by threatening me into treating his soon-to-be ex-wife. A no win situation for both of us. We also need to remember to take care of ourselves first and work within the limits of what we can do, what we know and what we know about the patient adhering to our recommendations.

From the example in the Scenario, it is not enough to do a thorough examination, it is everything and thensome. Because we are not looking at just anatomy and teeth, we are learning about the person who brought them to us. We all have our stories to tell. When a patient tells me a story like the one I just recanted, it is time to listen with all my senses. I want to serve the patient in the best way I know how, but there are some things that are beyond hurting oneself for in the process. Please learn from my example. There are many more stories like this one with much older people who are very set in their ways. All we can do is document, document, document and find the best solution for that patient without compromising our values, our limits of what we can honestly do or tolerate and protecting our sense of self.

10.6 Putting It All Together: Tips and Skills

The essence of "putting things all together" is a direct one-on-one, face-to-face conversation. The recipe for success is not just the ingredients one puts into making the treatment "tasty", but also adding in a little "extra" something to ensure that the final product is edible and digestible as well. What we should be aware of in this process:

- Have all your information in hand and reviewed prior to the patient being there.
- Familiarize yourself with the historical information as well as the clinical aspects of what the patient brought with them and your intended recommendation for treatment. Review your treatment notes and plan(s), including alternate treatment recommendations. Try to have a timed agenda for your treatment planning consultation and tell the patient and guests what it is. (I allot at least 1-2 hours for the session, depending upon the complexity of the case.)
- Do not assume anything.
- Be prepared for a two-way, or more, simultaneous transmission of thoughts, information and feelings in communicating with the older person, who may bring his/her caregiver(s) or possibly

his/her immediate family members, one of whom holds the Power of Attorney.

- Have enough space, good lighting, organized clinical materials, such as mounted study models, a wax-up of the reconstruction you intend to recommend using a dark inlay wax so the patient can see it in contrast to white plaster or yellow stone models, radiographs, charts, commercial study models illustrating disease and restorative issues. A notepad for each participant and pen or pencil for taking notes or writing down questions to ask. (I like to use a white board to draw examples of my treatment plan and then photograph it for the records.)
- Make sure to greet the patient yourself in the reception room and walk with them to your private consultation room. Make sure the space has adequate room for wheelchair, walker and other assisted aids access which the patient may bring with them. Ask if they would like a glass of water or if they need to use the restroom first. Sit at the same level so you both can see eye to eye. Kindness and thoughtfulness will get you a long way and is a major ingredient in your recipe for success. I call it mutual respect.
- Have a dedicated staff person in the room with you before you start to discuss the case presentation and the projected treatment recommendations. This person needs to be knowledgeable about dental treatment and able to take copious notes from each party and what was discussed as well as the questions that were asked.
- Determine if the patient is visually oriented, kinesthetically oriented or acoustically oriented before this meeting. That way you can be prepared for how you need to illustrate your findings and recommendations to the patient.
- Stay positive even in the face of adversity.
- Stop after each discussion point and ask if the patient and accompanying guests understand what is being said and if they have questions at that juncture. Have them repeat what they heard as active listening verifies their ability to hear, absorb, learn and understand.
- Make copies of the treatment plan(s) for the patient and his/her guardian. Give them an informed consent to sign for all intended procedures to return at their convenience prior to treatment should they elect to do anything.

For the dental practitioner, the entire scenario of doing the examination, the clinical work-up, the treatment plan(s) and addressing what the patient brings with him/her is akin to problem solving or a major component of clinical diagnosis and treatment planning of the geriatric patient.[4]

There is a specific knowledge base that one needs to master before such action occurs, like performing a geriatric evaluation and treatment plan for presentation, that allows the practitioner to understand the issues at hand that does not fully depend on developing new technical skills but rather specific information that gives insight into working with this cohort of people. These may be as follows:

1. An understanding of the "normal" aging process.
2. An understanding of pathological or abnormal aging.
3. An understanding of the medical issues brought with a geriatric patient that can and do affect the proposed treatment with respect to these medical conditions.
4. A knowledge of the pharmacology commonly used with geriatric patients and the possibility of the presence of a drug-induced dental disease or aberrant medical issue.
5. Essential interpersonal skills needed to communicate with the patient, their family members and other healthcare providers regarding the specific older patient.
6. Having the ability to know and use specific communication techniques required in working with older individuals who have sensory deficits, physical abnormalities and frailness and those that suffer from cognitive decline. These being in tune with the disabilities of the patient, the inability of the patient to understand and the practitioners own inability to express what needs to be conveyed as well as being able to actively listen to what the older patient is saying both in words, actions and tone of voice.
7. Having the experience in the practical aspects of clinical decision-making and the ability to relay these decisions on treatment in an understandable and acceptable way with respect to the

issues the older patient brings with them to your discussions and subsequent treatment sessions. In addition to having the knowledge, being able to relay this information in a simple and direct manner to both the patient and their family.

8. Having the ability to make the projected dental treatment comfortable, expedient, pain-free, workable, successful and acceptable for the older compromised patient and a positive experience overall for both the patient and the dental staff.

All these listed steps lead to mutual understanding and acceptance of facts, but not necessarily the treatment at hand. The specifics of treatment need to be verified by acknowledgment from the patient, their caregiver and family members, especially, the person with the power of attorney in order to proceed in good order. The practitioner must also acknowledge his/her willingness to do the treatment and not rationalize that he or she can do it when they do not have all the skill sets to make treatment successful. Honesty is the best policy at this juncture.

According to high-powered business executives, "Successful negotiation is not about getting to 'Yes'; it is about mastering 'No' and understanding what the path to an agreement is...".

When an older, self-indulgent, depressed, opinionated person makes a remark like, "I can't afford it", or says nothing at all, one must wait in silence and look at him or her with intent and respect. The person who waits in silence the longest is said to be the one who comes out on top. Manipulation is fair game for older people because for them, it may be habit from doing it for so long and getting away with it, or it may be a fun game for them! We need to either accept this or move on eventually to another patient, until this one has a conference with the family, or not, and the family makes the decision for the patient. In essence, we have done our job, if we follow the ideal treatment conference regimen and present the information in an educated, open, honest and understandable fashion.

Shay has suggested in the literature a systematic approach to planning oral care for the older adult, which he called "OSCAR" (Table 10.1), to be used to determine the needs of a specific patient.[4,5] He believed practitioners could utilize OSCAR as a way of fully understanding all the factors that could impact an older adult's eventual treatment process. This method can be used for those dental practitioners who are just beginning to adventure into treating the older adult, who in turn, may have a gamut of medical issues to consider as well and lots of questions.

Berkey *et al.*[6] proposed a different model based upon four domains of dental need as follows (Table 10.2).

Looking at the alternatives in Tables 10.1 and 10.2 and the questions asked and answered as previously mentioned, one can determine the patients' needs based upon the weight these all carry with respect to treatment needs and again, gain insight from the Five Levels of Care extrapolated by Berkey *et al.*[6] into a rational model of care with respect to the challenges the patient brings with them for treatment (Table 10.3).

Table 10.1 OSCAR – A geriatric dental assessment

O	Oral	Evaluates teeth, restorative treatment, periodontium, status of pulp, oral mucosa, occlusion and saliva.
S	Systemic	Evaluates normal age changes, medical diagnosis, drugs and interdisciplinary communications.
C	Capability	Evaluates functional ability: self-care, oral hygiene, caregivers, needs for transportation and mobility.
A	Autonomy	Evaluates ability to give informed consent or dependence on others.
R	Reality	Evaluates prioritization of oral health care, financial limitations, and anticipated life-span.

Table 10.2 The four domains of dental need

A	Function	Relates to the ability to chew and eat an adequate diet.
B	Sympto-matology	Relates to comfort while chewing and being free of pain, adequate saliva to speak, taste, swallow, etc.
C	Pathology	Relates to not having any oral discomfort or lesions in the mouth.
D	Aesthetic	Relates to perceived needs to improve their appearance or smile.

Table 10.3 The five levels of care

1	Very extensive care with complex needs, including rehabilitation of the dentition with fixed prosthodontics and the ability to accept this care.
2	Extensive care, which may be solved by a combination of fixed and removable prosthodontics and the ability to withstand the care.
3	Intermediate care, which requires some alternatives to traditional therapies.
4	Limited care: these patients cannot tolerate extensive time in the dental chair and need short appointments and a simplified treatment plan.
5	Very limited care: these patients should be treated for pain relief and infection control only.

To achieve the goals in Tables 10.1, 10.2, 10.3, the authors[4-6] suggested a series of questions that should be asked, possibly at the treatment conference. These need to be answered prior to treatment itself. They are:

1. The patient's desires and expectations.
2. The type and severity of dental need.
3. The impact on quality of life.
4. The probability of positive outcomes.
5. Reasonable treatment alternatives
6. The ability to tolerate the stress of treatment.
7. The capability to maintain oral health.
8. Financial and other resources.
9. The dentist's capabilities.
10. Other issues may be personal, familial or social in nature.

I find these 10 questions very germane and a good set of guidelines to go by when working up a treatment plan for an older patient. These can assist you in making the decisions you need to make about whether you can restore or want to restore anything for the specific older patient who brings you a myriad of medical and dental issues that they want you to solve for them.

Discussions of treatment planning, by necessity, cannot be complete without rigorously evaluating the role of evidence-based dental care and geriatric minimal intervention. Today, Minimally Invasive Dentistry (MID) is the Standard of Care, especially if one is a conscientious practitioner. Again, I have mentioned the "KISS" method of treatment when it comes to geriatric dentistry and that is "Keep It Simple Stupid". One can do marvelous treatment with advanced techniques, but at the same time keeping it simple for the sake of the older, more compromised individual. With the technology we have today in Dentistry, it is possible to do this kind of treatment with success and longevity.

A modified model of decision-making for older adults developed by Ettinger and Beck[7] elucidates a simple equation for analyzing the input gained through the patients own traits, wants, desires, physical and mental abilities and the restrictions inherent in their medical conditions and ability to treat them by the practitioner (Fig. 10.32).

Even in the face of all these decision-making algorithms to organize one's thought processes in dealing with the complexities of working with an older, compromised patient, does it say that the practitioner **must** treat them. There have been many times for myself when I was confronted with a dilemma to treat or not to treat an older individual. When I realized that certain older adults were inflexible in their thinking about dental disease and only wanted a "patch job" for something that was infected, causing them pain and suffering, that I might have said this is not for me to treat. We all have our ideals and our treatment ethics. Our oath states, "Do No Harm". Deciding to treat someone with multiple issues and advanced medical conditions on many medications, and whose life may be shortened by leaving something alone or "patched" when it should be treated, is a difficult enough of a situation to want to treat them, but not at the expense of harming them by doing a treatment that does not really help them in the long run. And I know that they will continue with the same symptoms, or worse when they see the next dental practitioner, perhaps complaining about me. So, we must be clear and honest at the onset about our own sense of ethics and experience levels. I have learned not to compromise my sense of integrity and professionalism in my almost 50 years of practice. If I need to refer to a physician or dental specialist, who can validate my concerns and the patient wants to come back and let me do what I suggested in the first place, I will accept them for treatment with a specific informed consent. However, one may never

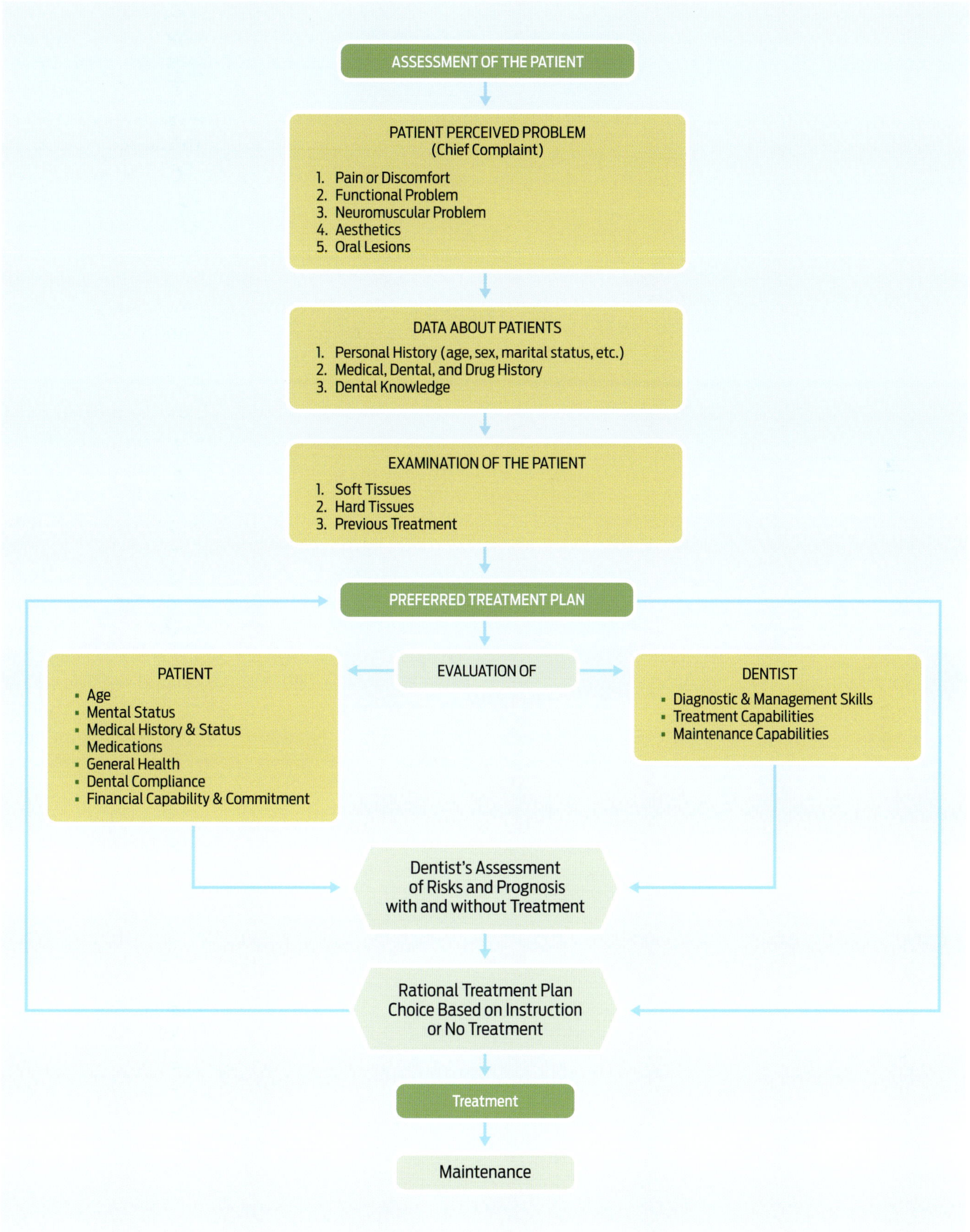

Fig. 10.32 Model of decision-making for older adults. (Modified by Dr. Eric Z. Shapira from Ettinger and Beck.)[7]

know what that dismissed patient will do if they do not call your office again for care. To say the least, it is emotionally painful for me to see this happen.

"I never give advice to patients, I give information-straight and simple. No one wants advice and even if they pay for it, they may never take you up on what you have charged them for. Information about oneself (the patient) is the best medicine. I charge for this too. However, we cannot force people, especially older more infirm people, to swallow it. All we can do is hold our hand out to them and offer them a way to ease their pain and suffering. The ultimate choice is theirs and we cannot make that for them, only guide them in the right direction."

Dr. Eric Zane Shapira

The Rational Evaluation of Patients[7] in Figure 10.32 is a simple, visual aid as a series of steppingstones across a creek. One foot in front of the other and a visual ladder leads the practitioner into a series of self-directed questions and issues as to which is the right way to move in order to get to the other side. Inputting all the collected information one has about the patient will assist us in gaining both confidence and results in the long run. Keeping the wants and desires of the patient at the forefront of the adventure, with both their goals and yours, incorporating the medical and dental challenges and integrating your proposed treatment plan to solve any issues, and moving along this ladder with confidence in setting up a treatment regimen for the patient can and will be an organized, systematic road map of successful events.

Never stop asking yourself questions about what you are doing, what you must consider, what you must incorporate and what changes should be made, if any. Include these same aspects of treatment questions from the patient as well. For it is the patient that we serve, and we must be aware that this is not a "one-man, one-sided journey".

The most important tip I can give anyone working with the older patient is to **be prepared**. Have all your information at your fingertips, know where you are headed, have a clear vision in your mind for each treatment plan you may speak about and make sure the recipients of your discussion are comfortable, able to hear, see, respond and understand what it is you are trying to convey. Sometimes, even with our best intentions put forth, we may not be successful. But if you are honest and open in a tone of voice that is caring and not cajoling, a body language that is open and not defensive or closed and eye contact that is direct and not askew, we may find success in all that we do. Make sure you ask questions and wait for the answers. If there are no answers forthcoming, then ask if there is an issue around what it is you stated. Many times, one may find that the recipients did not hear you, nor did they understand what you may have told them because your jargon was too scientific or "dentally specific" for them to understand. Keep things simple and direct on a level your patient can respectfully understand and respond. Always show respect and check-in periodically to make sure they are still with you or have questions. **Mutual respect allows others to have thoughts, information and feelings that are different than your own.** Never lose sight of this when working with older individuals and their representatives. This is the recipe for success, and it will work with most all age groups, but especially with our older patients.

"Remember, nothing is written in stone... Change is constant, and things are constantly changing. Live in the moment. Love yourself, be happy with what you have and the gifts you can give to others through your care and teachings, as well as by keeping an open mind. Learn to adapt. Keep on learning daily as no one can take your knowledge away, except 'Father Time.' These are the ingredients of a perfect recipe for success in all that you aspire to accomplish."

Dr. Eric Zane Shapira

References

1. Reed KL. *Basic management of medical emergencies: recognizing a patient's distress.* J Am Dent Assoc. 2010 May;141 Suppl 1:20S-4S.
2. Norris LH. *Early recognition limits in in-office emergencies.* J Mass Dent Soc. 1994 Summer;43(3):19-23.
3. Ramanayake RP, Ranasingha S, Lakmini S. *Management of emergencies in general practice: role of general practitioners.* J Family Med Prim Care. 2014 Oct-Dec;3(4):305-8.
4. Ettinger RL. *Treatment planning concepts for the ageing patient.* Aust Dent J. 2015 Mar;60 Suppl 1:71-85.
5. Shay K. *Identifying the needs of the elderly dental patient. The geriatric dental assessment.* Dent Clin North Am. 1994 Jul;38(3):499-523.
6. Berkey DB, Berg RG, Ettinger RL, Mersel A, Mann J. *The old-old dental patient: the challenge of clinical decision-making.* J Am Dent Assoc. 1996 Mar;127(3):321-32.
7. Ettinger RL, Beck JD, Martin WE. *Clinical decision making in evaluating patients: a process study.* Spec Care Dentist. 1990 May-Jun;10(3):78-83.

EPILOG

Caring for an Aging Nation

"In the end, it's not the years in your life that count. It's the life in your years."
Abraham Lincoln,
16th President of the United States of America

Geriatric dentistry is at the heart of dentistry itself. It is a subspecialty of Dentistry at present, rather than a stand-alone specialty in Dentistry, yet it stands in all its glory providing special and unique information, clinical excellence, new horizons, and vistas on modern treatment for older and more compromised adults and the people it serves. The number of Americans alone, 65 years and older, is expected to nearly double in the next 40 years. According to the U.S. Census Bureau, it has estimated that at least 10,000 people a day pass their 65th birthday and that more than 94.6 million people will be 65 or older in 2069! This is a staggering number and more than outweighs the number of younger persons within that same time segment due to decreased birth rates. In the same vein, the percentage of older adults aged 85 and over needing personal care was more than twice the percentage for adults ages 75-84 and five times the percentage for adults ages 65-74 within the last several years.

Considering this information, geriatric dentistry will play a significant role in "Engaging our Aging Population" in the future. But the "future" is already here in tomorrow and the tomorrow after that. Our population will demand that dental practitioners see the older, compromised individual as a "special" patient with special needs, in some cases, and place them on a pedestal as an example of living a long life through their successes and losses, through illness and injury, through rough times and joyful times and maintaining their vigil of keeping their oral and physical health in check, which will stand them as a beacon of light to follow and to guide those cohorts of theirs meandering in the fog of dismay without proper care, to a dental health system that will treat them in good faith and fashion.

In my many years of treating the older patient and teaching geriatric dentistry to both dental students, hygienists, and practitioners alike, I have learned much more from my older patients, than I could have ever taught them about themselves or me, considering their medical and dental health. Through their life stories, I have learned to appreciate my own life, the people around me and my own family and their values. As time goes by, the elders in my family have slowly left our World for some other place, some with a full complement of teeth in good condition, leaving me, as a metamorphic youth turning grey in the fall wind, to take their place in line, in the breezes of time.

The human being moves through phases of medical and dental care with respect to their age and living life. Many things are based on age in our society, but the mind can stay youthful forever, hopefully, if we nurture it, feed it, use it regularly and are lucky enough to enjoy the time we have left to do what we will. Our societies values, our values, methods of primary care including dentistry, will change in the future with each passing day; as change is constant, as is time. It does not stop for us in this life, so we must make the best use of it with every moment we have and with every fiber of our bodies and minds.

My wish is that I can live long enough to continue teaching my students, my patients, my family and friends, whoever they may be, as well as continuing to be creative in this venture. Discovering new ways to provide care for the older population and new methods of treating patients, utilizing new inventions and things that we have not even realized yet, would be a good goal for me to investigate.

Sketch of a Robotic Assistant

I once wrote an article, over 30 years ago, about the future of dentistry visualizing robots as assistants in dental offices and clinics. We now live in a robotic world. There is AI (Artificial Intelligence), whose information is employed by robots to perform operations in medicine and dentistry. "Robotic AI" machines that now place implants in the mouth, guided and supervised by the dental practitioner and supervised by their staff, are already being used in practice. The unthinkable is and has been here all along. There are massive computers used for medical purposes whereby one can feed it information on a specific disease or person who has this disease, and it can analyze the genetic structure of each entity and spew out a formula to treat that person in the best possible way, with the most prudent method to cure the disease and the analysis of the medicine used to combat the disease. It is beyond one's imagination as to what comes next. Maybe we should ask "Watson", the know-it-all medical giant AI computer, that may already have the answer in predicting the future to the "T."

We will be living longer as a Nation and as a World population. It is important that we acknowledge that all people should live in peace and harmony and that we all have the same basic needs, one of which is good oral health. Oral health with respect to oral disease stands as a pandemic around the world, especially in less fortunate areas where people live in poverty; however, with our assistance and our knowledge we can share helpful information about disease, effective treatment and good care with others for the benefit of all Mankind, especially the aging population.

Dentistry for the older population will be in the forefront of treatment needs in the future, once practitioners and the public understand the need for such a commodity. The practitioners that are in their youth and prime now will be part of the older segment of society in the future. Growing old with one's patients is a wonderful thing. Teaching and learning from each other along the way will help to improve the way we function in a doctor-patient relationship. This is the one thing that I tried to impress upon practitioners in this textbook. How to relate to our patients and how to allow them to be on an equal plane with us as people assisting people in the context of having dentistry done, to not only enhance their function and esthetics, but longevity. Throughout time into the 21st Century, our longevity has improved across the world. I attribute this, in part, not only to good medicine, but to even better health practice and the sharing of important advancements in clinical care, especially that of oral care.

The mouth is a nidus for disease and, as we are still learning today, oral diseases, specifically periodontal disease and tooth decay, can be the focus of systemic disease. This systemic disease can become our demise causing death from various cancers, starvation, suicide, intolerable pain, infection and more. It behooves all dental practitioners to take care of themselves as a living example for our aging patients and teach them your "secrets" about how you do it. Share your knowledge, give your gifts away. I always advocate that "we don't know what gifts we have until we give them away". Yet, we do not really think about that. It is rote for us as practitioners to tell someone that they need to improve their care, without first telling them what you do, how you do it and how you desire to stay healthy so that you will be around to assist them with their dental needs as you age together.

I have given several lectures on the "Geriatric Patient and the Aging Dentist". In these lectures I discuss how we are all susceptible to the changes of aging with the loss of our eyesight, our hearing, our dexterity, our ability to think properly, memory loss, generalized weakness and more. We are all of *Homo Sapiens* material, we are Human, making us vulnerable and fragile in the scheme of things. However, we can defend ourselves with the shield of knowledge by preparing for being one of those aging persons who are engaged in both medical and dental knowledge and self-care, which in turn, will help us live a longer, happier, and a more productive lives. It is our sworn duty as dental practitioners to teach our patients, not just treat them without discussion of the importance of "why" we are doing something to assist them in some way.

> *"The main object of teaching is not to give explanation, but to knock at the doors of the mind."*
>
> *Rabindranath Tagore, Philosopher*

To open one's mind to new ideas, new methods of care, to living a longer, healthier life is to engage life itself. Each of us has a duty to open the minds of our patients to helping themselves, but not before we help ourselves understand why this is so important. It is not for us to be concerned about making mistakes along the path we have chosen in Dentistry. I tell my students that "There are no mistakes in life, only experience: good judgment comes from experience and experience comes from 'bad' judgment". This is how we learn. Embrace your relationships with your older patients and friends and learn from them. In the long run you will be a much better practitioner and healer.

Geriatric dentistry is here to stay. I am sure that one day soon, the future will bring it forth as its own specialty in dentistry. I hope I am here to see it and part of the change-makers involved. And I hope that those reading this textbook have found it a learning experience and a helpful guide into improving your practices and enhancing your level of geriatric care and treatment. I have tried to give you a "feel" for some of the experiences I have had, both good and bad, successful, and not, as well as a taste of what it is like to treat this cohort of the population in a "Humanistic" way. I am hopeful that you will have taken away something useful, as well as found this text most beneficial for you personally in validating what you already know and do in your practices. May your staff and your patients be enlightened as well in the same or similar vein.

I wish you all the best in your future endeavors...

> *"Don't cry because it's over, smile because it happened."*
>
> *Dr. Seuss*

> *Carpe Diem....*
> *"Seize the Day" and enjoy it!*
>
> *Dr. Eric Zane Shapira*

Appendix

Sample Consent Forms

SAMPLE CONSENT FORM

Patient Name: Date:

Treatment recommendations:

The benefit of recommended treatment:

Risks and possible complications:

Approximate duration of treatment phases:

Estimated cost of treatment:

Alternate treatment recommendations:

Risks and possible complications (of alternative treatment):

(Patient Name) I have reviewed and discussed the recommended treatments and alternative treatment recommendations with Dr. ____________________. I understand that no dental treatment is risk free, the risks have been explained to me and that the dentist will take reasonable steps to limit any complications. Dr. [____________________] has answered my questions about my treatment.

I have provided an accurate and complete medical history including medications I am taking and any known allergies.

I wish to proceed with the treatment recommendations.

Signed Patient Date

Signed Dentist

Signed Witness

Fig. 1 Dental Consent Form from the American Dental Association.

DENTAL PATIENT CONSENT FORM

This information is provided to help you understand the treatment I am recommending for you. Before I begin treatment, I want to be certain that I have provided you with enough information in a way you can understand, so that you're well informed and confident that you wish to proceed. This form will provide some of the information. I will also have a discussion with you.

PLEASE BE SURE TO ASK ANY QUESTIONS YOU WISH!

It's better to ask them now than wonder about it after we start the treatment.
Nature of the Recommended Treatment:

____

____

I am recommending the following treatment(s) for you:

____

____

I base this recommendation on the visual examination(s) I have performed, on any X-rays, models, photos and other diagnostic tests I have taken, and on my knowledge of your medical and dental history. I have also taken into consideration any information you have given me about your needs and wants. The treatment is necessary because:

____

____

Fig. 2 Involved Consent Form. (*From MedPro Group Inc.*)

The benefits of this treatment are:

____

____

The prognosis, or chance of success, of the treatment is:

____

____

I expect that it will take approximately ____________________ to complete the treatment, but it could be shorter or longer based on what we experience as the treatment progresses.

I expect it to cost about $ ____________________ and I will let you know as soon as possible if the cost estimate increases or if it can be reduced.

ALTERNATIVE TREATMENTS

There are many ways to treat dental problems. I have chosen the one that I think best suits your needs. However, them are other ways that your condition can be treated, including:

____

____

Fig. 2 *(continued)*

(continued)

If you have any questions about these alternatives, or about any other treatments you have heard or thought about, please ask.

RISKS OF THE RECOMMENDED TREATMENT

No dental treatment is completely risk free. I will take reasonable steps to limit any complications of the treatment I have recommended. However, there are some complications that tend to occur with some regularity.

These include:

____

____

If you have any questions about these complications, or about any other complications you have heard or thought about, please ask. I believe that the treatment will be most successful when you understand as much as possible about it, because you will be able to provide more information to me and to ask better questions. No question is too simple to ask, and I have as much time to answer them as you need. When you feel you can make on educated decision about this recommendation, then we can get started with treatment.

ACKNOWLEDGMENT

I, ____________________ , have received information about the proposed treatment.

Fig. 2 *(continued)*

I have discussed my treatment with the undersigned Treating Dentist and have been given an opportunity to ask questions and have them fully answered. I understand the nature of the recommended treatment, alternate treatment options, and the risks of the recommended treatment and hold the Treating Dentist, and any of his/her associates, harmless of any wrongdoing in connection with the treatment. Provided that any complications did not arise due to negligence.

Furthermore, I wish to proceed with the recommend treatment.

Patient or Guardian

Signature: ____________________

Date: ____________________

Treating Dentist

Signature: ____________________

Date: ____________________

Witness

Signature: ____________________

Date: ____________________

Fig. 3 Advanced Consent Form. (*From MedPro Group Inc.*)

Treatment Planning Forms

Last Name First Name

Address

Phone# DOB

1	2	3	4	5	6	7	8	9	10	11	12	13	14	15	16

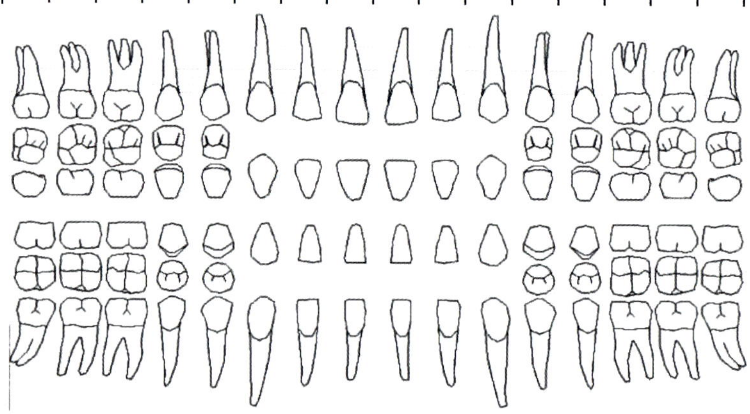

32	31	30	29	28	27	26	25	24	23	22	21	20	19	18	17

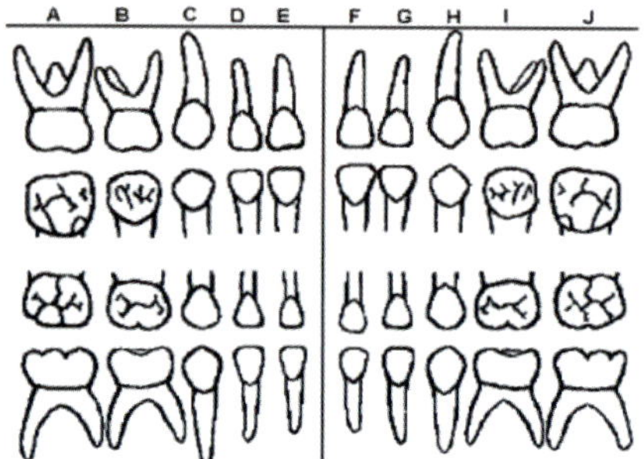

Medical alerts

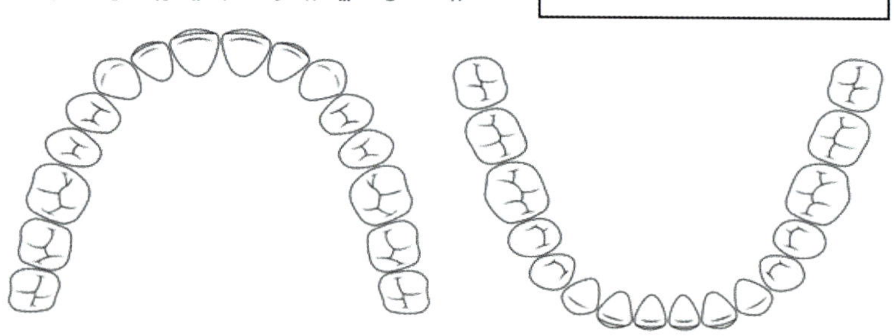

Remarks

MOULD

TEETH	Upper	Lower
Centrals		
Laterals		
Cuspids		
Posteriors		

SHADE

TEETH	Upper	Lower
Centrals		
Laterals		
Cuspids		
Posteriors		

DENTAL HISTORY

Chief Complaint

Date of last Visit

X-Rays Prophy

Face/Neck/Glands

Lips/Cheeks

Palate/Pharynx

Floor of mouth/Tongue/Frenum

General Condition of Teeth

Esthetics

Sensitivity Cold Hot Sweets

Abrasion Areas

General Condition of Restorations

Overhangs

Open Contacts

Food Traps

Occlusion/Interferences

Previous Orthodontics

General Periodontal Health

Previous Periodontal Treatment

Plaque	1	2	3	4
Inflammation	1	2	3	4
Calculus	1	2	3	4
Stain	1	2	3	4
Oral Hygiene	1	2	3	4

Summary of treatment

Fig. 4 A treatment plan form, useable for an outline of a treatment proposal.

ERIC ZANE SHAPIRA M.S. D.D.S.

HEAD AND NECK SCREENING EXAM

NAME DATE BLOOD PRESSURE UPDATE

Facial Symmetry WNL
Nose Chin Jaw

Eyes WNL Color Perla Yes/No
Pterygiums Right/Left Arcus Right/Left
Astigmatism Right/Left Pigment Right _____ Left _____

Skin WNL Pierced ears Right #____ Left #____
Freckles Yes/No
Dry Oily

Lymph Nodes WNL
Submandibular Pre & Post Auricular
Supraficialcervical Sub-Occipital
Cervical Buccal
Bi-lat moveable palpable firm soft

Thyriod Glands WNL

Lips WNL
Fordyce Granules upper/lower
Scars ___________ upper/lower, right/mid/left
Chapped yes/no
Abrasion lower/upper

Frenum Attachment
Max High Low Short Double Mand

Mucosa WNL
Linea Alba (check bite line) RT/L
Hyperkeratotic RT/L

Tongue WNL Coating yes/no Wide/Narrow
Tongue-tied yes/no
Papillae WNL
Sublingual Vericosities yes/no
Scalloped / fissured / geographic

Tonsils Yes/No Anterior/Posterior Uvala WNL

Palate
high wide narrow shallow normal
Middle Torus yes/no Boney Suture line yes/no

Floor of Mouth WNL Mandibular Tori right/left
Narrow/Wide Shallow/Deep

Salivary Glands WNL Saliva Viscous/Serous
Xerostomia/Siallorhea Sublingual WNL
Cheek WNL Submandibular WNL

Gingivae WNL grafts present yes/no #____________________
pigment recession - gen / localized
Stippling Color Shape

Missing Teeth Nos.

Removable Dental Appliances
Maxillary
Mandibular
Other

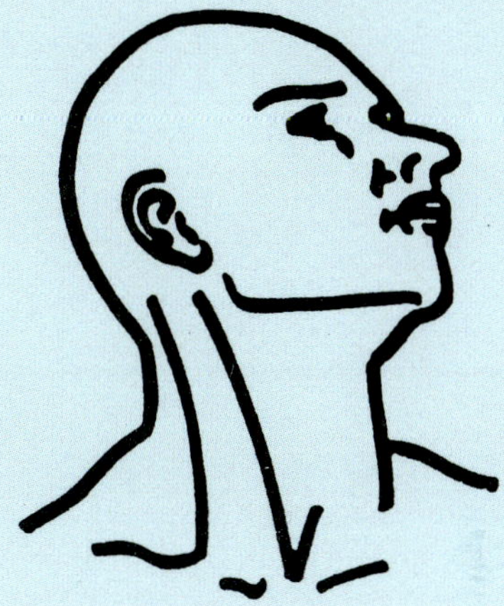

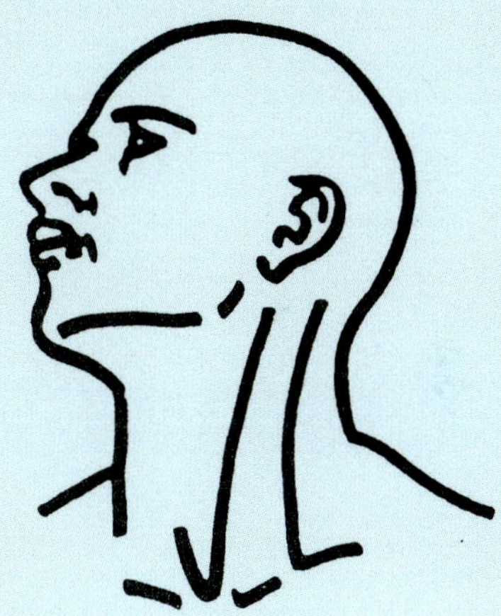

WNL - WITHIN NORMAL LIMITS
F - FLAT
R - RAISED
NP - NON-PIGMENTED
PN - PIGMENTED NEVUS
K - KERATOSIS
S - SCAR
SK - SEBACEOUS KERATOSIS
V - VESSEL
RT - RIGHT
L - LEFT
MUC - MUCOSA
VB - VERMILLION BORDER

Fig. 5 Head and Neck Screening Examination Sheet. (©Dr. Eric Z. Shapira)

ERIC ZANE SHAPIRA, M.S., D.D.S. **REFERRAL**

TO:

PATIENT'S NAME ________________________________ AGE ________

ADDRESS ________________ HOME PHONE ________________ WORK PHONE ________________

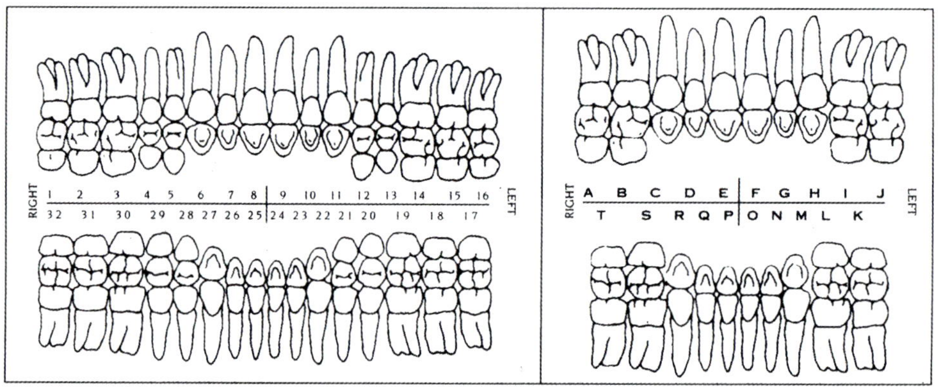

Chief complaint ________________________________

Previous Treatment and Medical History Considerations ________________________________

History of Present Condition ________________________________

Prognosis / Plan ________________________________

Evaluation / Comments ________________________________

Radiographs ARE / ARE NOT Available
- ☐ Sent with Patient
  (Please return to our office after treatment)

Plaque Control
- ☐ Excellent
- ☐ Good
- ☐ Fair
- ☐ Poor

Perio Chart ☐ enclosed ☐ mailed

Perio Recall _____ mos.

Periodontal Classification I II III IV
- ☐ Active
- ☐ Deteriorating
- ☐ Stable
- ☐ Improving

Home Care Routine
- ☐ Brush ☐ Floss ☐ Proxybrush
- ☐ Stimulator ☐ Flouride
- ☐ Electric T.B. ☐ 2-row T.B.
- ☐ Irrigation ☐ End tuft T.B.
- ☐ Rubber Tip ☐ Other

SIGNATURE OF REFERRING DOCTOR .... DATE ....

Fig. 6 Personal Referral Form. (©Dr. Eric Z. Shapira)

TEMPROMANDIBULAR JOINT & OCCLUSAL EVALUATION

(All measurements in millimeters)

Mandibular Range of Motion (limitation of opening)

- **0** - none
- **1** - slight (30-40)
- **2** - moderate (20-30)
- **3** - mod.-sev. (10-20)
- **4** - severe (0-10)
- **5** - joint laxity

Discomfort in R O M : Class

- **0** - no discomfort
- **1** - slight (pain at maximum opening only)
- **2** - Mod.(pain in last 1/2 of opening)
- **3** - mod.-sev. (pain in full R O M)
- **4** - pain prevents opening

R **0 1 2 3 4** L **0 1 2 3 4**

Deviation of opening R__ L__
Midline Deviation R__ L__
A. Disk(s) can be captured R__ L__
Loose Ligaments (excessive opening) R__ L__

Joint Sounds (Description of sounds)

- **1** - click
- **2** - crepitation R **1 2 3** L **1 2 3**
- **3** - rubbing

Timing: Opening R L Late/Early
Closing R L Late/Early

Loudness:

- **0** - no sound
- **1** - palpable
- **2** - audible w/ stethoscope
- **3** - audible
- **4** - loud
- **5** - reducible
- **6** - non reucible

R **0 1 2 3 4 5 6** L **0 1 2 3 4 5 6**

Previous Locking Open/Closed

JOINT & MUSCLE PALPATATION

- **1** - Awareness
- **2** - Discomfort
- **3** - Pain (pt. flinches and pulls away)
- **4** - Can't palpate
- **5** - Enlarged External

External

Masseter	-Superficial	R___ L___
	-Deep	R___ L___
Temporalis	-ant	R___ L___
	-mid	R___ L___
	-post	R___ L___
Sterno-Cl-Mast		R___ L___
Post. Cervicals		R___ L___
Trapezlus		R___ L___
Splenius Capitus		R___ L___
Semispinalis Capitus		R___ L___
Vertex		R___ L___

Internal

Medial Pterygoid	R___ L___
Lateral Pterygoid	R___ L___
Digastric	R___ L___
Anterior	R___ L___
Posterior	R___ L___
Mylohyoid	R___ L___
Infrhyoids	R___ L___

ALIGNMENT

Midline ________ mm
Overjet ________ mm
Overbite ________ mm
X-bite #_____ Shift Shift
Protrusive ________ mm Right _____ Left _____

Occlusion (class)
Right ______ Left ______

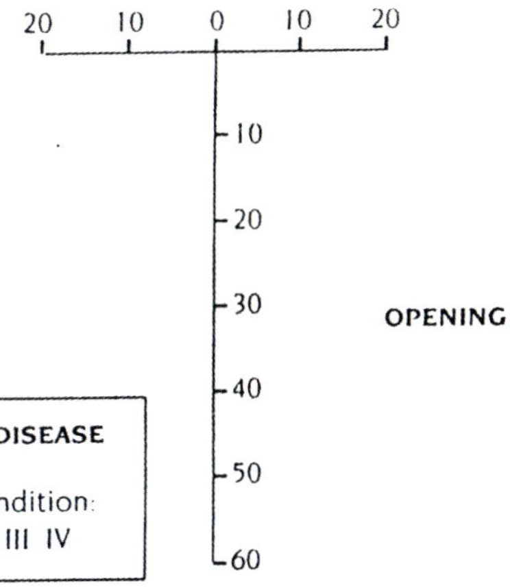

OCCLUSAL DISEASE

General condition:
Type I II III IV

MANDIBULAR MOVEMENT

Protrusive	1	2	3	4	5	6	7	8	9	10	11	12	13	14	15	16
	32	31	30	29	28	27	26	25	24	23	22	21	20	19	18	17
L.Lateral	1	2	3	4	5	6	7	8	9	10	11	12	13	14	15	16
	32	31	30	29	28	27	26	25	24	23	22	21	20	19	18	17
R.Lateral	1	2	3	4	5	6	7	8	9	10	11	12	13	14	15	16
	32	31	30	29	28	27	26	25	24	23	22	21	20	19	18	17

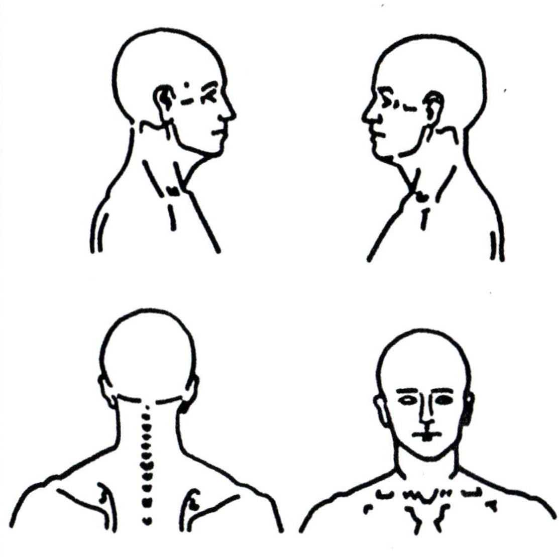

SHAPIRA PAPERS

Fig. 7 Temporomandibular Joint Screening Form. (©Dr. Eric Z. Shapira)

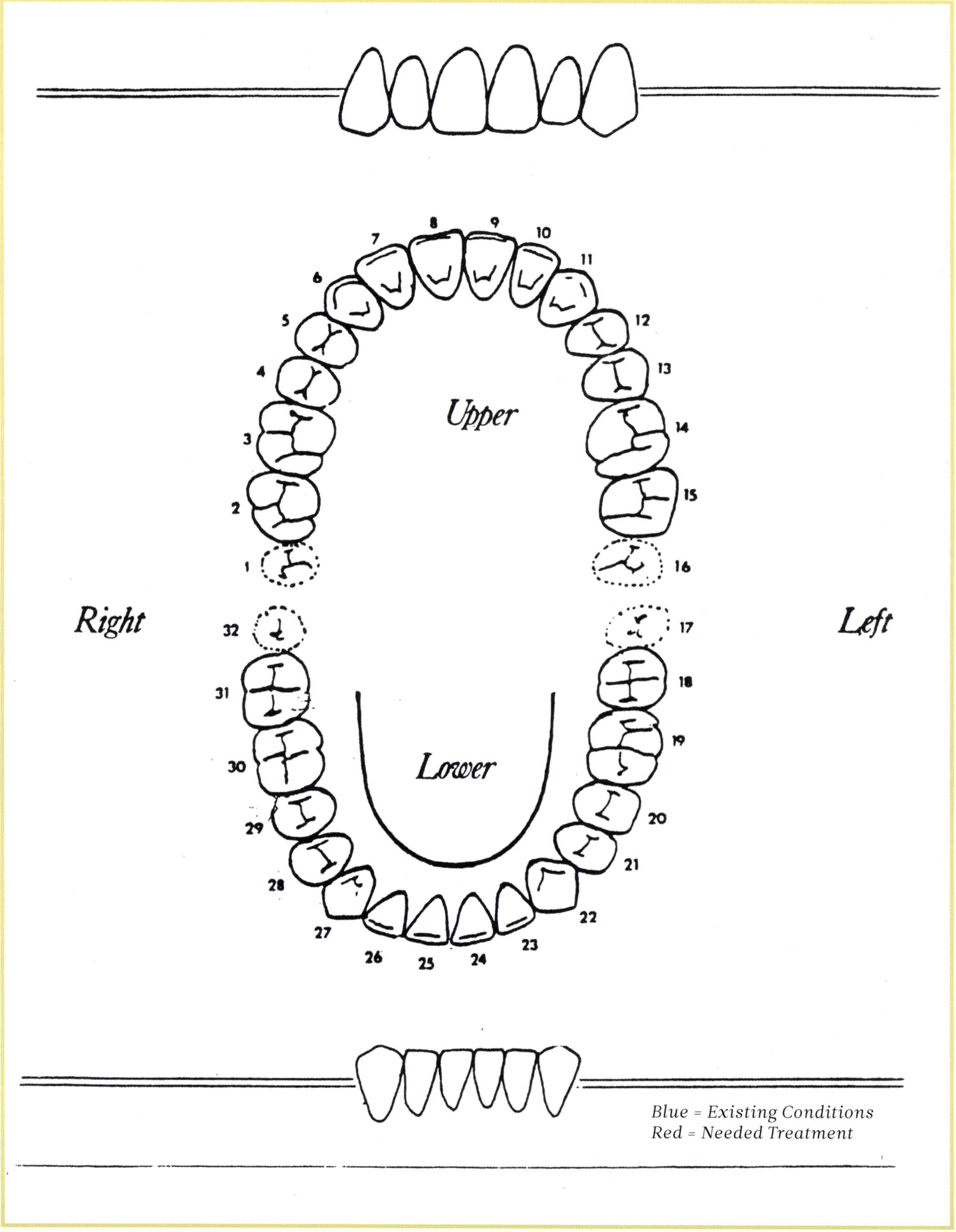

Fig. 8 Abbreviated chart for quick recall charting of existing and needed treatment. (From the practice of Dr. Eric Z. Shapira)

TMJ HISTORY

Yes No

- ☐ ☐ Do you clench or grind your teeth?
- ☐ ☐ Do you have pain or clicking upon opening or closing your mouth?
- ☐ ☐ Have you had a severe head or face injury?
- ☐ ☐ Do you suffer from frequent sore neck or headaches?
- ☐ ☐ Is there any difficulty in chewing or swallowing food?
- ☐ ☐ Have you ever worn an occlusal splint, night guard or bite plane?
- ☐ ☐ Have you had your bite adjusted?
- ☐ ☐ Is there restricted jaw motion?
- ☐ ☐ Is the restricted motion worse in the moming?
- ☐ ☐ Is the restricted motion worse in the evening?
- ☐ ☐ Do you have a clicking or popping noise in the right joint?
  How long ______
- ☐ ☐ Do you have pain in the right joint?
  How long ______
- ☐ ☐ Do you have a clicking or popping noise in the left joint?
  How long ______
- ☐ ☐ Do you have pain in the left joint?
  How long ______
- ☐ ☐ Does the pain come and go?
- ☐ ☐ Is the pain always present?
- ☐ ☐ ... upon awakening?
- ☐ ☐ ... when eating?
- ☐ ☐ ... when yawning?
- ☐ ☐ ... when sneezing?
- ☐ ☐ ... at the end of the day?
- ☐ ☐ Does the pain go to the jaw?
- ☐ ☐ ... to your teeth?
- ☐ ☐ ... to your head?
- ☐ ☐ ... to your eyes?
- ☐ ☐ ... to your ear?
- ☐ ☐ ... to your temple?
- ☐ ☐ ... to the back of your neck?
- ☐ ☐ ... to your shoulders?

Yes No

- ☐ ☐ Does the pain interfere with your sleep?
- ☐ ☐ ...make you fatigued?
- ☐ ☐ ...make you irritable?
- ☐ ☐ Have you been treated for depression?
- ☐ ☐ Have you ever suffered from rheumatoid arthritis?
  where ______
- ☐ ☐ Have you ever suffered from degenerative (osteo) arthritis?
  where ______
- ☐ ☐ Has any one in your family had arthritis?
  who ______
- ☐ ☐ Have you ever had a blow to the jaw?
  when ______
- ☐ ☐ Has your jaw ever locked wide open?
- ☐ ☐ Has it locked at just open?
- ☐ ☐ Has it locked closed?
- ☐ ☐ Does it lock so you cannot close your teeth together?
- ☐ ☐ Have you ever had cervical traction?
- ☐ ☐ Have your wisdom teeth been extracted?
- ☐ ☐ Have you ever been seen by an otolaryngologist (ear/nose Dr.)?
- ☐ ☐ Have you ever had an ear infection?
- ☐ ☐ Have you ever had ringing in your ears?
- ☐ ☐ Have you ever had pain in your ears?
- ☐ ☐ Are you in pain now?
  What kind of pain?
  ☐ sharp cutting
  ☐ deep aching
  Where is the pain? ______
  In your own words, please describe your problem: ______
  ______
  ______
  ______
  ______
  When did you first notice the problem?
  ______

Fig. 9 Temporomandibular Joint History Form and Exam Notes. (©Dr. Eric Z. Shapira)

DATE:

NAME:

COMPREHENSIVE PERIODONTAL ASSESSMENT

MISC.
(+/-) GING. CREST
FACIAL

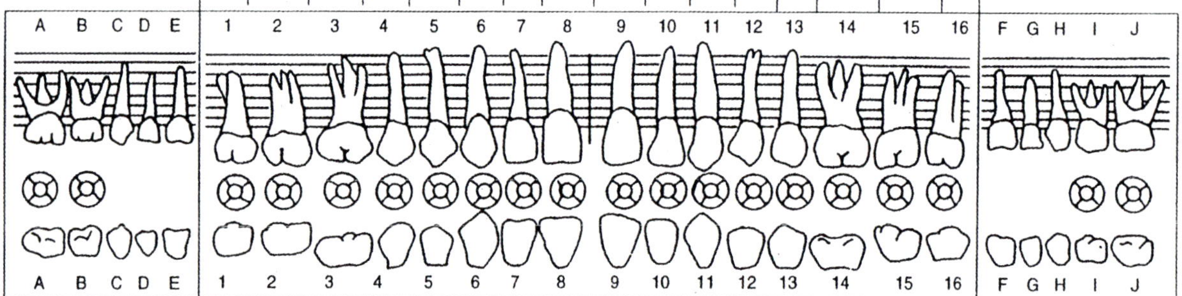

LINGUAL
(+/-) GING. CREST
MISC.

PLAQUE L M H
SUPRA CALC L M H
SUB CALC L M H
STAIN L M H

MISC.
(+/-) GING. CREST
LINGUAL

GINGIVAL:
COLOR - PINK/RED
R/B B/P
CONS - FIRM/SPONGY
FIBR./BULB.

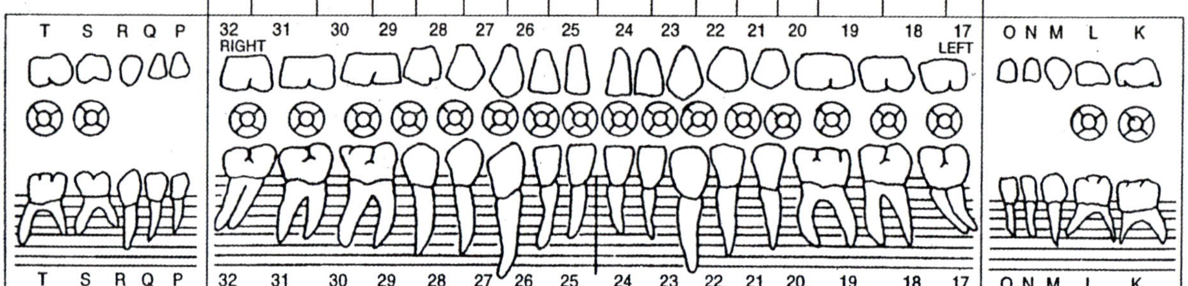

FACIAL
(+/-) GING. CREST
MISC.

GINGIVAL SHAPE:
◡ Cratered
⌒ Bulbous
— Flat

Circle Probe # in Red= Bleeding S=Suppuration Furcations= ΛCL 1, ΔCL 2, ▲CL 3
M = Min. Attached Gingiva NA = No Attachment MGP = Mucogingival Involvement

DIAGNOSIS:

Fig. 10 Periodontal Screening Form. (©Dr. Eric Z. Shapira)

PATIENT'S NAME ____
Last First

	DATE	TOOTH #	TREATMENT

Fig. 11 Typical Progress and Note Sheet.